Personalized Nutrition

Personalized Nutrition

Special Issue Editors

George Moschonis
Katherine Livingstone
Jessica Biesiekierski

MDPI • Basel • Beijing • Wuhan • Barcelona • Belgrade

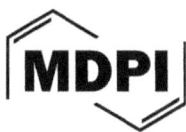

Special Issue Editors
George Moschonis
La Trobe University
Australia

Katherine Livingstone
Deakin University
Australia

Jessica Biesiekierski
La Trobe University
Australia

Editorial Office
MDPI
St. Alban-Anlage 66
4052 Basel, Switzerland

This is a reprint of articles from the Special Issue published online in the open access journal *Nutrients* (ISSN 2072-6643) from 2018 to 2019 (available at: https://www.mdpi.com/journal/nutrients/special_issues/Personalized_Nutrition).

For citation purposes, cite each article independently as indicated on the article page online and as indicated below:

LastName, A.A.; LastName, B.B.; LastName, C.C. Article Title. *Journal Name* **Year**, *Article Number*, Page Range.

ISBN 978-3-03921-445-7 (Pbk)
ISBN 978-3-03921-446-4 (PDF)

© 2019 by the authors. Articles in this book are Open Access and distributed under the Creative Commons Attribution (CC BY) license, which allows users to download, copy and build upon published articles, as long as the author and publisher are properly credited, which ensures maximum dissemination and a wider impact of our publications.

The book as a whole is distributed by MDPI under the terms and conditions of the Creative Commons license CC BY-NC-ND.

Contents

About the Special Issue Editors vii

Jessica R. Biesiekierski, Katherine M. Livingstone and George Moschonis
Personalised Nutrition: Updates, Gaps and Next Steps
Reprinted from: *Nutrients* **2019**, *11*, 1793, doi:10.3390/nu11081793 1

Bárbara Brayner, Gunveen Kaur, Michelle A. Keske and Katherine M. Livingstone
FADS Polymorphism, Omega-3 Fatty Acids and Diabetes Risk: A Systematic Review
Reprinted from: *Nutrients* **2018**, *10*, 758, doi:10.3390/nu10060758 6

Elie Chamoun, Nicholas A. Carroll, Lisa M. Duizer, Wenjuan Qi, Zeny Feng, Gerarda Darlington, Alison M. Duncan, Jess Haines, David W.L. Ma and the Guelph Family Health Study
The Relationship between Single Nucleotide Polymorphisms in Taste Receptor Genes, Taste Function and Dietary Intake in Preschool-Aged Children and Adults in the Guelph Family Health Study
Reprinted from: *Nutrients* **2018**, *10*, 990, doi:10.3390/nu10080990 17

Kerstin Kempf, Martin Röhling, Katja Niedermeier, Babette Gärtner and Stephan Martin
Individualized Meal Replacement Therapy Improves Clinically Relevant Long-Term Glycemic Control in Poorly Controlled Type 2 Diabetes Patients
Reprinted from: *Nutrients* **2018**, *10*, 1022, doi:10.3390/nu10081022 30

Enza D'Auria, Mariette Abrahams, Gian Vincenzo Zuccotti and Carina Venter
Personalized Nutrition Approach in Food Allergy: Is It Prime Time Yet?
Reprinted from: *Nutrients* **2019**, *11*, 359, doi:10.3390/nu11020359 46

Edyta Adamska-Patruno, Lucyna Ostrowska, Joanna Goscik, Joanna Fiedorczuk, Monika Moroz, Adam Kretowski and Maria Gorska
The Differences in Postprandial Serum Concentrations of Peptides That Regulate Satiety/Hunger and Metabolism after Various Meal Intake, in Men with Normal vs. Excessive BMI
Reprinted from: *Nutrients* **2019**, *11*, 493, doi:10.3390/nu11030493 62

Mads F. Hjorth, George A. Bray, Yishai Zohar, Lorien Urban, Derek C. Miketinas, Donald A. Williamson, Donna H. Ryan, Jennifer Rood, Catherine M. Champagne, Frank M. Sacks and Arne Astrup
Pretreatment Fasting Glucose and Insulin as Determinants of Weight Loss on Diets Varying in Macronutrients and Dietary Fibers—The POUNDS LOST Study
Reprinted from: *Nutrients* **2019**, *11*, 586, doi:10.3390/nu11030586 73

Theresa Drabsch and Christina Holzapfel
A Scientific Perspective of Personalised Gene-Based Dietary Recommendations for Weight Management
Reprinted from: *Nutrients* **2019**, *11*, 617, doi:10.3390/nu11030617 85

George Moschonis, Maria Michalopoulou, Konstantina Tsoutsoulopoulou, Elpis Vlachopapadopoulou, Stefanos Michalacos, Evangelia Charmandari, George P. Chrousos and Yannis Manios
Assessment of the Effectiveness of a Computerised Decision-Support Tool for Health Professionals for the Prevention and Treatment of Childhood Obesity. Results from a Randomised Controlled Trial
Reprinted from: *Nutrients* **2019**, *11*, 706, doi:10.3390/nu11030706 99

Edyta Adamska-Patruno, Joanna Godzien, Michal Ciborowski, Paulina Samczuk, Witold Bauer, Katarzyna Siewko, Maria Gorska, Coral Barbas and Adam Kretowski
The Type 2 Diabetes Susceptibility PROX1 Gene Variants Are Associated with Postprandial Plasma Metabolites Profile in Non-Diabetic Men
Reprinted from: *Nutrients* **2019**, *11*, 882, doi:10.3390/nu11040882 116

Jessica R Biesiekierski, Jonna Jalanka and Heidi M Staudacher
Can Gut Microbiota Composition Predict Response to Dietary Treatments?
Reprinted from: *Nutrients* **2019**, *11*, 1134, doi:10.3390/nu11051134 130

About the Special Issue Editors

George Moschonis is Associate Professor and Head of the discipline Dietetics and Human Nutrition at La Trobe University. During the last 15 years, he has built a strong research profile that is internationally recognised, mainly due to his roles as Project Manager and Key Investigator in nine interdisciplinary multicentre studies funded by the European Union. His main research interests are the identification of determinants or predictors (starting from very early life stages) of obesity and obesity-related cardiometabolic complications and the design, implementation, and evaluation of the effectiveness of personalised nutrition and lifestyle optimisation intervention programs which aim to tackle obesity and related co-morbidities (i.e., type 2 diabetes, cardiovascular disease, etc.) in children and adults.

Katherine Livingstone is Lecturer in Population Nutrition in the School of Exercise and Nutrition Sciences at Deakin University. Prior to being appointed as Lecturer, Dr Livingstone received two international fellowships to establish her research program in dietary patterns, determinants of dietary choices, and links to cardiometabolic health. Since completing her Ph.D. in 2013, Dr Livingstone has published >50 peer-reviewed journal articles which have amassed over 1000 citations. She has supervised a number of Masters, Honours, and Ph.D. students in these areas. Dr Livingstone also leads the research in better understanding the potential for personalised nutrition approaches to improve dietary patterns and overall dietary behaviours, and has collaborated on a pan-European personalised nutrition intervention.

Jessica Biesiekierski is Lecturer and Research Fellow in Dietetics and Human Nutrition at La Trobe University. She has international research expertise in the dietary effects on gastrointestinal physiology in health and disease, having completed her Ph.D. in the dietary management of gastrointestinal disorders and postdoctoral research exploring gastric nutrient sensing, including gastrointestinal motility, regulation of food intake, signalling pathways, and gut–brain interactions. Dr Biesiekierski's most notable research achievements include twice being awarded the international Rome Foundation's Award for the Most Cited Paper on Functional Gastrointestinal and Motility Disorders (most recently in 2015 and also in 2013) for her seminal work on gluten sensitivity.

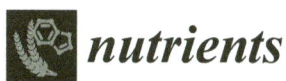

Editorial

Personalised Nutrition: Updates, Gaps and Next Steps

Jessica R. Biesiekierski [1,*], Katherine M. Livingstone [2] and George Moschonis [1]

[1] Department of Dietetics, Nutrition and Sport, School of Allied Health, Human Services and Sport, La Trobe University, Bundoora VIC 3086, Australia
[2] Institute for Physical Activity and Nutrition (IPAN), School of Exercise and Nutrition Sciences, Deakin University, Geelong VIC 3125, Australia
* Correspondence: j.biesiekierski@latrobe.edu.au

Received: 29 July 2019; Accepted: 1 August 2019; Published: 2 August 2019

1. Introduction

Personalised nutrition approaches provide healthy eating advice tailored to the nutritional needs of the individual. Although there is no one definition for personalised nutrition, advice has typically been based on the individual's behaviours, biological characteristics, and their interactions [1]. The objective of personalised nutrition is to improve dietary habits for the prevention or treatment of chronic disease, ultimately contributing to improvements in public health [2].

Two levels of the personalisation of nutrition advice have been conceived, which are based on the analysis of current behaviours, phenotypic characteristics and biological responses to diet [3]. The first level of personalised nutrition incorporates current behaviours and phenotypic characteristics (such as adiposity) to develop tailor-made dietary recommendations. The second level of personalised nutrition builds on the first layer but also takes into consideration the different responses to foods and/or nutrients that are dependent on genotypic or other biological characteristics [3].

Although there is some randomised controlled trial (RCT) evidence for the effectiveness of personalised nutrition advice [4], the scientific basis for personalisation of dietary advice is still in its infancy. The studies in this special issue of "Nutrients" bring together a series of recent clinical trials and review articles that present new data and update critical thinking to the current scientific basis that underpins personalised nutrition.

1.1. Behavioural Level of Personalised Nutrition

The first level of personalisation of nutrition advice requires the collection of information on an individual's current eating habits, behaviours and phenotypic characteristics [3]. These data are combined to provide personalised dietary advice tailored to these characteristics.

Maintaining sustained behavioural changes in personalised nutrition interventions is critical. Recent advances in technology have led to the development of behavioural tools to better facilitate adherence to personalised nutrition interventions. An example of this is demonstrated by Moschonis et al., who developed a computerised decision-support tool (DST) for use by paediatric healthcare professionals. The authors conducted an RCT designed to provide appropriate personalised nutrition meal plans and lifestyle recommendations in 35 overweight children and their families with healthcare professional support [5]. After three months of intervention, the group receiving advice through the DST showed improved changes in dietary patterns and body weight composition compared to the control group that received general recommendations [5].

1.2. Biological Levels of Personalised Nutrition

A number of studies in this special issue contributed to the scientific basis for personalisation based on biological characteristics (i.e., biomarkers, genotype, and microbiota). This includes understanding of the biological response due to dietary modifications, ranging from high-carbohydrate or high-fat meal challenges to whole diet interventions, and indicators of health and disease risk, including diabetes, obesity and appetite regulation.

1.2.1. Biomarkers

Hjorth et al. utilised fasting plasma glucose, fasting insulin and a homeostatic model assessment of insulin resistance (HOMA-IR) as prognostic markers of long-term weight loss. These biomarkers were assessed in 811 overweight adults following diets differing in carbohydrate, fat, and protein content [6]. After 24 months of dietary intervention, subjects with normal glycemia lost the most weight on the low-fat/high-protein diet, subjects with high HOMA-IR had the highest weight loss on the high-fat/high protein diet, and subjects with prediabetes and low fasting insulin benefited most from higher intakes of dietary fibre (≥35 g/10 MJ) [6].

Glycemic control was also investigated by Kempf et al., who conducted a 12-week RCT in adults with type 2 diabetes risk (T2D) with poorly controlled glucose levels (HbA1c ≥ 7.5%). Individuals were randomised to either a two- or three-meal replacement therapy. In weeks 2–4 of the intervention, both groups reintroduced a low carbohydrate lunch based on individual adaption to self-monitoring of blood glucose (SMGB), followed by breakfast reintroduction after week four and a final follow-up period at week 12 [7]. The findings showed that the individualised meal replacement accompanied with SMBG demonstrated beneficial reduction in HbA1c and other cardiometabolic risk factors in T2D [7]. Furthermore, the initiation of such an approach led to clinically relevant long-term improvements in HbA1c, compared to an observational control group that had standard care [7].

Further insights into the effective design of personalised meal plans was reported in a study led by Adamska-Patruno et al. [8]. The authors conducted a crossover trial in 23 normal-weight and 23 overweight/obese adult males using meal challenges containing meals comprised of either a high-carbohydrate, normal carbohydrate or high-fat content [8]. Results showed that normal-weight men had higher adiponectin and lower total ghrelin response after the high-carbohydrate meal and the overweight/obese men showed higher fasting and postprandial leptin levels overall [8]. These findings demonstrate how differences in postprandial gastric hormone levels are dependent on macronutrient meal composition and baseline body weight [8], highlighting the importance of regulating satiation and appetite sensations in the design of personalised interventions.

1.2.2. Genetics

Adamska-Patruno et al. conducted an acute meal-challenge study exploring gene variants and metabolites for T2D [9]. A total of 28 non-diabetic men were divided into either high risk or low risk according to carriage of the rs340874 SNP in the prospero-homeobox 1 (PROX1) gene [9]. A high or normal carbohydrate meal identified differences in postprandial metabolites associated with inflammatory and oxidative stress pathways, and bile acid signalling and lipid metabolism in PROX1 high-risk genotype men [9].

A systematic review performed by Brayner et al. evaluated the association between the FADS polymorphism, plasma long chain n-3 polyunsaturated fatty acids (PUFA) concentrations and risk of developing T2D [10]. Evaluation of five human observational studies and RCTs showed that FADS polymorphism may alter plasma fatty acid composition, therefore playing a protective role in the development of T2DM, while plasma n-3 PUFA levels were not associated with T2DM risk [10].

Taste receptor genes were investigated in an acute study in in 44 families to investigate taste function and dietary intake [11]. Chamoun et al. found key differences between children and parents as to which SNP in each of the sweet, fat, salt, umami and sour taste receptor genes was significantly associated with taste preference [11]. Furthermore, a multiple trait analysis of taste preference and nutrient composition of diet in the children revealed that rs9701796 in the TAS1R2 sweet taste receptor gene was associated with both sweet preference and percent energy from added sugar in the diet [11]. These findings suggest that for each taste preference, certain genetic variants are associated with taste function and thus, may be implicated in eating patterns.

1.2.3. Microbiota

A review of gut microbiota composition as a prediction tool for the clinical response after dietary intervention was reported by Biesiekierski et al. [12]. Although there are data to show that the gut microbiota composition and inter-individuality in response to diet are linked, this review highlighted that current data are too limited and inconsistent to support specific microbial signatures predicting response to dietary interventions [12]. This was true for both weight loss and/or glycaemic response in obesity, and symptom improvement in irritable bowel syndrome.

2. Remaining Challenges and Future Steps

There are a number of remaining research questions that require elucidation before the implementation of personalised nutrition advice can be effectively and confidently incorporated into clinical practice. This special issue identified that the many factors responsible for inter-individual differences vary in response to diet and that there is a paucity of RCTs that incorporate all of these factors into the one personalised nutrition offering.

The existing literature and abovementioned studies show a predominate focus on weight management and markers for T2D and obesity. There remain many other disease cohorts that are yet to be explored in relation to the appropriateness of personalised nutrition approaches. One area is individualised allergen avoidance advice. D'Auria et al. contributed a review addressing this, and highlighted that although personalised nutritional management of IgE mediated food allergy has improved, especially with increased understanding of allergy phenotypes, more research is required [13].

To further assess genotype-based personalised nutrition, Drabsch and Holzapfel reported an overall lack of strong clinical evidence for using genetic variants for personalised dietary recommendations for weight management [14]. The authors highlighted the lack of evidence supporting the use of genetic direct-to-consumer tests by evaluating a number of commercial companies offering gene-based dietary recommendations for weight loss [14]. Multidisciplinary intervention studies are necessary to provide the appropriate evidence on the effectiveness of these commercial tests.

The findings presented in this special issue will help inform the development and implementation of personalised nutrition approaches. The suggested sequence for implementation should follow a step wise approach beginning with the simplest level of personalising dietary advice, based on dietary intake and behavioural and phenotypical characteristics, before progressing to the more complex level that includes the addition of biomarkers, genotypic and microbiota data [1]. Given the complexity of continually changing behavioural and biological information that are both influenced by diet and influence response to dietary interventions, the finer details of how best to implement such an approach are still to be elucidated through advances in big data and digital science.

Future research to strengthen the evidence for personalised nutrition should include larger RCTs of longer intervention duration that aim to assess the effectiveness of personalised nutrition on long-term improvements in a variety of health outcomes. Moreover, future research should aim to address the current lack of consistency in the design of personalised advice across studies and their chosen methodologies [12]. This special issue will aid researchers in the design of more effective and comprehensive personalised nutrition research based on behavioural and biological characteristics.

3. Key Messages

This special issue on personalised nutrition presents a dynamic selection of reviews and original research in the ongoing development of evidence informing personalised nutrition strategies. Despite gaps in the scientific evidence, the future holds bright for the continued advancement of personalised nutrition, and ultimately how behavioural and biological characteristics can be integrated into step wise nutritional solutions specific to the needs of the individual for maintaining health and preventing disease.

Author Contributions: J.R.B., K.M.L. and G.M. conceptualised and co-wrote this article.

Conflicts of Interest: The authors declare no conflict of interest.

References

1. Celis-Morales, C.; Livingstone, K.M.; Marsaux, C.F.; Forster, H.; O'Donovan, C.B.; Woolhead, C.; Macready, A.L.; Fallaize, R.; Navas-Carretero, S.; Wim, H.M.; et al. Design and baseline characteristics of the Food4Me study: A web-based randomised controlled trial of personalised nutrition in seven European countries. *Genes Nutr.* **2015**, *10*, 450. [CrossRef] [PubMed]
2. Gibney, M.; Walsh, M.; Goosens, J. *Personalized Nutrition: Paving the Way to Better Population Health, in Good Nutrition: Perspectives for the 21st Century*; Eggersdorfer, M., Kraemer, K., Cordaro, J.B., Fanzo, J., Gibney, M., Kennedy, E., Labrique, A., Steffen, J., Eds.; Karger Publishers: Basel, Switzerland, 2016; pp. 235–248.
3. Ordovas, J.M.; Ferguson, L.R.; Tai, E.S.; Mathers, J.C. Personalised nutrition and health. *BMJ* **2018**, *361*, bmj.k-2173. [CrossRef] [PubMed]
4. Celis-Morales, C.; Livingstone, K.M.; Marsaux, C.F.; Macready, A.L.; Fallaize, R.; O'Donovan, C.B.; Woolhead, C.; Forster, H.; Walsh, M.C.; Navas-Carretero, S. Effect of personalized nutrition on health-related behaviour change: Evidence from the Food4me European randomized controlled trial. *Int. J. Epidemiol.* **2016**, *46*, 578–588. [CrossRef] [PubMed]
5. Moschonis, G.; Michalopoulou, M.; Tsoutsoulopoulou, K.; Vlachopapadopoulou, E.; Michalacos, S.; Charmandari, E.; Chrousos, G.P.; Manios, Y. Assessment of the Effectiveness of a Computerised Decision-Support Tool for Health Professionals for the Prevention and Treatment of Childhood Obesity. Results from a Randomised Controlled Trial. *Nutrients* **2019**, *11*, 706.
6. Hjorth, M.F.; Bray, G.A.; Zohar, Y.; Urban, L.; Miketinas, D.C.; Williamson, D.A.; Ryan, D.H.; Rood, J.; Champagne, C.M.; Sacks, F.M. Pretreatment Fasting Glucose and Insulin as Determinants of Weight Loss on Diets Varying in Macronutrients and Dietary Fibers—The POUNDS LOST Study. *Nutrients* **2019**, *11*, 586. [CrossRef] [PubMed]
7. Kempf, K.; Röhling, M.; Niedermeier, K.; Gärtner, B.; Martin, S. Individualized Meal Replacement Therapy Improves Clinically Relevant Long-Term Glycemic Control in Poorly Controlled Type 2 Diabetes Patients. *Nutrients* **2018**, *10*, 1022. [CrossRef] [PubMed]
8. Adamska-Patruno, E.; Ostrowska, L.; Goscik, J.; Fiedorczuk, J.; Moroz, M.; Kretowski, A.; Gorska, M. The Differences in Postprandial Serum Concentrations of Peptides That Regulate Satiety/Hunger and Metabolism after Various Meal Intake, in Men with Normal vs. Excessive BMI. *Nutrients* **2019**, *11*, 493. [CrossRef] [PubMed]
9. Adamska-Patruno, E.; Godzien, J.; Ciborowski, M.; Samczuk, P.; Bauer, W.; Siewko, K.; Gorska, M.; Barbas, C.; Kretowski, A. The Type 2 Diabetes Susceptibility PROX1 Gene Variants Are Associated with Postprandial Plasma Metabolites Profile in Non-Diabetic Men. *Nutrients* **2019**, *11*, 882. [CrossRef] [PubMed]
10. Brayner, B.; Kaur, G.; Keske, M.; Livingstone, K. FADS Polymorphism, Omega-3 Fatty Acids and Diabetes Risk: A Systematic Review. *Nutrients* **2018**, *10*, 758. [CrossRef] [PubMed]
11. Chamoun, E.; Carroll, N.; Duizer, L.; Qi, W.; Feng, Z.; Darlington, G.; Duncan, A.; Haines, J.; Ma, D. The Relationship between Single Nucleotide Polymorphisms in Taste Receptor Genes, Taste Function and Dietary Intake in Preschool-Aged Children and Adults in the Guelph Family Health Study. *Nutrients* **2018**, *10*, 990. [CrossRef] [PubMed]
12. Biesiekierski, J.R.; Jalanka, J.; Staudacher, H.M. Can Gut Microbiota Composition Predict Response to Dietary Treatments? *Nutrients* **2019**, *11*, 1134. [CrossRef] [PubMed]

13. D'Auria, E.; Abrahams, M.; Zuccotti, G.; Venter, C. Personalized Nutrition Approach in Food Allergy: Is It Prime Time Yet? *Nutrients* **2019**, *11*, 359. [CrossRef] [PubMed]
14. Drabsch, T.; Holzapfel, C. A Scientific Perspective of Personalised Gene-Based Dietary Recommendations for Weight Management. *Nutrients* **2019**, *11*, 617. [CrossRef] [PubMed]

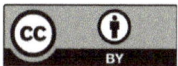

© 2019 by the authors. Licensee MDPI, Basel, Switzerland. This article is an open access article distributed under the terms and conditions of the Creative Commons Attribution (CC BY) license (http://creativecommons.org/licenses/by/4.0/).

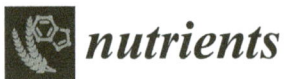

Review

FADS Polymorphism, Omega-3 Fatty Acids and Diabetes Risk: A Systematic Review

Bárbara Brayner [1], Gunveen Kaur [2], Michelle A. Keske [2] and Katherine M. Livingstone [2,*]

1. Laboratory of Nutritional Biochemistry, Centre of Health Science, Federal University of Rio de Janeiro, Rio de Janeiro 21941-902, Brazil; barbara_vitorinobrayner@hotmail.com
2. Institute for Physical Activity and Nutrition (IPAN), Deakin University, Geelong 3220, Australia; gunveen.kaur@deakin.edu.au (G.K.); michelle.keske@deakin.edu.au (M.A.K.)
* Correspondence: k.livingstone@deakin.edu.au

Received: 11 May 2018; Accepted: 11 June 2018; Published: 13 June 2018

Abstract: The role of *n*-3 long chain polyunsaturated fatty acids (LC *n*-3 PUFA) in reducing the risk of type 2 diabetes (T2DM) is not well established. The synthesis of LC *n*-3 PUFA requires fatty acid desaturase enzymes, which are encoded by the FADS gene. It is unclear if FADS polymorphism and dietary fatty acid intake can influence plasma or erythrocyte membrane fatty acid profile and thereby the risk of T2DM. Thus, the aim of this systematic review was to assess the current evidence for an effect of FADS polymorphism on T2DM risk and understand its associations with serum/erythrocyte and dietary LC *n*-3 PUFA. A systematic search was performed using PubMed, Embase, Cochrane and Scopus databases. A total of five studies met the inclusion criteria and were included in the present review. This review identified that FADS polymorphism may alter plasma fatty acid composition and play a protective role in the development of T2DM. Serum and erythrocyte LC *n*-3 PUFA levels were not associated with risk of T2DM, while dietary intake of LC *n*-3 PUFA was associated with lower risk of T2DM in one study only. The effect of LC *n*-3 PUFA consumption on associations between FADS polymorphism and T2DM warrants further investigation.

Keywords: FADS polymorphism; omega-3 fatty acids; type 2 diabetes

1. Introduction

Type 2 diabetes mellitus (T2DM) is a chronic disease that is characterized by an elevation of blood glucose levels (fasting glucose >7 mmol/L or HbA1c >6.5%) [1]. T2DM is often preceded by an insulin resistant state, where the normal biological response to the hormone insulin is impaired and insulin production is disregulated (compensatory hyperinsulinemia) to maintain normoglycemia [2,3]. The prevalence of T2DM and insulin resistance is increasing globally, affecting more than 400 million people worldwide [4]. This is leading to increasing rates of co-morbidities, such as neuropathy, hypertension and cardiovascular disease, and their associated healthcare costs [4].

The determinants of T2DM include genetic risk, poor diet and a sedentary lifestyle. It is estimated that 40% of first-degree relatives of patients with T2DM develop this disease, however the incidence in the general population worldwide is approximately 6% [5,6]. Dietary and exercise-based interventions have resulted in delayed progression of T2DM in as many as 50–60% of people with insulin resistance or pre-diabetes [7,8]. Moreover, the amount and quality of fatty acid consumption has been linked to risk of developing T2DM [9].

High intakes of saturated fatty acids and *n*-6 polyunsaturated fatty acids (PUFA) have been linked with impaired glucose tolerance and insulin resistance [9,10]. This is likely to be due to accumulation of excess lipids in liver, muscle and adipose tissue and an increase in pro-inflammatory compounds, such as the eicosanoids prostaglandin E2 and leukotriene B4, which are products of omega-6 fatty acid (arachidonic acid (AA)) [11]. In contrast, long chain omega-3 fatty acids (LC *n*-3 PUFA) such as docosahexaenoic acid (DHA) and eicosapentaenoic acid (EPA) are precursors of anti-inflammatory products, including resolvins, docosatriens and protectins [11,12], which have been shown to improve glucose tolerance and insulin sensitivity [12,13]. In a recent meta-analysis investigating the effect of LC n-3 PUFA in T2DM patients, the consumption of n-3 fatty acids, especially EPA and DHA, was shown to decrease serum triglyceride levels. In addition, the longer the intervention lasted, the better its effect on glucose control and lipid levels [14]. Given the association between LC n-3 PUFA and improved insulin sensitivity, it is important to understand if this translates to a reduced risk of developing T2DM. Foods and nutrients are not consumed in isolation, making it important to consider the role n-3 fatty acid intakes play within the context of the overall diet, i.e., dietary patterns [15]. Studies have shown that dietary patterns high in oily fish consumption have been linked to lower risk of T2DM [16], yet the impact of these dietary patterns on associations between the FADS polymorphism, plasma LC n-3 PUFA concentrations and risk of developing T2DM is unclear. In addition, little is known about how endogenous LC n-3 PUFA production and genetic risk influence these relationships.

The concentration of LC n-3 PUFA in red blood cells and plasma is dependent on both dietary intake and adequate endogenous production of these fatty acids [17]. LC n-3 PUFA can be endogenously synthesized via metabolism of the essential fatty acid alpha-linolenic acid (ALA). This endogenous production is mediated by the enzymes delta-5-desaturase (D5D) and delta-6-desaturase (D6D), which are encoded by the genes fatty acid desaturase 1 (FADS1) and fatty acid desaturase 2 (FADS2), respectively [18,19] (Figure 1).

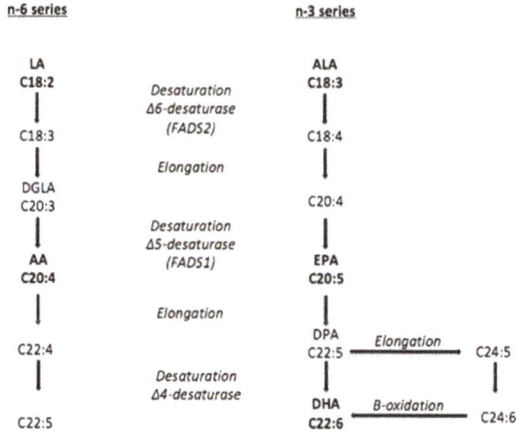

Figure 1. Pathway of desaturation and elongation of n-3 and n-6 fatty acids. The enzymes Δ6 and Δ5 desaturase are encoded by FADS2 and FADS1, respectively. LA: linoleic acid; DGLA: dihomo-gamma linolenic acid; AA: arachidonic acid; ALA: alpha-linolenic acid; EPA: eicosapentaenoic acid; DPA: docosapentaenoic acid; DHA: docosahexaenoic acid.

Single nucleotide polymorphisms (SNP) in the FADS gene have been linked to variations in fatty acid composition in various human compartments, such as erythrocyte membrane, plasma and breast milk [20–22]. However, little is known about which SNPs are responsible for these alterations [23]. A genetic variation in the FADS gene is linked to lower expression and activity of D5D and D6D, thereby increasing concentrations of the precursors linoleic acid (LA) and ALA but not of their downstream fatty acids AA, EPA and DHA [24–26]. The impact of dietary intakes and its potential to attenuate differences between major and minor allele carriers of the FADS polymorphism remains unclear [26,27].

Few studies have investigated whether LC n-3 PUFA intake is able to mitigate differences in plasma fatty acid profile among carriers of the FADS minor allele. Moreover, very little is known about how the FADS polymorphism and plasma concentrations and dietary intakes of n-3 fatty acids or dietary patterns high in n-3 fatty acids interact to influence an individual's risk of T2DM. The aim of this review was thus to systematically evaluate evidence on associations between the FADS polymorphism, plasma LC n-3 PUFA concentrations and risk of developing T2DM and understand the role of dietary fatty acid intakes on these associations.

2. Materials and Methods

2.1. Study Selection

This review includes publications from human observational studies and randomized controlled trials. Animal and in vitro studies were excluded. In order to be included in this review, the studies were required to include information on (i) FADS polymorphisms; (ii) omega-3 fatty acid intakes; (iii) plasma or erythrocyte membrane omega-3 fatty acid concentrations and (iv) whether participants presented with or were at risk of T2DM. Only publications in English were considered.

2.2. Search Strategy

Published studies between inception and February 2018 were identified from a literature search of four electronic databases: PubMed, Embase, Scopus and Cochrane Library. A manual search of the reference lists of relevant articles was also conducted to identify any additional papers that were not returned by the initial search. The search strategy involved combining three search themes using the Boolean operator 'and'. The first theme was ('FADS' OR 'Fatty acid desaturase'), the second theme was ('fatty acid*' OR 'n-3' OR 'n-3 fatty acid*' OR 'alpha linolenic acid' OR 'ala' OR 'eicosapentaenoic acid' OR 'epa' OR 'docosahexaenoic acid' OR 'dha' OR 'docosapentaenoic acid' OR 'dpa' OR 'long chain fatty acid*' OR 'diet' OR 'dietary pattern*' OR 'dietary fat*') and the third theme was ('type 2 diabetes' OR 'pre diabetes' OR 'insulin resistance' OR 'impaired glucose tolerance' OR 'glucose intolerance'). The search results were exported to a Reference Manager software, and were saved in a master file. Duplicates were removed via an in-built function within the software. A detailed record of all stages of the protocol was kept. This systematic review was undertaken in accordance with PRISMA guidelines and has been registered with PROSPERO, the International Prospective Register of Systematic Reviews (registration number: CRD42018084831).

2.3. Study Selection and Screening

Two reviewers independently assessed the article titles and abstracts for eligibility according to the inclusion and exclusion criteria. If both reviewers deemed the study suitable, the full text was retrieved for further evaluation. If there was disagreement, a third independent reviewer was used.

2.4. Data Extraction and Quality Assessment

Data extraction was performed by one reviewer using a standardized excel form developed by the researchers. A second reviewer checked the extraction for accuracy and consistency. The following information was extracted: (i) intervention characteristics: study design, sample size and country (ii) participant characteristics: age and sex (iii) FADS polymorphism (iv) fatty acids intakes and concentrations: dietary fatty acid intakes (saturated fatty acids, monounsaturated fatty acids, polyunsaturated fatty acids, eicosapentaenoic acid, docosapentaenoic acid and docosahexaenoic acid) and plasma or erythrocyte membrane n-3 fatty acid concentrations and (v) T2DM risk: defined by blood glucose levels; HbA1c levels; glucose tolerance; insulin sensitivity or type 2 diabetes. Two independent reviewers assessed the quality of the studies using the Cochrane Risk of Bias Tool [28]. A third reviewer was consulted if there was a discrepancy. The quality of each study was assessed according to the following criteria: measurement protocols, blinding, incomplete data outcome and selective reporting.

3. Results

The initial search identified a total of 2015 potential studies. After removal of duplicates, titles and abstracts of 1871 papers were screened. Based on this screening process, 1859 articles were excluded for not meeting our pre-defined inclusion criteria. The 12 articles selected after the screening process were then assessed in more depth using the full-text article. As detailed in Figure 2, six of those 12 articles did not have information on dietary intake and were therefore excluded from this review. One article did not report information on type 2 diabetes and was thus also excluded. In total, five articles were deemed eligible and were included in the present review.

The characteristics of the studies included in this review are presented in Table 1. The first study had a cross-sectional design [29], the second was a prospective cohort [30], the third was a randomized controlled trial [31], the fourth was a case-control study and the fifth was a prospective cohort study [32]. Most of the studies included both male and female participants, except for the cross-sectional study, which only included men [29]. The sample size ranged from 208 [31] to 2114 [30]. All of the studies were conducted with adult participants and the mean age ranged from 31 [31] to 63 years [33]. Three studies investigated the risk of developing T2DM: one by physician diagnosis during the cohort study (using International Classification of Diseases criteria) [30], one by past physician diagnosis (using World Health Organization criteria) [33] and the last one using an oral glucose tolerance test [32]. Two studies [29,31] analyzed fasting glucose and insulin and from that calculated insulin resistance/insulin sensitivity by the homeostasis model assessment (HOMA). All five studies investigated polymorphisms in the FADS gene cluster. Three studies collected information on serum fatty acid composition [29,32,33] and two of those assessed the desaturase enzymes activity [32,33]. One study analyzed erythrocyte membrane fatty acid composition and also investigated desaturase enzymes activity [30]. Three studies used food frequency questionnaires to collect dietary information [30,31,33], one used a 3-day food record [33] and the other used three 24-h recalls, which assessed intake on two typical week days and one atypical day (weekend or holiday) [29]. Dietary intakes reported included intakes of key nutrients and select food groups only. No studies reported overall dietary patterns.

The majority of the studies included in this systematic review were considered to have low risk of bias in their measurement protocols, blinding of volunteers and personnel, outcomes and selective reporting. Only one study [33] did not provide clear information on the blinding protocol for the participants (performance bias) and the outcome assessment (detection bias) (see supplementary Table S1).

Kim et al. [29] investigated cross-sectional associations between FADS gene polymorphism (SNPs rs174537, rs174575, rs1000778) and insulin resistance as well as serum fatty acid composition. Findings showed that HOMA-IR was higher in carriers of the minor FADS allele when individuals had higher serum concentrations of DGLA ($\geq$1.4% in total serum phospholipids (p for interaction = 0.009) or AA ($\geq$4.6% in total serum phospholipids, p for interaction = 0.047). No significant association was found between n-3 fatty acid levels in serum phospholipids, FADS polymorphism and HOMA-IR. Regarding dietary lipid intake, no significant association was found between different FADS polymorphisms. Additionally, individuals with this polymorphism had significantly higher fasting insulin (mean 9.7 $\pm$ 5.9 µIU/mL) than individuals who were homozygous for the major allele (mean 8.7 $\pm$ 3.8 µIU/mL) (p < 0.05) [29].

In a prospective cohort, Kroger et al. [30] identified that the fatty acid profiles of erythrocyte membrane phospholipids and the activity of desaturase enzymes, but not dietary fatty acids, were strongly linked to the incidence of T2DM. Results showed that high proportions of LA in erythrocyte membrane fatty acid were linked with lower risk of developing T2DM (relative risk (RR) for the highest versus the lowest quintiles of LA concentrations = 0.8 (95% CI: 0.5, 1.1)). In contrast, high proportions of gamma-linolenic acid (18:3n-6) and DGLA (20:3n-6) predicted increased risk of T2DM (RR for the highest versus the lowest quintiles of gamma-linolenic acid = 2.0 (95% CI: 1.4, 2.9); 1.72 (95% CI: 1.2, 2.5), respectively). The concentration of n-3 PUFA was not significantly associated with risk of T2DM development. Furthermore, lower activity of D6D enzyme predicted lower risk of T2DM in carriers of the minor FADS allele (SNP rs174546), compared to individuals without (RR for individuals homozygous for the minor allele TT genotype = 0.60 (95% CI: 0.4, 0.9) vs. heterozygous for the CT genotype = 0.75 (95% CI: 0.6, 1.0)). Dietary fatty acid intake was not significantly associated with T2DM incidence in this study [30].

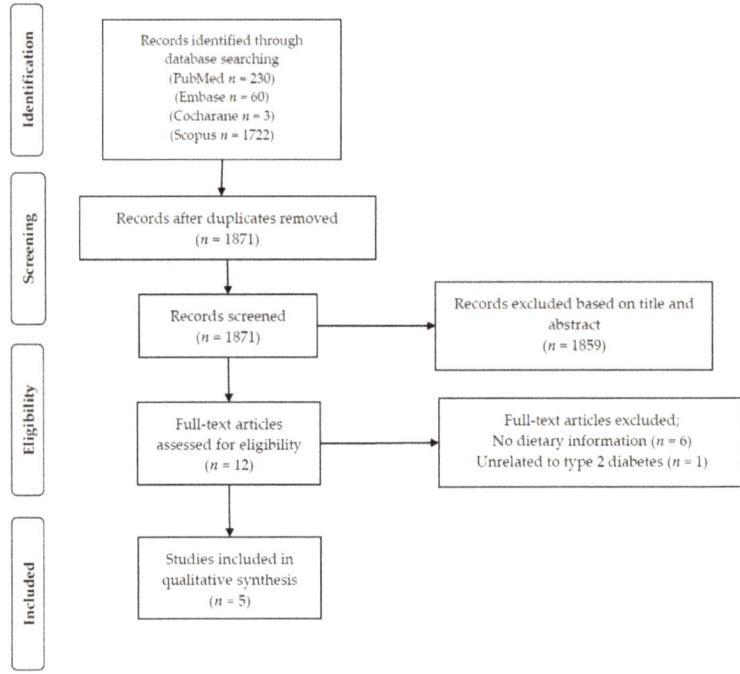

Figure 2. Study selection for inclusion in the systematic review based on the Preferred Reporting Items for Systematic Reviews and Meta-analyses (PRISMA) statement.

In a randomized controlled trial, Cormier et al. [31] demonstrated that the SNP rs482548 had an interaction effect on the relationship between LC n-3 PUFA supplementation and fasting glucose levels. This interaction effect led to higher levels of fasting glucose after supplementation in carrier of the FADS polymorphism (p interaction = 0.008). In addition, several SNPs were associated with decreased HOMA-IR in response to LC n-3 PUFA supplementation (rs7394871 p = 0.03; rs174602 p = 0.01; rs174570 p = 0.03; rs7482316 p = 0.05).

Yao et al. [33] identified that minor allele carriers of the SNP rs174616 were associated with decreased risk of T2DM in a case-control study. Despite other investigated SNPs not being associated with T2DM development, they were associated with serum PUFA composition; individuals who were carriers of the minor allele had higher serum PUFA and lower LC-PUFA composition. T2DM patients, who were carriers of the minor allele of rs174545 and rs2072114, had lower levels of EPA (p = 0.000; p = 0.002) and DPA (p = 0.006; p = 0.0024), respectively. For the SNP rs2072114 concentration of LA was also higher in carriers of the minor allele (p = 0.004). The minor allele of rs175602 was associated with lower concentrations of EPA (p = 0.007) in T2DM individuals. In addition, desaturase activity of D5D, measured by EPA/ALA ratio, was lower (p = 0.009), while D6D, measured by AA/LA ratio, was higher (p < 0.001) in T2DM individuals. Moreover, dietary saturated fatty acid intake (p < 0.0014) was higher in T2DM cases, whilst PUFA intake was lower (p > 0.054) [33].

Table 1. Characteristics of the five studies that met the inclusion criteria of this systematic review.

Author, Year	Country, Age (Mean, SD)	n	Study Design	Exposure	Outcome	Results	Conclusion
Kim et al., 2011 [29]	Korea, 30–69 years (48.7, 9.3)	576	Cross-sectional study	FADS polymorphisms: rs174537, rs174575, rs1000778	T2DM risk: fasting glucose (mg/dL), fasting insulin (μIU/mL) and HOMA-IR Fatty acid concentration: serum phospholipid FA composition (relative %): SFA, MUFA, PUFA (ALA, LA, AA, EPA, DGLA, DPA, DHA) Insulin Resistance (HOMA)	HOMA-IR and serum FA composition or FA ratios were associated with the FADS SNPs (rs174575) minor allele carriers had higher HOMA-IR when they had higher concentrations of DGLA ($\geq 1.4\%$ in total FA, p for interaction = 0.009) or of AA ($\geq 4.6\%$, p for interaction = 0.047). No significant association was found between n-3 FA serum composition, FADS polymorphism and HOMA-IR.	FADS SNPs were associated with higher HOMA-IR, when individuals had higher serum LC n-6 PUFA. No significant association was found for serum n-3 FA.
Kroger et al., 2011 [30]	Germany, 35–65 years (Controls 50, 8.9 and cases 55.1, 7.4)	Controls: 2114; cases: 673	Prospective cohort, 7 year follow up	Dietary intake: SFA (% of total fat intake), MUFA (% of total fat intake), n-3 PUFA (% of total fat intake), n-6 PUFA (% of total fat intake), total PUFA (% of total fat intake) FADS polymorphism: rs174546 Desaturase activity Fatty acid concentration: erythrocyte membrane phospholipids FA (% of total FA), AA/DGLA (D5D) and ALA/LA (D6D) ratios	T2DM risk: clinical diagnosis of T2DM	Risk of T2DM differed according to FA profile of erythrocyte membrane phospholipids. Higher proportions of LA were associated with lower risk of T2DM (RR for extreme quintiles = 0.76 (95% CI: 0.54, 1.08); whereas higher proportions of GLA and DGLA predicted increased T2DM risk (RR for extreme quintiles = 2.00 (95% CI: 1.38, 2.88); RR = 1.72 (95% CI: 1.18, 2.53), respectively). Activity of desaturase enzymes was linked to incidence of T2DM. Lower activity of D6D predicted lower risk of T2DM in carriers of the minor allele compared to those without (RR CT genotype = 0.75 (95% CI: 0.59, 0.96); TT genotype = 0.64 (95% CI: 0.43, 0.94). Dietary FA intake was not associated with T2DM.	T2DM incidence was higher in individuals with higher proportions of LC n-6 PUFA and lower D6D activity. No association was found with dietary n-3 FA intake.
Cormier et al., 2013 [31]	Canada, 18–50 years (30.8, 8.7)	208	Randomized controlled trial, 6 week duration	Dietary intake: 3–3.3 g/day of fish oil (1.9–2.2 g of EPA + 1.1 of DHA) FADS polymorphism: rs174556, rs174627, rs482548, rs2072114, rs12807005, rs174448, rs2845573, rs7394871, rs7942717, rs7482316, rs174602, rs498793, rs174546, rs174570, rs174579, rs174611, rs174616, rs968567	Fasting Glucose (mM), Fasting Insulin (p/L), HOMA-IR	SNPs involved in the FADS gene cluster were associated with glycemic control parameters (a supplementation * genotype interaction effect on FG levels was observed for rs482548 (p = 0.008)), mainly decreased HOMA-IR, in response to a high dose intervention with n-3 PUFA (supplementation * genotype interaction effect for rs174602 (p = 0.01); rs174570 (p = 0.03); rs7394871 (p = 0.03))	FADS SNPs were associated with lower HOMA-IR and higher fasting glucose in response to a high dose n-3 PUFA supplementation.

Table 1. Cont.

Author, Year	Country, Age (Mean, SD)	n	Study Design	Exposure	Outcome	Results	Conclusion
Yao et al., 2015 [33]	China, (Controls: 51.38, 11.27 years; cases: 63.24, 10.43 years)	Controls: 421; cases: 331	Case-control study	Dietary intake: total fat (%E), SFA (%E), MUFA (%E), PUFA (%E). FADS polymorphism: rs174545, rs2072114, rs174602, rs174616. Desaturase activity. Fatty acid concentration: serum PUFA composition (% of total FA), EPA/ALA (D5D) and AA/LA (D6D) ratios	T2DM risk *	Minor allele carriers of the rs174616 are associated with a decreased risk of T2DM ($p = 0.023$). Desaturase activity of D5D was decreased ($p = 0.009$), while D6D was increased ($p < 0.001$) in T2DM individuals. Dietary saturated fatty acid ($p < 0.0014$) was significantly higher in T2DM cases, whilst PUFA intake was lower ($p > 0.054$)	Higher PUFAs intake, desaturase activity and SNP rs174616 are associated with decreased risk of T2DM.
Takkunen et al., 2016 [32]	Finland, 40–65 years (55.4, 7.14)	407	Prospective cohort, 6 year follow up	Dietary intake: total fat (g/day), SFA (g/100 g of total fat), MUFA (g/100 g of total fat), PUFA (g/100 g of total fat). Desaturase activity: AA/DGLA (D5D) and ALA/LA (D6D) ratios using FADS polymorphism (rs174550) for validation. Fatty acid concentration: 20 serum FA (mol%)	T2DM incidence OGTT (mmol/L)	Total serum LC n-3 PUFA ($p = 0.001$) and estimated D5D activity ($p = 0.011$) predicted lower incidence of T2DM.	Lower incidence of T2DM was associated with serum LC n-3 PUFA, proportions of marine n-3 FA and estimated D5D activity.

FADS: fatty acid desaturase; HOMA: homeostasis model assessment; OGTT: oral glucose tolerance test; FG: fasting glucose; FA: fatty acids; SNP: single nucleotide polymorphism; T2DM: type 2 diabetes mellitus; AA: arachidonic acid; ALA: alpha-linolenic acid; LA: linoleic acid; DGLA: dihomo gamma-linolenic acid; EPA: eicosapentaenoic acid; DHA: docosahexaenoic acid; GLA: gamma-linolenic acid; D5D: delta 5 desaturase; D6D: delta 6 desaturase; SFA: saturated fatty acid; MUFA: monounsaturated fatty acid; %E: percentage of total energy intake; PUFA: polyunsaturated fatty acid; LC-PUFA: long chain polyunsaturated fatty acid; RR: relative risk; CI: confidence interval. * This study looked at T2DM as an exposure and an outcome.

Takkunen et al. [32] demonstrated that total serum LC n-3 PUFA concentration ($p = 0.001$) and D5D activity ($p = 0.011$) were associated with lower incidence of T2DM in a prospective cohort. In addition, serum concentrations of EPA ($p = 0.016$) and DPA ($p = 0.024$) were positively associated with insulin sensitivity.

4. Discussion

This is the first review to systematically evaluate the evidence regarding the association between FADS polymorphism, plasma or erythrocyte membrane LC n-3 PUFA fatty acid concentrations and T2DM risk, and if those relationships are influenced by dietary fatty acid intakes. After conducting a systematic search across four databases, five articles were identified that were eligible for inclusion in this review. The main findings were that FADS polymorphism and higher D5D and lower D6D activity may alter plasma and erythrocyte fatty acid composition, thereby playing a protective role in the development of T2DM. While two studies showed no association between serum n-3 PUFA concentration [29] or erythrocyte n-3 PUFA concentration [30] and risk of T2DM, these studies did show that higher concentrations of some of the n-6 PUFA in serum/erythrocytes (DGLA, 18:3n-6 and 20:3n-6) were associated with higher risk of T2DM, while 18:2n-6 was associated with lower risk of T2DM. In addition, dietary consumption of LC n-3 PUFA had a protective association with T2DM in one study [32], but no association was observed in others [29,30,33]. Supplementation with high doses of LC n-3 PUFA improved HOMA-IR in some variants of FADS polymorphism but increased fasting glucose levels in carriers of the minor allele for rs482548 (FADS2) [31].

The literature suggests there is an association between serum fatty acid composition and FADS SNPs. The cross-sectional study by Kim et al. [29], conducted with 576 Korean men, showed that the serum fatty acid composition varied in individuals with different SNPs of FADS gene. However, these variations were only significant for n-6 fatty acids (18:2n-6, AA and DGLA levels in serum phospholipids). Another study investigated this correlation in Caucasian individuals in Germany, with a sample of 727 subjects [20]. The SNPs investigated in this study explained 28% of the variance in AA in the individuals with polymorphism and 12% of its fatty acids precursors. In this study, LC n-3 PUFA concentrations also varied between different genotypes: DPA and EPA were lower whilst its precursor ALA was higher in individuals with a polymorphism in the FADS gene [20], suggesting that FADS polymorphism does influence fatty acids levels in blood. Similarly, Malerba et al. [21], genotyped 658 Italian subjects from the Verona Heart Project and measured fatty acid composition not only in serum but also in erythrocyte membrane. This study confirmed that the substrates of D5D and D6D (LA, ALA) were higher in serum and erythrocyte membranes of minor allele carriers, whilst their products (AA, EPA, DPA) were lower.

Studies have also investigated the relationship directly between the activity of desaturase enzymes and T2DM [30,33]. A prospective cohort of 2114 subjects from Germany investigated associations between dietary fatty acid intakes, T2DM risk and desaturase activity. Higher proportion of LA in erythrocytes predicted lower risk of T2DM development, whilst higher proportions of GLA and DGLA were associated with a higher risk of T2DM development. Additionally, in individuals with this polymorphism, lower D6D activity was related to lower T2DM incidence [30]. Furthermore, a study evaluating the influence of FADS1 and FADS2 genetic variants on desaturase activity and lipid concentrations in 820 T2DM patients identified that FADS1 rs174547 and FADS2 rs2727270 genotypes were significantly correlated to lower levels of D5D and D6D activity in T2DM patients [34]. Another prospective cohort carried out in 407 subjects from Finland found that total serum LC n-3 PUFA, proportions of marine n-3 FA and the estimated activity of D5D predicted lower incidence of T2DM, which is likely to be due to higher insulin sensitivity [32]. Therefore, it is likely that the FADS polymorphism, which influences D5D and D6D activity, may modulate the risk of developing T2DM.

Our findings suggest that serum and erythrocyte fatty acid composition may be affected by dietary intake of n-3 PUFA. Similarly, there is some research suggesting that the consumption of n-3 PUFA may have a beneficial effect on glycemic control and insulin sensitivity [12–14], however, the effect of n-3 PUFA on risk of T2DM is still unclear. A meta-analysis of prospective studies that focused on dietary n-3 PUFA sources, biomarker levels of n-3 PUFA and the incidence of T2DM, concluded that the evidence was mixed [35]. Only dietary intake of ALA from plant-based food was found to be modestly associated with lower risk of developing T2DM [35]. The relationship between n-3 PUFA intake and T2DM is further complicated when considering the role of FADS polymorphism. Cormier et al. [31] identified that the FADS SNPs were significantly associated with glycemic control, including lower HOMA-IR in response to the fish oil supplementation in Canadian subjects. These findings suggest that LC n-3 PUFA supplementation may play a protective role against T2DM in carriers of the minor allele for FADS gene. These findings are consistent with Yao et al. [31] which observed that Chinese individuals who were carriers of the minor allele of the FADS SNP (rs174616) had a lower risk of developing T2DM. Furthermore, higher intake of PUFA appeared to have had a protective effect on this relationship [33]. The protective role of dietary LC n-3 PUFA in the development of T2DM has been observed more often in Asian populations than in European/North Americans. Besides cultural differences in the preparation of foods that are rich sources of LC n-3 PUFA (raw/steamed vs. deep-fried), genetic factors are likely to strongly influence this association [36].

The mechanism as to how FADS polymorphism and dietary LC n-3 PUFA intake affects T2DM development remains unclear [29,31]. However, a possible explanation is that this genetic variant has been linked to lower D6D activity and lower concentrations of AA in plasma, red blood cells and adipose tissue [18,20,22]. This compound is the precursor of pro-inflammatory metabolites, which are related to an increase in overall inflammatory state [11]. Importantly, LC n-3 PUFA dietary intake is associated with the production of anti-inflammatory compounds [12] and the FADS polymorphism may lead to lower AA levels in plasma and red blood cells. As a result, this may lead to greater availability of cyclooxygenase and lipoxygenase enzymes to metabolize LC n-3 PUFA into their anti-inflammatory metabolites, thereby lowering inflammation and having a positive effect on T2DM risk. While this mechanism is plausible, further clinical research is needed to better understand this potential mechanism of action. In addition, dietary information collected in these studies focused on nutrient intakes only; the role n-3 fatty acid intake within the context of dietary patterns remains unclear.

5. Conclusions

This review was the first to systematically evaluate the role of FADS polymorphism on n-3 fatty acid concentration in plasma or erythrocyte membrane and on T2DM risk, and to identify if those relationships could be influenced by dietary intake. Given the heterogeneity in the study designs and the small number of studies eligible for inclusion in this review, our ability to draw firm conclusions was limited. Nonetheless, this review identified that the FADS polymorphism may influence plasma and erythrocyte fatty acid composition as well as T2DM risk markers, such as HOMA-IR and fasting glucose. All five studies demonstrated that there was a significant positive association between carrying the FADS polymorphism and T2DM risk. However, dietary LC n-3 PUFA intake was only associated with lower T2DM risk in one study. When considering which FADS SNPs are involved in these associations, the majority of the studies investigated different SNPs and therefore it was not possible to identify the role of any single SNP on risk of T2DM. Future research, preferably randomized controlled trials, is necessary to understand the mediation effect of dietary fatty acid intake on associations between FADS polymorphism, plasma or erythrocyte fatty acid and risk of developing T2DM. In addition, with an increasing focus on understanding diet as whole, the role of dietary patterns on these relationships warrants further investigation.

Supplementary Materials: The following are available online at http://www.mdpi.com/2072-6643/10/6/758/s1, Table S1: Quality Assessment.

Author Contributions: Conceptualization, B.B., G.K., M.A.K. and K.M.L.; Data curation, B.B., G.K., M.A.K. and K.M.L.; Methodology, B.B., G.K., M.A.K. and K.M.L.; Investigation, B.B.; Project administration G.K., M.A.K., K.M.L.; Resources, G.K., M.A.K., K.M.L.; Writing-Original Draft Preparation, B.B, G.K., M.A.K. and K.M.L.;

Writing-Review & Editing, G.K., M.A.K. and K.M.L.; Visualization B.B., G.K., M.A.K. and K.M.L.; Validation, G.K., M.A.K. and K.M.L.; Supervision, G.K., M.A.K. and K.M.L.

Funding: This research received no external funding.

Conflicts of Interest: The authors declare no conflict of interest.

References

1. American Diabetes Association. Available online: http://www.diabetes.org/diabetes-basics/diagnosis/?loc=db-slabnav (accessed on 1 March 2018).
2. Beale, E.G. Insulin signaling and insulin resistance. *J. Investig. Med.* **2013**, *61*. [CrossRef] [PubMed]
3. Guo, S. Insulin signaling, resistance, and the metabolic syndrome: Insights from mouse models to disease mechanism. *J. Endocrinol.* **2014**, *220*. [CrossRef] [PubMed]
4. World Health Organization. Available online: http://www.who.int/diabetes/en/ (accessed on 3 January 2018).
5. Wu, Y.; Ding, Y.; Tanaka, Y.; Zhang, W. Risk factors contributing to type 2 diabetes and recent advances in the treatment and prevention. *Int. J. Med. Sci.* **2014**, *6*, 1185–2000. [CrossRef] [PubMed]
6. Hivert, M.F.; Vassy, J.L.; Meigs, J.B. Susceptibility to type 2 diabetes mellitus—From genes to prevention. *Nat. Rev. Endocrinol.* **2014**, *10*, 189–205. [CrossRef] [PubMed]
7. Knowler, W.C.; Barrett-Connor, E.; Folwer, S.E.; Hamman, R.F.; Lachin, J.M.; Walker, E.A.; Nathan, D.M. Reduction in the incidence of type 2 diabetes with lifestyle intervention or metformin. *N. Engl. J. Med.* **2002**, *346*, 393–403. [CrossRef] [PubMed]
8. Tuomilehto, J.; Lindstrom, J.; Eriksson, J.G.; Valle, T.T.; Hämäläinen, H.; Ilanne-Parikka, P.; Keinänen-Kiukaanniemi, S.; Laakso, M.; Louheranta, A.; Rastas, M.; et al. Prevention of type 2 diabetes mellitus by changes in lifestyle among subjects with impaired glucose tolerance. *N. Engl. J. Med.* **2001**, *344*, 1343–1350. [CrossRef] [PubMed]
9. Sears, B.; Perry, M. The role of fatty acids in insulin resistance. *Lipids Health Dis.* **2015**, *14*, 121–129. [CrossRef] [PubMed]
10. Moloney, F.; Yeow, T.P.; Mullen, A.; Nolan, J.J.; Roche, H.M. Conjugated linoleic acid supplementation, insulin sensitivity, and lipoprotein metabolism in patients with type 2 diabetes mellitus. *Am. J. Clin. Nutr.* **2004**, *80*, 887–895. [CrossRef] [PubMed]
11. Fritsche, K.L. The science of fatty acids and inflammation. *Adv. Nutr.* **2015**, *6*, 293S–301S. [CrossRef] [PubMed]
12. Olalla, L.M.S.; Muniz, F.J.S.; Vaquero, M.P. N-3 fatty acids in glucose metabolism and insulin sensitivity. *Nutr. Hops.* **2009**, *24*, 113–127.
13. Lardinois, C.K.; Starich, G.H. Polyunsaturated fats enhance peripheral glucose utilization in rats. *J. Am. Coll. Nutr.* **1991**, *10*, 340–345. [CrossRef] [PubMed]
14. Chen, C.; Yu, X.; Shao, S. Effects of omega-3 fatty acid supplementation on glucose control and lipid levels in type 2 diabetes: A meta-analysis. *PLoS ONE* **2015**, *10*, e0139565. [CrossRef] [PubMed]
15. Tapsell, L.C.; Neale, E.P.; Satija, A.; Hu, F.B. Foods, nutrients and dietary patterns: Interconnections and implications for dietary guidelines. *Adv. Nutr.* **2016**, *7*, 445–454. [CrossRef] [PubMed]
16. Zhang, M.; Picard-Deland, E.; Marette, A. Fish and marine omega-3 polyunsaturated fatty acid consumption and incidence of type 2 diabetes: A systematic review and meta-analysis. *Int. J. Endocrinol.* **2013**, *2013*, 1–11. [CrossRef]
17. Calder, P.C. Mechanism of action of (*n*-3) fatty acids. *J. Nutr.* **2012**, *142*, 592S–599S. [CrossRef] [PubMed]
18. Lattka, E.; Illig, T.; Koletzko, B.; Heinrich, J. Genetic variants of the FADS1-FADS2 gene cluster as related to essential fatty acid metabolism. *Curr. Opin. Lipidol.* **2010**, *21*, 64–69. [CrossRef] [PubMed]
19. Merino, D.M.; Ma, D.W.L.; Mutch, D.M. Genetic variation in lipid desaturases and its impact on the development of human disease. *Lipids Health Dis.* **2010**, *9*, 63–77. [CrossRef] [PubMed]
20. Schaeffer, L.; Gohlke, H.; Muller, M.; Heid, I.M.; Palmer, L.J.; Kompauer, I.; Demmelmair, H.; Illig, T.; Koletzko, B.; Heinrich, J. Common genetic variants of the FADS1 FADS2 gene cluster and their reconstructed haplotypes are associated with the fatty acid composition in phospholipids. *Hum. Mol. Genet.* **2006**, *15*, 1745–1756. [CrossRef] [PubMed]

21. Malerba, G.; Schaeffer, L.; Xumerle, L.; Klopp, N.; Trabetti, E.; Biscuola, M.; Cavallari, U.; Galavotti, R.; Martinelli, N.; Guarini, P.; et al. SNPs of the FADS gene cluster are associated with polyunsaturated fatty acids in a cohort of patients with cardiovascular disease. *Lipids* **2008**, *43*, 289–299. [CrossRef] [PubMed]
22. Xie, L.; Innis, S.M. Genetic variants of the FADS1 FADS2 gene cluster are associated with altered (*n*-6) and (*n*-3) essential fatty acids in plasma and erythrocyte phospholipids in women during pregnancy and in breast milk during lactation. *J. Nutr.* **2008**, *138*, 2222–2228. [CrossRef] [PubMed]
23. Minihane, A.M. Impact of the genotype on EPA and DHA status and responsiveness to increased intakes. *Nutrients* **2016**, *8*, 123. [CrossRef] [PubMed]
24. Simpoulos, A.P. Genetic variants in the metabolism of omega-6 and omega-3 fatty acids: Their role in the determination of nutritional requirements and chronic disease risk. *Exp. Biol. Med.* **2010**, *235*, 785–795. [CrossRef] [PubMed]
25. Barman, M.; Nilsson, S.; Naluai, A.T.; Sandin, A.; Wold, A.E.; Sandberg, A.S. Single Nucleotide polymorphism in the FADS gene cluster but no ELOVL2 gene are associated with serum polyunsaturated fatty acid composition and development of allergy (in a Swedish Birth Cohort). *Nutrients* **2015**, *7*, 10100–10115. [CrossRef] [PubMed]
26. Ralston, J.C.; Matravadia, S.; Garudio, N.; Holloway, G.P.; Mutch, D.M. Polyunsaturated fatty acid regulation of adipocyte FADS1 and FADS2 expression and Function. *Obesity* **2015**, *23*, 725–728. [CrossRef] [PubMed]
27. Sholtz, S.A.; Kerling, E.H.; Shaddy, D.J.; Li, S.; Thodosoff, J.M.; Colombo, J.; Carlson, S.E. Docosahexaenoic acid (DHA) supplementation in pregnancy differentially modulates arachidonic acid and DHA status across FADS genotypes in pregnancy. *Prostaglandins Leukot. Essent. Fat. Acids* **2015**, *94*, 29–33. [CrossRef] [PubMed]
28. Higgins, J.P.T.; Green, S. (Eds.) *Cochrane Handbook for Systematic Reviews of Interventions*, Version 5.1.0 [updated March 2011]; The Cochrane Collaboration, 2011. Available online: http://handbook.cochrane.org (accessed on 2 March 2018).
29. Kim, O.Y.; Lim, H.H.; Yang, L.I.; Chae, J.S.; Lee, J.H. Fatty acid desaturase (FADS) gene polymorphism and insulin resistance in association with serum phospholipid polyunsaturated fatty acid composition in healthy Korean men: Cross-sectional study. *Nutr. Metab.* **2011**, *8*, 24. [CrossRef] [PubMed]
30. Kroger, J.; Zietemann, V.; Enzenbach, C.; Weikert, C.; Jansen, E.H.J.M.; Doring, F.; Joost, H.G.; Boeing, H.; Schulze, M.B. Erythrocyte membrane phospholipids fatty acids, desaturase activity, and dietary fatty acids in relation to risk of type 2 diabetes in the European Prospective Investigation into Cancer and Nutrition (EPIC)-Potsdam Study. *Am. J. Clin. Nutr.* **2011**, *93*, 127–142. [CrossRef] [PubMed]
31. Cormier, H.; Rudkowska, I.; Thifault, E.; Lemieux, S.; Couture, P.; Vohl, M.C. Polymorphism in fatty acid desaturase (FADS) gene cluster: Effects on glycemic controls following an omega-3 polyunsaturated fatty acids (PUFA) supplementation. *Genes* **2013**, *4*, 485–498. [CrossRef] [PubMed]
32. Takkunen, M.J.; Schwab, U.S.; Mello, V.D.F.; Eriksson, J.G.; Lindstrom, J.; Tuomilehto, J.; Uusitupa, M.I.J. Longitudinal associations of serum fatty acid composition with type 2 diabetes risk and markers of insulin secretion and sensitivity in the Finish Diabetes Prevention Study. *Eur. J. Nutr.* **2016**, *55*, 967–979. [CrossRef] [PubMed]
33. Yao, M.; Li, J.; Xie, T.; He, T.; Fang, L.; Shi, Y.; Hou, L.; Lian, K.; Wang, R.; Jiang, L. Polymorphism of rs174616 in the FADS1-FADS2 gene cluster is associated with a reduced risk of type 2 diabetes mellitus in northern Han Chinese people. *Diabetes Res. Clin. Pract.* **2015**, *109*, 206–212. [CrossRef] [PubMed]
34. Huang, M.C.; Chang, W.T.; Chang, H.Y.; Chung, H.F.; Chen, F.P.; Huang, Y.F.; Hsu, C.C.; Hwang, S.J. FADS gene polymorphism, fatty acid desaturase activities, and HDL-C in type 2 diabetes. *Int. J. Environ. Res. Public Health* **2017**, *14*, 572. [CrossRef] [PubMed]
35. Wu, J.H.Y.; Micha, R.; Imamura, F.; Pan, A.; Biggs, M.L.; Ajaz, O.; Dujousse, L.; Hu, F.B.; Mozaffarian, D. Omega-3 fatty acids and incident type 2 diabetes: A systematic review and meta-analysis. *Br. J. Nutr.* **2012**, *107*, S214–S227. [CrossRef] [PubMed]
36. Wallin, A.; Di Giuseppe, D.; Orsini, N.; Patel, P.S.; Forouhi, N.G.; Wolk, A. Fish consumption, dietary long-chain *n*-3 fatty acids and risk of type 2 diabetes: Systematic review and meta-analysis of prospective studies. *Diabetes Care* **2012**, *35*, 918–929. [CrossRef] [PubMed]

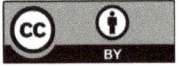

© 2018 by the authors. Licensee MDPI, Basel, Switzerland. This article is an open access article distributed under the terms and conditions of the Creative Commons Attribution (CC BY) license (http://creativecommons.org/licenses/by/4.0/).

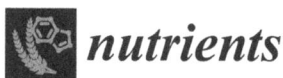

Article

The Relationship between Single Nucleotide Polymorphisms in Taste Receptor Genes, Taste Function and Dietary Intake in Preschool-Aged Children and Adults in the Guelph Family Health Study

Elie Chamoun [1], Nicholas A. Carroll [1], Lisa M. Duizer [2], Wenjuan Qi [3], Zeny Feng [3], Gerarda Darlington [3], Alison M. Duncan [1], Jess Haines [4], David W.L. Ma [1,*] and the Guelph Family Health Study [5]

[1] Department of Human Health and Nutritional Sciences, University of Guelph, Guelph, ON N1G 2W1, Canada; echamoun@uoguelph.ca (E.C.); ncarro03@uoguelph.ca (N.A.C.); amduncan@uoguelph.ca (A.M.D.)
[2] Department of Food Science, University of Guelph, Guelph, ON N1G 2W1, Canada; lduizer@uoguelph.ca
[3] Department of Mathematics and Statistics, University of Guelph, Guelph, ON N1G 2W1, Canada; wqi@uoguelph.ca (W.Q.); zfeng@uoguelph.ca (Z.F.); gdarling@uoguelph.ca (G.D.)
[4] Department of Family Relations and Applied Nutrition, University of Guelph, Guelph, ON N1G 2W1 Canada; jhaines@uguelph.ca
[5] University of Guelph, Guelph, ON N1G 2W1, Canada; guelphfamilyhealthstudy@gmail.com
* Correspondence: davidma@uoguelph.ca; Tel.: +1(519)-824-4120 (ext. 52272)

Received: 9 July 2018; Accepted: 27 July 2018; Published: 29 July 2018

Abstract: Taste is a fundamental determinant of food selection, and inter-individual variations in taste perception may be important risk factors for poor eating habits and obesity. Characterizing differences in taste perception and their influences on dietary intake may lead to an improved understanding of obesity risk and a potential to develop personalized nutrition recommendations. This study explored associations between 93 single nucleotide polymorphisms (SNPs) in sweet, fat, bitter, salt, sour, and umami taste receptors and psychophysical measures of taste. Forty-four families from the Guelph Family Health Study participated, including 60 children and 65 adults. Saliva was collected for genetic analysis and parents completed a three-day food record for their children. Parents underwent a test for suprathreshold sensitivity (ST) and taste preference (PR) for sweet, fat, salt, umami, and sour as well as a phenylthiocarbamide (PTC) taste status test. Children underwent PR tests and a PTC taste status test. Analysis of SNPs and psychophysical measures of taste yielded 23 significant associations in parents and 11 in children. After adjusting for multiple hypothesis testing, the rs713598 in the *TAS2R38* bitter taste receptor gene and rs236514 in the *KCNJ2* sour taste-associated gene remained significantly associated with PTC ST and sour PR in parents, respectively. In children, rs173135 in *KCNJ2* and rs4790522 in the *TRPV1* salt taste-associated gene remained significantly associated with sour and salt taste PRs, respectively. A multiple trait analysis of PR and nutrient composition of diet in the children revealed that rs9701796 in the *TAS1R2* sweet taste receptor gene was associated with both sweet PR and percent energy from added sugar in the diet. These findings provide evidence that for bitter, sour, salt, and sweet taste, certain genetic variants are associated with taste function and may be implicated in eating patterns. (Support was provided by the Ontario Ministry of Agriculture, Food, and Rural Affairs).

Keywords: taste; genetics; diet; health; children; adults

1. Introduction

The prevalence of obesity and associated co-morbidities is rising internationally despite ongoing prevention and intervention efforts [1,2]. Therefore, new strategies are warranted to promote the development of effective obesity prevention initiatives. As about half of the risk of developing obesity is heritable [3,4], characterizing the genetic component of obesity and incorporating this information into obesity prevention efforts may be a key part of the complex solution to this global problem. Excess intake of calories due to poor eating habits has been widely recognized as a major factor in the development of obesity, and these habits are established in the earliest years of life [5]. While the genetic basis of these adverse behaviors is not clear, taste preferences have been shown to vary due in part to genetics and to be associated with poor eating habits [6]. Characterizing the genetic factors that predispose to certain taste preferences may therefore provide a tool to tailor eating patterns to promote healthy eating habits.

The relationship between genetic variation and taste has previously been investigated by examining single nucleotide polymorphisms (SNPs) with outcomes of sensory tests. In particular, studies have focused on the link between taste receptor gene SNPs and measures of taste sensitivity, taste preference, and dietary intake [7–16]. However, previous studies typically analyze very few SNPs and only measure sensitivity, preference or dietary intake related to one type of taste. In this study, 93 SNPs spanning taste receptor genes that elicit fat, sweet, salt, sour, umami, and bitter tastes were examined for their associations with measures of taste sensitivity and taste preference. SNPs determined to be significantly associated with taste were then examined for potential associations with dietary intake in children. As a result of this comprehensive analysis, SNPs that are associated with taste perception can subsequently be assessed for their effect on the intake of dietary components related to that same type of taste.

2. Methods

2.1. Participants

Forty-nine families, including 72 children and 81 adults, were recruited from the Guelph Family Health Study—an existing family-based cohort study. Exclusion criteria included smoking, diagnosis of hypogeusia or ageusia, and having undergone bariatric surgery. Children under the age of 3 years were not recruited due to the potential difficulty in understanding and performing sensory tasks. This study was approved by the Research Ethics Board at the University of Guelph (REB#16-12-629).

2.2. Anthropometry, Body Composition, and Blood Pressure Measurements

Parents and their children arrived at the University of Guelph in the Body Composition Lab having fasted for at least two hours. Among both parents, height was measured to the nearest 0.1 cm using a wall-mounted stadiometer (Medical Scales and Measuring Devices; Seca Corp, Ontario, CA, USA) and measured in children to the nearest 0.1 cm using a pediatric length board (Weigh and Measure, LLC; ShorrBoard®, Olney, MD, USA). Body weight was measured while wearing tight-fitting clothing and no shoes using the BOD POD™ digital scale (Cosmed Inc., Concord, CA, USA). Body mass index (kg/m^2) was calculated from the weight and height measurements. The BOD POD™ was used to determine body composition of adult participants using air displacement plethysmography. Fat mass % in children was determined using bioelectric impedance analysis. Trained research assistants used the Quantum IV – Body Composition AnalyzerTM (RJL Systems, Clinton Township, MI, USA) using single-frequency, with electrodes placed on the right hand and foot. Total body water (TBW) was determined using the Kushner equation [17], then TBW was divided by an age- and sex-specific hydration factor to obtain fat mass %. Among both parents and children, blood pressure and heart rate were measured from the right brachial artery using an automated oscillometric device (HBP-1300 OMRON, Mississauga, Ontario, CA, USA). Cuff size was determined based on arm circumference. Among adults and children, three rested measurements of blood pressure (systolic and diastolic) and heart rate were obtained via an automatic reading while participants were seated in an upright position. The average of the final two measurements for each participant was used in subsequent analyses.

2.3. SNP Selection and Genotyping

A PubMed SNP search was conducted for the following genes previously implicated in taste detection: *CD36, GPR120, GPR40, TAS1R1, TAS1R2, TAS1R3, TAS2R38, ENaC, TRPV1, GRM4,* and *KCNJ2*. The resulting SNPs from each gene were filtered by global minor allele frequency (MAF), and SNPs with a minor allele frequency below 5% were removed [18]. The resulting SNPs were filtered using HaploView 4.2 software to obtain tag SNPs (tSNPs). Each tSNP is considered independent due to low linkage disequilibrium ($r^2 < 0.05$).

Saliva was collected at the health assessment using the Oragene•DNA (OG-575) collection kit for Assisted Collection (DNA Genotek). Participants were fasted for a minimum of 30 minutes before the saliva sample was provided. Genetic material from saliva was extracted by ethanol precipitation according to the manufacturer's protocol (DNA Genotek). The DNA samples were sent to The Centre for Applied Genomics at The Hospital for Sick Children (Toronto, Canada) where they underwent genotyping using the Agena MassArray System.

2.4. Psychophysical Measurements

Psychophysical tests for adults were administered in sensory booths at the University of Guelph Sensory Laboratory ($n = 65$). Filter paper strips (Indigo Instruments – Cat#33814-Ctl; 47 mm × 6 mm × 0.3 mm) immersed in varying concentrations of tastants were used to determine suprathreshold sensitivity (ST) for the adults only. The tastants were: sucrose for sweet taste (Thermo Fisher Scientific, Rockford, IL, USA; S5-500), monosodium glutamate (MSG) (Thermo Fisher; ICN10180080) and inosine monophosphate (IMP) (Thermo Fisher; AC226260250) for umami taste, sodium chloride (NaCl) for salt taste (Thermo Fisher; S641-500), citric acid for sour taste (A940-500), oleic acid for fat taste (A195-500) (Thermo Fisher Scientific), and PTC for bitter taste (Indigo Instruments, Waterloo, Ontario, Canada,– Cat#33814-PTC). Oleic acid was homogenized in deionized water prior to immersing the filter paper, and all other tastants were dissolved in water at ambient temperature. Filter paper strips were immersed in the tastant solution for about one second before placing them on a drying rack to dry overnight at ambient temperature. This procedure was performed only once for all strips before the study commenced. Taste strips immersed in a solution with the same tastant and concentration were stored together at 4 °C in a small plastic re-sealable bag. Each time a strip was tested, participants placed the taste strip in the middle of their tongue, closed their mouths, and allowed at least five seconds for the tastants to be sensed by taste receptors. Participants were asked to rinse and expectorate with distilled water before beginning and following each strip. Within each taste modality, the range of tastant concentrations tested is shown in Table 1. Oral ST was determined using filter paper strips for a range of tastant concentrations by computing the area-under-the-curve (AUC) of intensity ratings on the general labeled magnitude scale (gLMS) [19], and preference (PR) was measured using a forced-choice paired comparison of hummus samples. Participants were presented with a range of taste strips in random order and were asked to rate the intensity of the strips from 0–100 on a gLMS where 0 = undetectable, 2 = barely detectable, 6 = weak, 18 = moderate, 35 = strong, 52 = very strong, and 100 = strongest imaginable sensation of any kind. For bitter taste, only one rating of PTC intensity was obtained.

In the PR test for adults, paired hummus samples labeled with random three-digit codes were presented simultaneously to participants in a small translucent sample cup. Each pair of hummus samples consisted of one sample with a standard study formulation and the other with an added ingredient to more strongly elicit a specific taste modality. The standard study hummus was formulated at the University of Guelph Formulation Laboratory. First, chickpeas (540 mL—ARZ Fine Foods) were rinsed in a strainer with cold water and poured into the three-quart polycarbonate bowl of the Robot Coupe Food Processor (Model# R2NCLR). Distilled water (92 mL—President's Choice), olive + canola oil mix (54 mL—Pur Oliva), lemon juice (10 mL—ReaLemon), tahini (35 mL—ARZ), and salt (5.5 g—Thermo Fisher; S641-500) were then added to the chickpeas. The mix was processed for 40 s, mixed with a spoon to allow chunks of chickpeas on the sides of the processor bowl to be re-incorporated, and processed again for 60 seconds. Five 150 g quantities of hummus were then set aside for the preparation of hummus samples with added ingredients. To elicit stronger fat, salt, sour, sweet, and umami taste, olive + canola oil mix (15 g), salt (0.5 g), lemon juice (7 g), sucrose (4 g), and MSG (4 g) were respectively added to a 150 g quantity of the standard study hummus and mixed thoroughly with a spoon. For each participant, ten sample cups containing five standard hummus samples as well as five hummus samples with added ingredients were prepared (8 g each). A random number generator was used by a research assistant to produce the three-digit codes with which to label the sample cups such that the sensory test administrator was blinded to the hummus formulations. In the PR test, each sample was tasted using a metal spoon following an oral rinse with distilled water. After the second hummus sample was tasted, participants were asked "Which of the two hummus samples did you prefer?" and responded by providing the sensory test administrator with the three-digit code of the preferred sample. Oral ST and PR for all taste modalities were measured during the same study visit.

Table 1. Range of tastant concentrations used for each psychophysical test.

Taste Modality (Stimulus)	Threshold/Suprathreshold (mM)	Preference (mM)
Sweet (sucrose)	2.5–500	6%–36% (w/v *)
Umami (MSG)	3.13–200	3.13–200
Umami (IMP)	0.313–20	0.313–20
Umami (MSG+IMP)	3.13–200 MSG + 0.5 IMP	3.13–200 MSG + 0.5 IMP
Salt (sodium chloride)	5–100	50–250
Sour (citric acid)	1–15	10–200
Fat (oleic acid)	30–100	50–100
Bitter (PTC)	3 µg/strip	-

Tastants were diluted in distilled water and filter papers were submerged in the solutions. * weight/volume. MSG: monosodium glutamate, IMP: inosine monophosphate, PTC: phenylthiocarbamide.

Children participated in a PR test and a PTC taster test only, following a 2-hour fast ($n = 60$). While the hummus formulations in the PR test were identical to the test with the adults, the forced-choice paired-comparison method was adapted for young children to ensure that the tasks of the procedure would be understood. Once the children provided verbal assent to participate, they joined the test administrator alone in a conference room that was void of any potential distractions. To confirm that the children understood the test, a mock forced-choice paired-comparison task was performed using hair elastic bands of various colors and two containers labeled with a happy face on one and a sad face on the other. The children were asked to choose a "favorite color" and report this color to the test administrator. The children were then presented with two bands, one of which was their favorite color and the other was a different color. The children were then instructed to choose their favorite hair band and place it inside the container labeled with a happy face. If the child placed the hair band with their favorite color into the appropriate container, then they were deemed capable of performing the preference test with the hummus samples. When choosing a preferred hummus sample, the children simply had to point to their preferred sample and the three-digit code of this sample was recorded by the test administrator. Instead of providing an intensity rating on the gLMS for the strip of PTC paper, the children participated in a yes-no task to determine PTC taster status. The children responded with a "yes" or a "no" to the question "Does that taste bad or have no taste at all?" If the children reported a bad taste, they were recorded as "PTC tasters" whereas children who reported no taste were recorded as "non-tasters".

2.5. Dietary Intake of Children

Parents completed a three-day food record for their children, including two weekdays and one weekend day. Parents documented a detailed description of each food or beverage (i.e., cooking method, brand name) and the amount consumed. Food records were inputted into a nutrient analysis program (ESHA Food Processor, Version 11.0.110, Salem, OR, USA). Calories from sugar, added sugar, total carbohydrates, fat, and protein were computed from an average of three days. Energy density of the whole diet as well as the relative contributions of energy density of sugar, added sugar, total carbohydrates, fat, and protein were also computed.

2.6. Statistics

With R Statistical Software Version 3.4.0 (R Foundation for Statistical Computing, Vienna, Austria), generalized estimating equations (GEE) were used first to estimate the regression coefficients for linear models of psychophysical measures of taste and SNPs. Secondly, SNPs significantly associated with a psychophysical measure of taste were then further analyzed using GEE to estimate the regression coefficients for logistic regression models of SNPs and trait pairs including one taste variable and one diet variable. A logistic regression was used as the alleles of each SNP were treated as binomial experiments with $n = 2$ [20–23]. Only SNPs initially found to be significantly associated with a taste preference in children, prior to the Bonferroni adjustment, were subsequently assessed for associations with dietary intake using logistic regression. Taste variables were generally only paired with diet variables whereby the nutrient elicits that type of taste. For example, SNPs significantly associated with sweet taste preference would only further investigated for associations with added sugar intake. As sour taste is not typically associated with sensing nutrients, it was paired with (1) percent energy from added sugar as sourness often accompanies sweetness in children's candies, and (2) total energy density of diet to examine any potential global effects of sour taste preference on the diet. GEEs were also used to estimate the regression coefficients for linear models to examine the associations between diet variables and covariates including age, sex, and BMI due to the potential moderating effect of BMI on taste perception [7,19,24–26]. Analyses for both parents and children account for correlated outcomes resulting from multiple siblings within some families and from sharing the same household. Regressions were only performed for SNPs located in a gene associated with the same taste modality as the taste outcome. Statistical significance was set to $p \leq 0.05$.

3. Results

3.1. Participant Characteristics

While 72 children and 81 adults from 49 families were recruited for the study, 60 children and 65 adults from 44 families completed the study. Five recruited families did not complete the study due to discontinued communication with the research personnel following recruitment. Adult participant characteristics are summarized in Table 2 and child participant characteristics are summarized in Table 3. Mothers ($n = 41$) and fathers ($n = 24$) had a mean age of 36.3 ± 4.3 years while boys ($n = 27$) and girls ($n = 33$) had a mean age of 4.1 ± 1.2 years. The mean BMI of adults (27.1 ± 5.6 kg/m^2) indicated overweight and the mean BMI z-score of children (0.30 ± 0.99) indicated normal weight.

Table 2. Adult participant characteristics in total and separated by sex.

Characteristic	Total	Female	Male
n	65	41	24
Age (years)	36.3 (4.3)	35.8 (4.5)	37.2 (4.0)
Systolic Blood Pressure (mmHg)	118.4 (19.1)	113.9 (9.9)	130.1 (12.5)
Diastolic Blood Pressure (mmHg)	72.9 (12.4)	70.3 (8.0)	79.6 (8.8)
Heart rate (beats/min)	69.8 (7.9)	69.9 (9.6)	69.8 (7.9)
BMI (kg/m^2)	27.1 (5.6)	26.4 (5.6)	28.1 (4.9)
% Body Fat	-	34.3 (8.9)	26.8 (9.0)
Ethnicity (%)			
Caucasian	85	-	-
Other	15	-	-

Means (SD) were computed for all characteristics except for ethnicities, which are presented as percentages.

Table 3. Child participant characteristics.

Characteristic	Total
n	60
Female	33
Male	27
Age (years)	4.1 (1.2)
Systolic Blood Pressure (mmHg)	102.5 (13.6)
Diastolic Blood Pressure (mmHg)	56.9 (11.2)
Heart rate (beats/min)	91.0 (12.4)
BMI z-score	0.30 (0.99)
% Body Fat	29.3 (6.1)
Ethnicity (%)	
Caucasian	81
Other	19

Means (SD) were computed for all characteristics except for sex and ethnicity, which are presented as frequencies and percentages, respectively. Sample size for each characteristic may vary due to incomplete information from 6 children.

3.2. Genetics and Taste Function/Preference

In total, 93 tSNPs were genotyped from thirteen taste-associated genes in both children and adults. Twenty tSNPs were genotyped from fat taste-associated genes (*CD36*, *GPR120*, and *GPR40*), eleven tSNPs were genotyped from sweet taste receptor genes (*TAS1R2* and *TAS1R3*), rs713598 was genotyped from the bitter taste receptor gene *TAS2R38*, twenty tSNPs were genotyped from salt taste-associated genes (*ENaC* and *TRPV1*), twenty-nine tSNPs were genotyped from umami taste receptor genes (*TAS1R1*, *TAS1R3*, and *GRM4*), and twelve tSNPs were genotyped from sour taste-associated genes (*ASIC1* and *KCNJ2*).

As summarized in Table 4, twenty-three tSNPs were associated with a taste outcome in adults before applying a statistical correction for multiple hypotheses. Following a Bonferroni adjustment for multiple hypothesis testing, the rs713598 and rs236514 SNPs remained significantly associated with taste outcomes. The C allele of the rs173598 SNP in the *TAS2R38* bitter taste receptor gene was significantly associated with PTC sensitivity. The A allele of the rs236514 SNP in the *KCNJ2* sour taste-associated gene was significantly associated with sour preference. As summarized in Table 5, eleven tSNPs were associated with a taste outcome in children before applying a statistical correction for multiple hypotheses. Two tSNPs remained significantly associated with a taste outcome in children after applying a Bonferroni adjustment. The C allele of the rs4790522 tSNP in the *TRPV1* salt taste-associated gene was associated with a significantly higher salt preference compared to the A allele in children. The T allele of the rs173135 tSNP in the *KCNJ2* sour taste-associated gene was associated with a significantly higher sour preference compared to the C allele in children. In both parents and children, the C allele of the rs236512 SNP from *KCNJ2* was associated with sour preference. In parents, the A allele of the rs150908 SNP in *TRPV1* was associated with both higher salt taste sensitivity and a lower preference for salt.

Table 4. Associations between single nucleotide polymorphisms (SNPs) in taste receptor genes and suprathreshold sensitivity and taste preference in adults.

SNP ID	(Gene)	Taste Modality	Outcome	p-Value
rs12137730	(TAS1R2)	Sweet	Suprathreshold	0.021
rs2499729	(GRM4)			0.031
rs3778045	(GRM4)		Suprathreshold	0.007
rs4908563	(TAS1R1)			0.022
rs11759763	(GRM4)			0.007
rs2451328	(GRM4)			0.021
rs2451361	(GRM4)	Umami		0.012
rs2499682	(GRM4)		Preference	0.020
rs2499729	(GRM4)			0.036
rs7772932	(GRM4)			0.015
rs937039	(GRM4)			0.046
rs9380406	(GRM4)			0.007
rs150908	(TRPV1)			0.043
rs161386	(TRPV1)	Salt	Suprathreshold	0.045
rs222745	(TRPV1)			0.036
rs150908	(TRPV1)		Preference	0.036
rs2301151	(GPR40)	Fat	Suprathreshold	0.016
rs3211816	(CD36)			0.014
rs713598	(TAS2R38)	Bitter	Suprathreshold	0.003 *
rs236512	(KCNJ2)			0.041
rs236514	(KCNJ2)	Sour	Preference	0.002 *
rs376184	(ASIC1)			0.019
rs643637	(KCNJ2)			0.011

Generalized estimating equations were used to estimate the regression coefficients of a linear model including suprathreshold sensitivity and taste preference with SNPs (n = 65). Regressions were only performed for SNPs located in a gene associated with the same taste modality as the taste outcome. Following a Bonferroni adjustment for multiple hypothesis testing, the rs713598 and rs236514 SNPs remained significantly associated with phenylthiocarbamide suprathreshold and sour preference, respectively. The Bonferroni adjustment of the reported p-values accounted for the number of hypotheses equal to the number of SNPs in genes associated with each taste modality. * $p \leq 0.05$ following a Bonferroni adjustment for multiple hypotheses.

Table 5. Associations between SNPs in taste receptor genes and taste preference in children.

SNP ID	(Gene)	Taste Modality	p-Value
rs7534618	(TAS1R2)	Sweet	0.026
rs9701796	(TAS1R2)		0.013
rs4713740	(mGluR4)	Umami	0.039
rs4790151	(TRPV1)		0.008
rs4790522	(TRPV1)	Salt	0.001 *
rs877610	(TRPV1)		0.010
rs17108968	(GPR120)	Fat	0.029

Table 5. Cont.

SNP ID (Gene)		Taste Modality	p-Value
rs173135	(KCNJ2)		<0.001 *
rs236512	(KCNJ2)	Sour	0.007
rs236513	(KCNJ2)		0.006
rs9890133	(KCNJ2)		0.006

Generalized estimating equations were used to estimate the regression coefficients of a linear model including taste preference with SNPs ($n = 60$). Regressions were only performed for SNPs located in a gene associated with the same taste modality as the taste outcome. The rs4790522 (TAS1R2) and rs173135 (KCNJ2) SNPs remained significant following a Bonferroni adjustment for multiple hypothesis testing. The Bonferroni adjustment of the reported p-values accounted for the number of hypotheses equal to the number of SNPs in genes associated with each taste modality. * $p \leq 0.05$ following a Bonferroni adjustment for multiple hypotheses.

3.3. Multiple Trait Analysis: SNPs, Taste and Dietary Intake

Results of the multiple trait analysis are summarized in Table 6. Age, sex, and BMI were not significantly associated with any of the diet variables. The rs9701796 SNP in the *TAS1R2* sweet taste receptor gene was associated with both sweet taste preference ($p = 0.022$) and percent energy from added sugar in the diet ($p = 0.05$). The rs9701796 SNP was also significantly related to sweet taste preference when included in a model with total energy density of diet ($p = 0.05$), however total energy density of diet was not statistically significant in the model. While the rs173135 SNP in the *KCNJ2* sour taste-associated gene was no longer significantly associated with sour taste preference, this SNP was significantly associated with total energy density of diet with sour taste preference included in the model ($p = 0.03$).

Table 6. Multiple trait analysis of SNPs in taste receptor genes, taste preferences and dietary intake in children.

SNP (Gene)	Taste Modality	Dietary Outcome	p-Value	
			Taste Preference	Diet
rs17108968 (GPR120)	Fat	Total energy density (kcal/g)	0.09	0.46
		Energy from fat (kcal)	0.10	0.69
		% Energy from fat	0.09	0.65
rs4790151 (TRPV1)	Salt	Sodium (mg)	0.92	0.30
rs4790522 (TRPV1)			0.29	0.44
rs877610 (TRPV1)			0.58	0.71
rs173135 (KCNJ2)	Sour	Total energy density (kcal/g)	0.20	0.03 *
		% Energy from added sugar	0.39	0.49
rs236512 (KCNJ2)		Total energy density (kcal/g)	0.64	0.36
		% Energy from added sugar	0.80	0.35
rs236513 (KCNJ2)		Total energy density (kcal/g)	0.34	0.11
		% Energy from added sugar	0.55	0.78
rs9890133 (KCNJ2)		Total energy density (kcal/g)	0.34	0.11
		% Energy from added sugar	0.55	0.78
rs7534618 (TAS1R2)	Sweet	% Energy from added sugar	0.47	0.11
		Total energy density (kcal/g)	0.32	0.39
rs9701796 (TAS1R2)		% Energy from added sugar	0.02 *	0.05 *
		Total energy density (kcal/g)	0.05 *	0.98
rs4713740 (GRM4)	Umami	Total energy density (kcal/g)	0.37	0.59
		% Energy from protein	0.37	0.99

Generalized estimating equations were used to estimate the regression coefficients of a logistic model including SNPs with trait pairs including a taste preference variable and a diet variable ($n = 60$). Regressions were only performed for SNPs determined to be significantly associated with taste preferences in the initial linear regressions. Taste variables were generally only paired with specific diet variables whereby the nutrient elicits that type of taste. * $p \leq 0.05$.

4. Discussion

This study examined associations between a comprehensive panel of SNPs in taste receptor genes and psychophysical measures of taste across all known taste modalities in both parents and their children. Overall, the findings in this study showed that SNPs in taste receptor genes from all of the different types of taste may contribute to inter-individual differences in psychophysical measures of taste. However, only four SNPs (rs173135, rs236514, rs4790522 and rs713598) were found to be significantly related to a taste outcome after applying a statistical correction for multiple hypothesis testing.

The rs4790522 SNP, located in the salt taste-associated gene *TRPV1*, was found to be significantly associated with preference for salt in children. Regulation of salt intake, or sodium, is due in part to variation in genes related to homeostatic sodium regulation [27–30] and to hedonic responses to the taste of salt [8]. Sodium intake is important to monitor due to its role in the development of hypertension, a risk factor for the development of cardiovascular disease [31–34]. The rs4790522 SNP has previously been shown to change the miRNA binding site of *TRPV1*, suggesting that this SNP may affect the stability of the mRNA precursor to *TRPV1* and prevent translation into its functional protein [35]. The potential decreased functionality of *TRPV1* may reduce salt taste sensitivity and therefore increase the preference of salt in carriers of this SNP. To the authors' knowledge, no associations have previously been found between the rs4790522 SNP and salt taste. Future studies should also consider examining the rs150908 SNP which exhibited significant associations with both salt sensitivity and salt preference in parents, increasing the potential relevance of this variant for salt taste. Studies with larger sample sizes are warranted to replicate these results in order to better understand the genetic basis for salt sensitivity, and therefore hypertension.

Sour taste is elicited by acidic substances through the depolarization of type III taste bud cells [36]. While sourness is conventionally considered a means to avoid the consumption of spoiled foods, many animals find mildly acidic foods to be palatable. Moreover, genetic factors may be more important than shared environment to determine the pleasantness and intensity of sour taste as 34–50% of the variation in pleasantness and use-frequency of sour foods is attributable to genetics [37]. With the knowledge that there is a genetic basis for the preference for sour foods in humans, Ye et al. (2016) proposed that sour taste is mediated by the potassium ion channel $K_{IR}2.1$, encoded by the *KCNJ2* gene [38]. The rs173135 and rs236514 SNPs in *KCNJ2* were found to be associated with the preference for sour in children and parents, respectively. Moreover, the rs236512 SNP was associated with sour preference in both children and adults. Observing associations with sour preference in two different cohorts suggests that this association may pertain to changes in sour taste function. The genetic basis of human sour taste has not previously been explored through examining *KCNJ2* SNPs. These novel findings provide a foundation for future studies to investigate the genetic basis of sour taste as well as sour food intake.

Variants in *TAS1R2* and *TAS1R3* sweet taste receptor genes have previously been associated with changes in taste sensitivity to sugar [39–46], the excessive consumption of which is an established risk factor for obesity and chronic disease [47–49]. Previous research has implicated SNPs in *TAS1R2* and *TAS1R3* in inter-individual differences in sugar sensitivity [7,10] and dietary intake [6,7,9,11,16]. However, this study is the first to find an association between a SNP in a sweet tasting gene with both sucrose preference and dietary sucrose intake. In an analysis of SNPs together with taste and diet, it was found that the rs9701796 SNP in the sweet taste receptor gene *TAS1R2* was both associated with sweet taste preference and percent energy from added sugar in the children. In a previous study in children and adolescents, rs9701796 was associated with increased waist-height ratio as well as with a higher chocolate powder intake in obese children [14]. In another study of children aged 7–12, rs9701796 was not associated with dental caries, a marker often related to excessive sweet food consumption [50]. More research pertaining to this variant is warranted, particularly to assess its relationship with the consumption of sweet foods. By establishing these types of associations in future studies, genetic loci can be considered risk factors for the overconsumption of sweet foods and be used clinically to indicate the risk of developing obesity and other chronic diseases.

The bitterness of green leafy vegetables including Brassica vegetables is related to the taste of thiol compounds and may be stronger in those homozygous for the C allele at the rs713598 locus in the TAS2R38 taste receptor gene. Non-carriers of the C allele may not taste PTC, and this may then influence the perceived bitterness of Brassica vegetables [51]. While parents in this study exhibited a strong association between rs713598 genotype and PTC tasting, no relationship was observed between rs713598 genotype and PTC taster status in children. Children would be expected to show a stronger genotype-phenotype relationship due to having less exposure to culture at their age; however, the lack of association in this study is likely an indicator of the poor reliability of measuring PTC taste sensitivity in this age group. Children between 3–8 years of age may not have an adequately developed understanding of the quality of bitterness. While the study personnel administered a simple yes-no task to determine PTC taster status in the children, this task may still have been too complex due to the unusual taste and paper format of the stimulus.

There are some limitations to consider in this study. Firstly, the data obtained by assessing taste sensitivity in parents, using isolated compounds on filter paper strips, cannot be used to make direct associations between genetics and food intake. This can also be considered a strength of the study as the observations made are accurate for specific taste modalities; however, salt taste was not accounted for when MSG taste was analyzed. The use of hummus as a food matrix in this study may have introduced uncertainty due to the perception of texture, temperature, and other matrix-specific qualities; however the use of a food as a stimulus increases the relevance of these results to food preferences and food selection. In addition, participants were tested for sensitivity and preference on only one occasion, but this should be repeated to confirm validity. Medication was not screened prior to the study, and it is possible that medications taken by the participants could have interfered with taste perception. While this study was powered to observe differences in sensory outcomes, the sample size was small and the likelihood of making type II errors would be lower with a larger sample. Finally, the genetic heterogeneity due to the presence of more than one ethnicity in this sample may hinder the interpretation of the results as the minor allele frequencies of SNPs differ depending on the population. However, the statistical methods used in this work account for correlated outcomes as parents share a household and siblings share household and genetics.

5. Conclusions

This study demonstrated that SNPs in taste receptor genes may contribute to inter-individual differences in taste sensitivity, taste preference and dietary intake. These findings, based on a comprehensive panel of genetic variants in adults and young children, support the relevance of genetics in explaining variation in taste function. The genetic determinants of taste function are important to understand as they may predispose individuals to developing poor eating patterns. In the future, effective strategies can be developed to improve eating habits and therefore risk of obesity through personalized nutritional recommendations based on unique taste preferences.

Author Contributions: E.C. conceived and designed the experiments, collected and analyzed data, and wrote the paper; N.A.C. helped with data collection and analysis; L.D. helped to design the sensory experiments and provided critical revision for the paper; Z.F. helped with the statistical analysis and provided critical revision for the paper; W.Q. helped with statistical analysis; G.D. helped with the statistical analysis and provided critical revision for the paper; A.M.D. helped with the dietary data and provided critical revision for the paper; J.H. provided critical revision for the paper; D.W.L.M. conceived and designed the experiments and provided critical revision for the paper.

Funding: This research was funded by the Ontario Ministry of Agriculture, Food, and Rural Affairs (grant# 030194)

Conflicts of Interest: The authors declare no conflict of interest.

References

1. World Health Organization. Obesity and Overweight. Available online: http://www.who.int/news-room/fact-sheets/detail/obesity-and-overweight (accessed on 5 May 2018).
2. Caballero, B. The global epidemic of obesity: An overview. *Epidemiol. Rev.* **2007**, *29*, 1–5. [CrossRef] [PubMed]
3. Borjeson, M. The aetiology of obesity in children. A study of 101 twin pairs. *Acta Paediatr. Scand.* **1976**, *65*, 279–287. [CrossRef] [PubMed]
4. Stunkard, A.J.; Foch, T.T.; Hrubec, Z. A twin study of human obesity. *JAMA* **1986**, *256*, 51–54. [CrossRef] [PubMed]
5. Skouteris, H.; McCabe, M.; Swinburn, B.; Newgreen, V.; Sacher, P.; Chadwick, P. Parental influence and obesity prevention in pre-schoolers: A systematic review of interventions. *Obes. Rev.* **2011**, *12*, 315–328. [CrossRef] [PubMed]
6. Chamoun, E.; Hutchinson, J.; Krystia, O.; Mirotta, J.; Mutch, D.; Buchholz, A.; Duncan, A.; Darlington, G.; Haines, J.; Ma, D.; et al. Single nucleotide polymorphisms in taste receptor genes are associated with snacking patterns of preschool-aged children in the Guelph family health study: A pilot study. *Nutrients* **2018**, *10*, 153. [CrossRef] [PubMed]
7. Dias, A.G.; Eny, K.M.; Cockburn, M.; Chiu, W.; Nielsen, D.E.; Duizer, L.; El-Sohemy, A. Variation in the tas1r2 gene, sweet taste perception and intake of sugars. *J. Nutrigenet. Nutrigenomics* **2015**, *8*, 81–90. [CrossRef] [PubMed]
8. Dias, A.G.; Rousseau, D.; Duizer, L.; Cockburn, M.; Chiu, W.; Nielsen, D.; El-Sohemy, A. Genetic variation in putative salt taste receptors and salt taste perception in humans. *Chem. Senses* **2013**, *38*, 137–145. [CrossRef] [PubMed]
9. Eny, K.M.; Wolever, T.M.; Corey, P.N.; El-Sohemy, A. Genetic variation in tas1r2 (ile191val) is associated with consumption of sugars in overweight and obese individuals in 2 distinct populations. *Am. J. Clin. Nutr.* **2010**, *92*, 1501–1510. [CrossRef] [PubMed]
10. Fushan, A.A.; Simons, C.T.; Slack, J.P.; Manichaikul, A.; Drayna, D. Allelic polymorphism within the tas1r3 promoter is associated with human taste sensitivity to sucrose. *Curr. Biol.* **2009**, *19*, 1288–1293. [CrossRef] [PubMed]
11. Han, P.; Keast, R.S.J.; Roura, E. Salivary leptin and tas1r2/tas1r3 polymorphisms are related to sweet taste sensitivity and carbohydrate intake from a buffet meal in healthy young adults. *Br. J. Nutr.* **2017**, *118*, 763–770. [CrossRef] [PubMed]
12. Hoppu, U.; Laitinen, K.; Jaakkola, J.; Sandell, M. The htas2r38 genotype is associated with sugar and candy consumption in preschool boys. *J. Hum. Nutr. Diet.* **2015**, *28*, 45–51. [CrossRef] [PubMed]
13. Keller, K.L.; Liang, L.C.; Sakimura, J.; May, D.; van, B.C.; Breen, C.; Driggin, E.; Tepper, B.J.; Lanzano, P.C.; Deng, L.; et al. Common variants in the cd36 gene are associated with oral fat perception, fat preferences, and obesity in African Americans. *Obesity. (Silver. Spring)* **2012**, *20*, 1066–1073. [CrossRef] [PubMed]
14. Pioltine, M.B.; de Melo, M.E.; Santos, A.S.; Machado, A.D.; Fernandes, A.E.; Fujiwara, C.T.; Cercato, C.; Mancini, M.C. Genetic variations in sweet taste receptor gene are related to chocolate powder and dietary fiber intake in obese children and adolescents. *J. Pers. Med.* **2018**, *8*, 7. [CrossRef] [PubMed]
15. Raliou, M.; Wiencis, A.; Pillias, A.M.; Planchais, A.; Eloit, C.; Boucher, Y.; Trotier, D.; Montmayeur, J.P.; Faurion, A. Nonsynonymous single nucleotide polymorphisms in human tas1r1, tas1r3, and mglur1 and individual taste sensitivity to glutamate. *Am. J. Clin. Nutr.* **2009**, *90*, 789S–799S. [CrossRef] [PubMed]
16. Ramos-Lopez, O.; Panduro, A.; Martinez-Lopez, E.; Roman, S. Sweet taste receptor tas1r2 polymorphism (val191val) is associated with a higher carbohydrate intake and hypertriglyceridemia among the population of west Mexico. *Nutrients* **2016**, *8*, 101. [CrossRef] [PubMed]
17. Kushner, R.F.; Schoeller, D.A.; Fjeld, C.R.; Danford, L. Is the impedance index (ht2/r) significant in predicting total body water? *Am. J. Clin. Nutr.* **1992**, *56*, 835–839. [CrossRef] [PubMed]
18. The international hapmap project. *Nature* **2003**, *426*, 789–796. Available online: https://www.nature.com/articles/nature02168 (accessed on 1 March 2016).
19. Pepino, M.Y.; Finkbeiner, S.; Beauchamp, G.K.; Mennella, J.A. Obese women have lower monosodium glutamate taste sensitivity and prefer higher concentrations than do normal-weight women. *Obesity (Silver Spring)* **2010**, *18*, 959–965. [CrossRef] [PubMed]

20. Feng, Z.; Wong, W.W.L.; Gao, X.; Schenkel, F. Generalized genetic association study with samples of related individuals. *Ann. Appl. Stat.* **2011**, *5*, 2109–2130. [CrossRef]
21. Zeny, F. A generalized quasi-likelihood scoring approach for simultaneously testing the genetic association of multiple traits. *J. R. Stat. Soc. Series C (Appl. Stat.)* **2014**, *63*, 483–498.
22. Wang, W.; Feng, Z.; Bull, S.B.; Wang, Z. A 2-step strategy for detecting pleiotropic effects on multiple longitudinal traits. *Front. Genet.* **2014**, *5*, 357. [CrossRef] [PubMed]
23. Yubin, S.; Zeny, F.; Sanjeena, S. A genome-wide association study of multiple longitudinal traits with related subjects. *Stat* **2016**, *5*, 22–44.
24. Park, D.C.; Yeo, J.H.; Ryu, I.Y.; Kim, S.H.; Jung, J.; Yeo, S.G. Differences in taste detection thresholds between normal-weight and obese young adults. *Acta Otolaryngol.* **2015**, *135*, 478–483. [CrossRef] [PubMed]
25. Stewart, J.E.; Feinle-Bisset, C.; Golding, M.; Delahunty, C.; Clifton, P.M.; Keast, R.S. Oral sensitivity to fatty acids, food consumption and bmi in human subjects. *Br. J. Nutr.* **2010**, *104*, 145–152. [CrossRef] [PubMed]
26. Stewart, J.E.; Feinle-Bisset, C.; Keast, R.S. Fatty acid detection during food consumption and digestion: Associations with ingestive behavior and obesity. *Prog. Lipid Res.* **2011**, *50*, 225–233. [CrossRef] [PubMed]
27. Gu, X.; Gu, D.; He, J.; Rao, D.C.; Hixson, J.E.; Chen, J.; Li, J.; Huang, J.; Wu, X.; Rice, T.K.; et al. Resequencing epithelial sodium channel genes identifies rare variants associated with blood pressure salt-sensitivity: The gensalt study. *Am. J. Hypertens.* **2017**, *31*, 205–211. [CrossRef] [PubMed]
28. Yang, X.; He, J.; Gu, D.; Hixson, J.E.; Huang, J.; Rao, D.C.; Shimmin, L.C.; Chen, J.; Rice, T.K.; Li, J.; et al. Associations of epithelial sodium channel genes with blood pressure changes and hypertension incidence: The gensalt study. *Am. J. Hypertens.* **2014**, *27*, 1370–1376. [CrossRef] [PubMed]
29. Rao, A.D.; Sun, B.; Saxena, A.; Hopkins, P.N.; Jeunemaitre, X.; Brown, N.J.; Adler, G.K.; Williams, J.S. Polymorphisms in the serum- and glucocorticoid-inducible kinase 1 gene are associated with blood pressure and renin response to dietary salt intake. *J. Hum. Hypertens.* **2013**, *27*, 176–180. [CrossRef] [PubMed]
30. Zhao, Q.; Gu, D.; Hixson, J.E.; Liu, D.P.; Rao, D.C.; Jaquish, C.E.; Kelly, T.N.; Lu, F.; Ma, J.; Mu, J.; et al. Common variants in epithelial sodium channel genes contribute to salt sensitivity of blood pressure: The gensalt study. *Circ. Cardiovasc. Genet.* **2011**, *4*, 375–380. [CrossRef] [PubMed]
31. Strazzullo, P.; D'Elia, L.; Kandala, N.B.; Cappuccio, F.P. Salt intake, stroke, and cardiovascular disease: Meta-analysis of prospective studies. *BMJ* **2009**, *339*, b4567. [CrossRef] [PubMed]
32. Cook, N.R.; Cutler, J.A.; Obarzanek, E.; Buring, J.E.; Rexrode, K.M.; Kumanyika, S.K.; Appel, L.J.; Whelton, P.K. Long term effects of dietary sodium reduction on cardiovascular disease outcomes: Observational follow-up of the trials of hypertension prevention (tohp). *BMJ* **2007**, *334*, 885–888. [CrossRef] [PubMed]
33. Liu, K.; Stamler, J. Assessment of sodium intake in epidemiological studies on blood pressure. *Ann. Clin. Res.* **1984**, *16*, 49–54. [PubMed]
34. Elliott, P.; Stamler, J.; Nichols, R.; Dyer, A.R.; Stamler, R.; Kesteloot, H.; Marmot, M. Intersalt revisited: Further analyses of 24 hour sodium excretion and blood pressure within and across populations. Intersalt cooperative research group. *BMJ* **1996**, *312*, 1249–1253. [CrossRef] [PubMed]
35. Zhang, J.; Zhou, Z.; Zhang, N.; Jin, W.; Ren, Y.; Chen, C. Establishment of preliminary regulatory network of trpv1 and related cytokines. *Saudi J. Biol. Sci.* **2017**, *24*, 582–588. [CrossRef] [PubMed]
36. Huang, Y.A.; Maruyama, Y.; Stimac, R.; Roper, S.D. Presynaptic (type iii) cells in mouse taste buds sense sour (acid) taste. *J. Physiol.* **2008**, *586*, 2903–2912. [CrossRef] [PubMed]
37. Tornwall, O.; Silventoinen, K.; Keskitalo-Vuokko, K.; Perola, M.; Kaprio, J.; Tuorila, H. Genetic contribution to sour taste preference. *Appetite* **2012**, *58*, 687–694. [CrossRef] [PubMed]
38. Ye, W.; Chang, R.B.; Bushman, J.D.; Tu, Y.H.; Mulhall, E.M.; Wilson, C.E.; Cooper, A.J.; Chick, W.S.; Hill-Eubanks, D.C.; Nelson, M.T.; et al. The k+ channel kir2.1 functions in tandem with proton influx to mediate sour taste transduction. *Proc. Natl. Acad. Sci. U.S.A.* **2016**, *113*, E229–E238. [CrossRef] [PubMed]
39. Drayna, D. Human taste genetics. *Annu. Rev. Genomics Hum. Genet.* **2005**, *6*, 217–235. [CrossRef] [PubMed]
40. Keskitalo, K.; Knaapila, A.; Kallela, M.; Palotie, A.; Wessman, M.; Sammalisto, S.; Peltonen, L.; Tuorila, H.; Perola, M. Sweet taste preferences are partly genetically determined: Identification of a trait locus on chromosome 16. *Am. J. Clin. Nutr.* **2007**, *86*, 55–63. [CrossRef] [PubMed]
41. Keskitalo, K.; Tuorila, H.; Spector, T.D.; Cherkas, L.F.; Knaapila, A.; Silventoinen, K.; Perola, M. Same genetic components underlie different measures of sweet taste preference. *Am. J. Clin. Nutr.* **2007**, *86*, 1663–1669. [CrossRef] [PubMed]

42. Keskitalo, K.; Tuorila, H.; Spector, T.D.; Cherkas, L.F.; Knaapila, A.; Kaprio, J.; Silventoinen, K.; Perola, M. The three-factor eating questionnaire, body mass index, and responses to sweet and salty fatty foods: A twin study of genetic and environmental associations. *Am. J. Clin. Nutr.* **2008**, *88*, 263–271. [CrossRef] [PubMed]
43. Kim, U.K.; Breslin, P.A.; Reed, D.; Drayna, D. Genetics of human taste perception. *J. Dent. Res.* **2004**, *83*, 448–453. [CrossRef] [PubMed]
44. Reed, D.R.; Bachmanov, A.A.; Beauchamp, G.K.; Tordoff, M.G.; Price, R.A. Heritable variation in food preferences and their contribution to obesity. *Behav. Genet.* **1997**, *27*, 373–387. [CrossRef] [PubMed]
45. Reed, D.R.; McDaniel, A.H. The human sweet tooth. *BMC. Oral Health* **2006**, *6*, S17. [CrossRef] [PubMed]
46. Reed, D.R.; Tanaka, T.; McDaniel, A.H. Diverse tastes: Genetics of sweet and bitter perception. *Physiol Behav* **2006**, *88*, 215–226. [CrossRef] [PubMed]
47. Gross, L.S.; Li, L.; Ford, E.S.; Liu, S. Increased consumption of refined carbohydrates and the epidemic of type 2 diabetes in the United States: An ecologic assessment. *Am. J. Clin. Nutr.* **2004**, *79*, 774–779. [CrossRef] [PubMed]
48. Bray, G.A.; Nielsen, S.J.; Popkin, B.M. Consumption of high-fructose corn syrup in beverages may play a role in the epidemic of obesity. *Am. J. Clin. Nutr.* **2004**, *79*, 537–543. [CrossRef] [PubMed]
49. Lustig, R.H.; Schmidt, L.A.; Brindis, C.D. Public health: The toxic truth about sugar. *Nature* **2012**, *482*, 27–29. [CrossRef] [PubMed]
50. Haznedaroglu, E.; Koldemir-Gunduz, M.; Bakir-Coskun, N.; Bozkus, H.M.; Cagatay, P.; Susleyici-Duman, B.; Mentes, A. Association of sweet taste receptor gene polymorphisms with dental caries experience in school children. *Caries. Res.* **2015**, *49*, 275–281. [CrossRef] [PubMed]
51. Kim, U.; Jorgenson, E.; Coon, H.; Leppert, M.; Risch, N.; Drayna, D. Positional Cloning of the Human Quantitative Trait Locus Underlying Taste Sensitivity to Phenylthiocarbamide. *Science* **2003**, *299*, 1221–1225. [CrossRef] [PubMed]

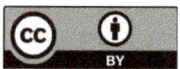

© 2018 by the authors. Licensee MDPI, Basel, Switzerland. This article is an open access article distributed under the terms and conditions of the Creative Commons Attribution (CC BY) license (http://creativecommons.org/licenses/by/4.0/).

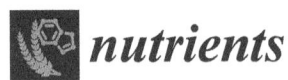

Article

Individualized Meal Replacement Therapy Improves Clinically Relevant Long-Term Glycemic Control in Poorly Controlled Type 2 Diabetes Patients

Kerstin Kempf [1,†], Martin Röhling [1,*,†], Katja Niedermeier [1], Babette Gärtner [1] and Stephan Martin [1,2]

1. West-German Centre of Diabetes and Health, Düsseldorf Catholic Hospital Group, Hohensandweg 37, 40591 Düsseldorf, Germany; kerstin.kempf@wdgz.de (K.K.); katjaniedermeier@web.de (K.N.); babette.gaertner@vkkd-kliniken.de (B.G.); stephan.martin@vkkd-kliniken.de (S.M.)
2. Faculty of Medicine, Heinrich Heine University Düsseldorf, 40225 Düsseldorf, Germany
* Correspondence: martin.roehling@vkkd-kliniken.de; Tel.: +49-(0)211-56-60-360-76; Fax: +49-(0)211-56-60-360-72
† Equal authorship.

Received: 14 June 2018; Accepted: 1 August 2018; Published: 4 August 2018

Abstract: *Background* Formula diets can improve glycemic control or can even induce remission in type 2 diabetes. We hypothesized that especially an individualized intense meal replacement by a low-carbohydrate formula diet with accompanied self-monitoring of blood glucose (SMBG) contributes to long-term improvements in HbA1c, weight, and cardiometabolic risk factors in poorly controlled type 2 diabetes. *Methods* Type 2 diabetes patients were randomized into either a moderate group (M-group) with two meal replacements/day (n = 160) or a stringent group (S-group) with three meal replacements/day (n = 149) during the first week of intervention (1300–1500 kcal/day). Subsequently, both groups reintroduced a low-carbohydrate lunch based on individual adaption due to SMBG in weeks 2–4. After week 4, breakfast was reintroduced until week 12. During the follow-up period, all of the participants were asked to continue replacing one meal per day until the 52-weeks follow-up. Additionally, an observational control group (n = 100) remained in routine care. Parameters were compared at baseline, after 12 and 52 weeks within and between all of the groups. *Results* 321 participants (83%) completed the acute meal replacement phase after 12 weeks and 279 participants (72%) the whole intervention after 52 weeks. Both intervention groups achieved improvements in HbA1c, fasting blood glucose, blood pressure, and weight (all p < 0.001) within 12 weeks. However, these results were not significantly different between both of the intervention groups. The estimated treatment difference in HbA1c reduction was (mean (95% confidence interval [CI]) -0.10% with 95% CI [−0.40; 0.21] also (p > 0.05) (S-group vs. M-group) not statistically different after 12 weeks. However, only the S-group showed a clinically relevant improvement in HbA1c of −0.81% [−1.06; −0.55] (p < 0.001) after 52 weeks of follow-up, whereas HbA1c was not statistically different between the M- and control group. *Conclusion* Individualized meal replacement with SMBG demonstrated beneficial effects on HbA1c and cardiometabolic parameters in type 2 diabetes. Furthermore, the initiation of a weight loss program with one week of full meal replacement (three meals per day) resulted in a clinically relevant long-term HbA1c reduction, as compared to an observational control group that had standard care.

Keywords: type 2 diabetes; low-carbohydrate diet; HbA1c; weight loss; formula diet

1. Introduction

Current type 2 diabetes mellitus guidelines recommend lifestyle intervention as basic treatment. However, patients often fail to improve their eating behavior, physical activity, body weight, and glycemic control in the long run. In this context, new strategies have been developed, such as technology-based approaches [1], to improve adherence to lifestyle interventions and to enable long-term benefits [2]. In contrast, a failing lifestyle intervention contributes to an initiation of a pharmaceutical co-intervention in the next step, however, anti-diabetic medication does not prevent the progression of type 2 diabetes [3]. Within 10 years after diagnosis, about 50% of type 2 diabetes patients start with insulin therapy [4]. This often results in additional weight gain, leading to an increased insulin dosage [5]. Thus, this vicious circle proceeds and disease remission had been unlikely until bariatric surgery demonstrated that type 2 diabetes is reversible [6]. After bariatric surgery, glycemic control improves within a few days, even before a decrease of body weight becomes apparent [7], but this treatment has several severe side-effects [8] and long-term effects are still unclear [9]. In this context, it is still unknown whether the magnitude of improvement is primarily due to caloric restriction or is unique to the surgical procedure [10]. Given the huge need for alternative approaches with long-term effects regarding HbA1c reduction and remission of diabetes, formula diets can be simple and effective measures [11]. Furthermore, the use of energy-restricted formula diets in obese persons with type 2 diabetes improved cardiometabolic endpoints, e.g., waist circumference, fat mass, blood pressure, insulin, or HbA1c, [12]. Moreover, intervention studies, especially those from a group in the United Kingdom (UK) [11,13–15], with a stringent and very low-calorie formula diet were even able to induce diabetes remission [13–15]. In previously published studies, we had already investigated the single or combined effect of low-carbohydrate formula diets and/or telemedicine in patients with type 2 diabetes inducing HbA1c, anti-diabetic medication, and body weight improvements [12,16]. Furthermore, we could also demonstrate the beneficial effect of individual meal prescription accompanied with self-monitoring of blood glucose (SMBG) in patients with type 2 diabetes [17]. However, there are hardly any studies investigating the dose-response relationship of an early intense and individualized low-carbohydrate and moderate-calorie meal replacement therapy by formula diet in patients with type 2 diabetes. Furthermore, a previous study revealed a high dropout rate of 32% for a stringent diet intervention with low-carbohydrate meal replacement [12]. We, therefore, conducted the current intervention by comparing two diet regimens, differing in treatment intensity, with a third observation control group that remained in routine care, in patients with type 2 diabetes.

2. Materials and Methods

2.1. Study Design

The present study consisted of two intervention groups and one observational control group. Volunteers were recruited in Germany by newspaper articles. Eligible type 2 diabetes patients were randomized according to an electronically generated randomization list into two parallel intervention groups with either a moderate (M-group, $n = 160$) or a stringent diet regime (S-group, $n = 149$). The observational group ($n = 100$) corresponds with the control group from our TeLiPro study (NCT02066831) [16]. The participants, the study nurse, and the outcome assessor were blinded for sequence of allocation concealment. The first participant was enrolled on 7 February 2012 and the last participant finished the intervention on 13 June 2014. The study was conducted at the West-German Centre of Diabetes and Health in Düsseldorf (WDGZ), Germany, in cooperation with family doctors and diabetologists around Germany and in accordance with the ethical standards that were laid down in the 1964 Declaration of Helsinki and its later amendments. Approval of the research protocol was obtained from the ethics committee of the Ärztekammer Nordrhein (No. 2011294) and it was registered at clinicaltrials.gov under the number NCT02230501, ClinicalTrials.gov. All of the participants gave written informed consent prior to their inclusion into the study.

2.2. Study Population

Patients with type 2 diabetes, aged 25–79 years with poorly controlled glucose levels (HbA1c $\geq$ 7.5%), and body mass index (BMI) $\geq$ 27 kg/m^2 were included in the study. Participants were excluded when one of the following exclusion criteria was existent: (i) acute infections; (ii) chronic diseases such as cancer, chronic obstructive pulmonary disease, asthma, dementia, chronic gut diseases, psychoses, liver cirrhosis, nephropathy, and kidney insufficiency with glomerular filtration rate < 30 mL/min/1.73 m^2; (iii) weight loss of >2 kg/week in the last month; (iv) smoking cessation or planned smoking cessation during the study; (v) drugs for active weight reduction; (vi) pregnancy or breast-feeding; and, (vii) known intolerance with components of the used formula diet.

2.3. Intervention

At the first contact, the design and intention of the study were explained to the participants by study nurses and trial physicians. A manual and a formula diet were handed out to the patients of the intervention groups. The manual included information about the preparation of the individualized meal replacement as well as general facts about low-carbohydrate meals and their interaction with the blood glucose level. Participants were instructed to perform self-monitoring of blood glucose (SMBG) and note down these values into the manual, the amount of meal replacement taken, the number of meals replaced, as well as their daily dose of anti-diabetic medication. Participants were advised to perform a seven-point blood glucose diurnal profile and they were urged to perform event-driven measurements, e.g., 1.5–2 h after no, low-, or high- carbohydrate consumption or in the fasting state in the morning when exercise had been done the evening before. The patients were encouraged to draw their own conclusions from the SMBG results and to adapt their meals and habits aiming to keep blood glucose levels within a normal range, which was individually prescribed and adapted during the study process. The manual provided guidance on how to change eating habits and how to react to elevated blood glucose levels with physical activity. Based on their own experience and in accordance with the prescriptions to adapt their blood glucose levels, participants were responsible for modifying their diet and received help in the case of nutrition-related uncertainties. In sum, meal replacement and SMBG were individually recommended and adopted to the personal preferences throughout the study. Based on these values, anti-diabetic therapy was monitored and then individually adjusted by trial physicians. This "personalized nutrition and treatment" was one of the main educative approaches in our study. At each visit, study nurses revised the manual and educated/instructed the participants in terms of low-carbohydrate diet, SMBG, physical activity, and self-motivation. Study visits took place after week 1, 4, and 12 and were accompanied with telephone calls or personal meetings. A detailed timeline of the study visits is shown in the Supplementary Figure S1. Participants of the control group only received a self-management guide, a weighing scale, as well as a step counter and they were advised to measure their steps and weight daily.

2.4. Outcomes and Measurements

Clinical and biochemical data were measured at baseline, after 12 weeks of intervention, and after 52 weeks of follow-up. Venous blood was collected after an overnight fast and abdication of medication of at least 10 h by inserting an intravenous cannula into the forearm vein, and laboratory parameters (HbA1c, fasting blood glucose, total cholesterol, high-density-lipoprotein (HDL), and low-density-lipoprotein (LDL) cholesterol) were analyzed at the local laboratory as described in detail elsewhere [16]. Validated questionnaires were used to assess eating behavior (German version of the 'Three-factor Eating Questionnaire' (TFEQ)) and quality of life ('Short Form-36' (SF36)), as previously described [16]. Anti-diabetic medication and changes throughout the study were documented. Adverse events were documented.

2.5. Diet Regimen

The chosen formula diet (Almased-Vitalkost; Almased-Wellness-GmbH, Bienenbüttel, Germany) contained 30.6 g carbohydrates and 1507 kJ (360 kcal) energy per 100 g powder and it was provided to all study probands during the whole study period. Participants of the intervention groups replaced breakfast, lunch, and dinner with 1 g Almased/kg normal body weight (defined as height in cm −100) per meal dissolved in 250 mL water during the first week and consumed 45 g of oil rich in omega-3-fatty acids (1665 kJ; 398 kcal) and 750 mL vegetable juice each day, as previously described [16]. No additional snacks were permitted. During weeks 2–4, the participants replaced breakfast and dinner with the formula diet and ate a low-carbohydrate lunch. The lunch should include 150–200 g of fish or meat, 500 g vegetables, and not more than 50 g of carbohydrates from wholegrain bread or brown rice. The low-carbohydrate nutrition had to be continued in the weeks 5–12, while only dinner was replaced by formula diet. Instructions were identical for the participants of both groups. The only difference between both intervention groups was that the M-group should only replace two meals per day during the first week. All of the participants were asked to continue replacing one meal per day during the follow-up period until the final visit at the 52-weeks follow-up. Both participant and study staff were responsible for the individualized treatment. SMBG as well as the personalized formula diet and the reintroduction of normal meals were interactively modified. Furthermore, the personalized formula diet depends on the current weight of each proband and is characterized by low-carbohydrate meals that are aiming to regulate a normal blood glucose level. We assessed protocol compliance by requiring the participants to note the frequency and amount of formula diet they used as well as the composition of their meals during the first 12 weeks. This information had to be sent back. Afterwards, they got another ration of formula diet for the next weeks. We chose this design with a very similar intervention program as the current study situation reveals that only intense behavioral lifestyle interventions can contribute to meaningful results [14], and we were interested in the dose-response pattern in initial treatment phase during the first week. Furthermore, we had seen in a previous study that a very stringent regime leads to high dropout rates, and we, therefore, wanted to test a gentler entry [12]. The control group remained in routine care (quarterly visits with their attending physician for routine health-care visits, as defined by the Disease Management Programs (DMP) for Type 2 Diabetes in Germany) and did not participate in the meal replacement program.

2.6. Statistics

Previous own data have indicated that with the use of a low-carbohydrate meal replacement a reduction in HbA1c of 0.7% could be achieved [12], while a reduction of $1.0 \pm 0.8\%$ for the S-group was assumed. To be able to measure differences between both of the intervention groups with a power of 80% and a level of significance of 5%, a sample size calculation revealed that at least 230 datasets would be needed. Since a dropout rate of about 25% was estimated, the plan was to recruit a total of 140 participants per group. Data are presented as means and standard deviations (mean $\pm$ SD), median and first and third quartiles (median (first; third quartiles)), means and 95% confidence intervals (mean [95% CI]), or percentages, as appropriate. Completer analyses were performed. Missing values were imputed by the 'last-observation-carried-forward' (LOCF) principle. As HbA1c is the primary parameter in the present study, LOCF was solely applied for other parameters.

Primary endpoint was the differences in Hba1c after 12 weeks between groups, secondary outcomes were the differences in body weight, BMI, cardiometabolic risk factors, eating behavior, quality of life, and frequency of anti-diabetic medication after 12 weeks of meal replacement intervention and 52 weeks of follow-up between the two intervention groups. Furthermore, the estimated treatment difference (ETD), as well as the proportion of weight loss in percentage, was determined. Non-parametric data were analysed with Mann-Whitney U, Wilcoxon, and Friedman test and parametric data with Student's *t*-test, paired *t*-test, and analysis of variance with repeated measures to determine the differences between groups following the intervention. Multivariable univariate regression analyses were carried out to investigate group differences while adjusting for baseline parameters. Dichotomous variables as well frequencies were compared by the Fishers exact test, McNemar test, or Cochrane Q test.

Tertiary outcomes focused on changes in all aforementioned parameters from baseline to week 12 and week 52 within both intervention groups. These were analyzed while using mixed models adjusting for repeated measurements, baseline values, and multiple testing.

Further analyses focused on differences between the intervention groups and the observational control group in regard to HbA1c and weight loss. These analyses were performed in accordance with the statistical approaches used for the determination of the primary endpoints. All statistical tests were two sided, and the level of significance was set at $\alpha = 0.05$. P values were adjusted for multiple comparisons using Bonferroni correction. All of the analyses were performed using SPSS 22.0 (SPSS Inc., Chicago, IL, USA) and GraphPad Prism 6.04 (GraphPad Software, San Diego, CA, USA).

3. Results

A total of 309 participants were randomized into the S-group ($n = 149$) or M-group ($n = 160$), and a control group of $n = 100$ were observed, as shown in Figure 1. Three hundred and twenty-one participants (83% [321:385], $n = 125$ M-group; $n = 122$ S-group; $n = 74$ control group) from the starting cohort finished the 12-weeks intervention, while 64 participants dropped out within the 12-weeks period. Follow-up data after 52 weeks were available from 279 participants (72% [279:385]). Reasons for dropouts were: (i) spontaneous intolerances (5%); (ii) health problems (25%); (iii) professional reasons (5%); (iv) personal reasons (60%); and, other reasons (5%). The demographical and clinical characteristics of the three groups are shown in Table 1. Participants who completed the intervention and follow-up phase and those who dropped out or were lost to follow-up did not differ significantly, apart from differences in diabetes duration, eating behavior, and quality of life between the groups (Supplementary Table S1). No adverse effects have been reported. Patients of the control group were more frequently treated with antidiabetic medication than those in the intervention groups, particularly, regarding insulin therapy. The individual antidiabetic drug classes are listed in Supplementary Table S2.

Table 1. Baseline characteristics of the participants who finished the 12-week diet intervention.

	M-Group ($n = 125$)	S-Group ($n = 122$)	Control Group ($n = 74$)
Sex (% male)	46.4	52.5	52.7
Age (years)	60 ± 10	59 ± 9	60 ± 8
Weight (kg)	110 ± 24	107 ± 20	111 ± 21
BMI (kg/m^2)	37.5 ± 7.6	36.1 ± 5.9	37.0 ± 6.7
HbA1c (%)	8.4 ± 1.1	8.4 ± 1.2	8.2 ± 1.2
Known diabetes duration (years)	9 ± 6	8 ± 7	11 ± 8 [‡,†]
FBG (mg/dL)	181 ± 53	178 ± 63	179 ± 54
SBP (mmHg)	135 ± 17	134 ± 14	134 ± 13
DBP (mmHg)	82 ± 8	80 ± 8	81 ± 9
Total cholesterol (mg/dL)	200 ± 52	198 ± 43	194 ± 48
HDL (mg/dL)	46 ± 10	47 ± 11	47 ± 11
LDL (mg/dL)	118 ± 32	119 ± 37	117 ± 36
Triglyceride (mg/dL)	383 ± 586	220 ± 157	194 ± 113
TFEQ [cognitive control] (au)	10 (7; 13)	10 (7; 13)	7 (6; 8) [#,‡‡]
TFEQ [suggestibility] (au)	7 (5; 10)	7 (4; 10)	5 (3; 6) [#,‡‡]
TFEQ [hunger] (au)	6 (4; 9)	5 (3; 9)	5 (4; 8)
SF36 [physical health] (au)	42 (35; 50)	42 (34; 51)	40 (31; 52)
SF36 [mental health] (au)	49 (38; 57)	49 (32; 57)	39 (35; 42) [#,‡‡]

Shown are means ± SD, median (1st; 3rd quartiles) or percentages. [#] CON vs. M-group, $p < 0.01$; [†] CON vs. M-group, $p < 0.05$; [‡‡] CON vs. S-group, $p < 0.01$; [‡] CON vs. S-group, $p < 0.05$; au, arbitrary units; FBG, fasting blood glucose; BMI, body mass index; DBP, diastolic blood pressure; HDL, high-density-lipoprotein; LDL, low-density-lipoprotein; SF36, short form-36; SBP, systolic blood pressure; TFEQ, three-factor eating questionnaire.

Modified CONSORT flow diagram for individual randomized controlled trials of nonpharmacologic treatments.
An extra box per intervention group relating to care providers and centers has been added.
IQR = interquartile range; max = maximum; min = minimum

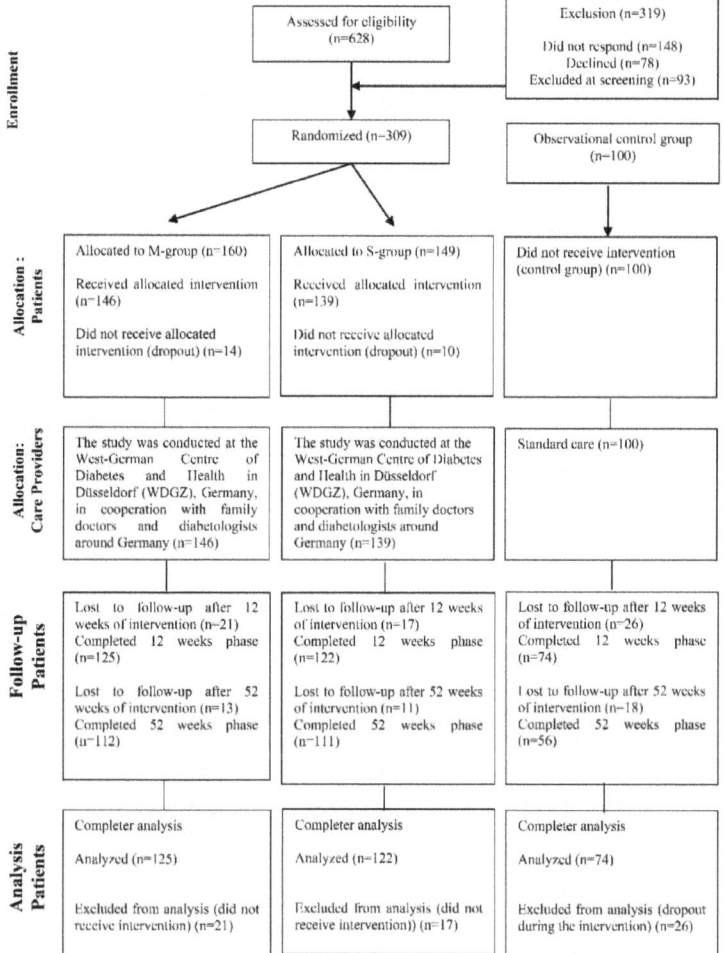

Figure 1. Flow chart.

Besides marginal differences in eating behavior and triglycerides, both intervention groups showed no significant differences in any parameter at week 12 or 52 (Table 2). The ETD in HbA1c reduction after 12 weeks between both intervention groups was −0.10% with 95% CI [−0.40; 0.21] ($p > 0.05$). Treatment superiority of the S-group vs. M-Group is not statistically significant after the 52-weeks follow-up with −0.22% [−0.56; 0.10] ($p = 0.15$). Furthermore, the proportion of weight loss between both of the intervention groups was not different from baseline to week 12 and week 52 (Figure 2).

Table 2. Group comparison between S-group and M-group after 12 and 52 weeks (primary endpoints).

	12 Weeks			52 Weeks		
	S-Group (n = 122)	M-Group (n = 125)	P	S-Group (n = 111)	M-Group (n = 112)	P
Sex (% male)	52.5	46.4	0.374	50.4	46.3	0.593
Age (years)	59 ± 9	60 ± 10	0.966	59 ± 9	60 ± 10	0.523
Weight (kg)	103 ± 22	103 ± 23	0.333	98 ± 17	101 ± 23	0.245
BMI (kg/m^2)	33.9 ± 5.6	35.1 ± 7.5	0.108	33.2 ± 5.1	34.8 ± 7.6	0.074
HbA1c (%)	7.5 ± 1.3	7.6 ± 1.1	0.539	7.6 ± 1.3	7.9 ± 1.4	0.085
Known diabetes duration (years)	7.7 ± 6.6	8.6 ± 6.4	0.265	7.3 ± 5.2	8.9 ± 6.6	0.053
FBG (mg/dL)	154 ± 54	157 ± 50	0.673	156 ± 51	165 ± 52	0.163
RR [syst] (mmHg)	128 ± 14	129 ± 16	0.404	128 ± 14	129 ± 13	0.507
RR [dia] (mmHg)	77 ± 8	79 ± 8	0.082	77 ± 8	78 ± 8	0.339
Total cholesterol (mg/dL)	191 ± 43	190 ± 38	0.829	198 ± 50	194 ± 48	0.571
HDL (mg/dL)	47 ± 10	46 ± 11	0.661	51 ± 36	47 ± 12	0.253
LDL (mg/dL)	116 ± 36	112 ± 31	0.357	120 ± 37	111 ± 33	0.054
Triglyceride (mg/dL)	193 ± 111	205 ± 193	0.564	190 ± 102	368 ± 534	0.025
TFEQ [cognitive control] (au)	13 (9; 16)	13 (9; 16)	0.590	13 (9; 16)	13 (9; 16)	0.704
TFEQ [suggestibility] (au)	5 (3; 8)	6 (3; 10)	0.313	6 (4; 8)	6 (4; 9)	0.189
TFEQ [hunger] (au)	3 (2; 6)	4 (2; 8)	0.131	3 (1; 6)	5 (2; 8)	0.034
SF36 [physical health] (au)	46 (38; 53)	46 (35; 52)	0.277	46 (37; 52)	42 (34; 52)	0.052
SF36 [mental health] (au)	51 (35; 58)	52 (38; 58)	0.330	49 (29; 56)	52 (37; 58)	0.074
No medication (%)	8.2	6.4	0.632	8.2	4.5	0.285
Metformin (%)	76.2	81.6	0.350	76.2	80.4	0.625
DPP4 inhibitors (%)	23.8	29.6	0.317	23.8	33.9	0.187
Sulfonylureas (%)	1.6	4.0	0.447	1.6	8.9	0.285
Glinides (%)	0	0	NA	0	2.7	0.622
Glitazone (%)	0	0	NA	0	0.9	0.990
Glucosidase inhibitors (%)	0	0	NA	0.9	0	0.990
GLP-1 receptor agonists (%)	9.0	11.2	0.674	9.0	11.6	0.661
Sodium-glucose co-transporter-2 (%)	0.8	0.8	0.990	0.9	0.9	0.990
Insulin (%)	18.9	13.6	0.302	18.9	15.3	0.140

Shown are means ± standard deviations, median (1st; 3rd quartiles) or percentages. Differences after 12 and 52 weeks between groups were analyzed using multivariable regression models adjusting for baseline values; au, arbitrary units; FBG, fasting blood glucose; BMI, body mass index; DBP, diastolic blood pressure; HDL, high-density-lipoprotein; LDL, low-density-lipoprotein; NA, not applicable; SBP, systolic blood pressure; SF36, short form-36; TFEQ, three-factor eating questionnaire; DDP4, dipeptidyl peptidase 4; GLP-1, glucagon-like peptide-1.

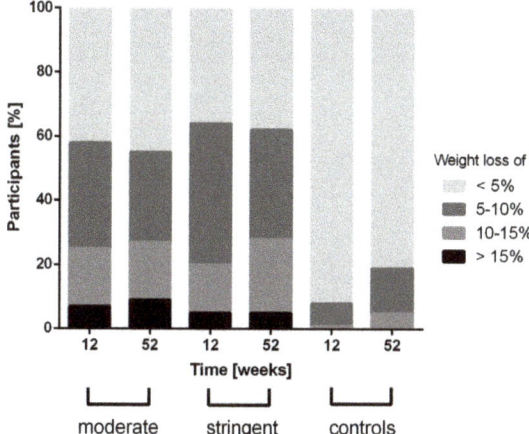

Figure 2. Weight change achieved after 12 and 52 weeks of intervention. Analyses of difference in frequency distribution of weight loss were calculated by using Fisher's exact test.

After 12 weeks of intervention, HbA1c was reduced by (mean [95% confidence interval (CI)]) −0.97% [−1.21 to −0.74] in the S-group and by −0.84% [−1.08 to −0.61] in the M-group (both $p < 0.001$) as shown in Table 3. These improvements were still significant after the Bonferroni correction for multiple testing. After 52 weeks of follow-up, the reduction of HbA1c lost its clinical relevance ($\geq 0.60\%$) [18] in the M-group with −0.55% [−0.80 to −0.29] when compared to the S-Group with −0.81% [−1.06 to −0.55]. Patients of the control group showed no improvement in HbA1c neither after 12 weeks nor after 52 weeks.

Changes of anthropometric, clinical, pharmaceutical, and behavioral parameters within both of the intervention groups after 12 and 52 weeks of intervention are shown in Table 3. Improvements in body weight, BMI, fasting blood glucose, systolic and diastolic blood pressure, as well as eating behavior were observed in the M- and S-group after 12 and 52 weeks of follow-up (all $p < 0.01$). These changes in HbA1c, weight, BMI, fasting blood glucose, systolic and diastolic blood pressure, as well as eating behavior were still significant after the Bonferroni correction for multiple testing (p value = 0.002) in the within-groups analysis. Doses of anti-diabetic medication was already adjusted within the first week of intervention. Frequencies of anti-diabetic drugs were not significantly changed within groups after Bonferroni correction.

Table 3. Changes of anthropometric, clinical, pharmaceutical, and behavioral parameters (secondary endpoints).

	M-Group (n = 125)	S-Group (n = 122)	p
HbA1c (%)	8.4 ± 1.1	8.4 ± 1.2	
Δ HbA1c (%) 12 weeks	−0.84 [−1.08; −0.61] ***,a	−0.97 [−1.21; −0.74] ***,a	0.538
Δ HbA1c (%) 52 weeks	−0.55 [−0.80; −0.29] ***,a	−0.81 [−1.06; −0.55] ***,a	0.149
Weight (kg)	110 ± 24	107 ± 20	
Δ Weight (kg) 12 weeks	−6.93 [−8.08; −5.78] ***,a	−6.91 [−8.07; −5.76] ***,a	0.999
Δ Weight (kg) 52 weeks	−7.30 [−8.65; −5.95] ***,a	−7.45 [−8.80; −6.10] ***,a	0.615
BMI (kg/m^2)	37.5 ± 7.6	36.1 ± 5.9	
Δ BMI (kg/m^2) 12 weeks	−2.38 [−2.78; −1.98] ***,a	−2.35 [−2.75; −1.95] ***,a	0.911
Δ BMI (kg/m^2) 52 weeks	−2.36 [−2.84; −1.88] ***,a	−2.50 [−2.98; −2.02] ***,a	0.536
FBG (mg/dL)	181 ± 53	178 ± 63	
Δ FBG (mg/dL) 12 weeks	−24 [−34; −13] ***,a	−25 [−36; −15] ***,a	0.791
Δ FBG (mg/dL) 52 weeks	−17 [−30; −5] **	−22 [−35; −10] ***,a	0.196
SBP (mmHg)	136 ± 17	134 ± 14	

Table 3. Cont.

	M-Group (n = 125)	S-Group (n = 122)	p
Δ SBP (mmHg) 12 weeks	−5.6 [−8.7; −2.5] ***,a	−6.6 [−9.7; −3.5] ***,a	0.512
Δ SBP (mmHg) 52 weeks	−6.0 [−9.3; −2.7] ***,a	−5.8 [−9.1; −2.5] ***,a	0.858
DBP (mmHg)	82 ± 8	80 ± 8	
Δ DBP (mmHg) 12 weeks	−2.9 [−4.5; −1.3] ***,a	−3.0 [−4.6; −1.4] ***,a	0.371
Δ DBP (mmHg) 52 weeks	−3.7 [−5.6; −1.9] ***,a	−2.9 [−4.8; −1.0] **	0.992
Total cholesterol (mg/dL)	200 ± 52	198 ± 43	
Δ Total cholesterol (mg/dL) 12 weeks	−11.1 [−18.9; −3.3] **	−7.0 [−14.7; 0.8]	0.565
Δ Total cholesterol (mg/dL) 52 weeks	−8.0 [−17.3; 1.3]	0.1 [−9.3; 9.4]	0.396
HDL (mg/dL)	46 ± 10	47 ± 11	
Δ HDL (mg/dL) 12 weeks	−0.1 [−1.6; 1.4]	−0.1 [−1.6; 1.4]	0.908
Δ HDL (mg/dL) 52 weeks	0.9 [−4.0; 5.9]	4.5 [−0.5; 9.5]	0.248
LDL (mg/dL)	118 ± 32	119 ± 37	
Δ LDL (mg/dL) 12 weeks	−6.6 [−10.9; −2.3] **	−3.3 [−7.6; 1.0]	0.144
Δ LDL (mg/dL) 52 weeks	−7.6 [−12.8; −2.4] **	1.8 [−3.4; 7.0]	0.012
Triglyceride (mg/dL)	383 ± 586	220 ± 157	
Δ Triglyceride (mg/dL) 12 weeks	−186 [−268; −104] ***,a	−27 [−109; 56]	0.041
Δ Triglyceride (mg/dL) 52 weeks	−35 [−86; 17]	−31 [−83; 21]	0.865
TFEQ [cognitive control] (au)	9.7 ± 3.9	10.0 ± 4.3	
Δ TFEQ [cognitive control] (au) 12 weeks	2.5 [1.7; 3.3] ***,a	2.5 [1.7; 3.3] ***,a	0.847
Δ TFEQ [cognitive control] (au) 52 weeks	2.3 [1.5; 3.1] ***,a	2.2 [1.4; 3.0] ***,a	0.633
TFEQ [suggestibility] (au)	7.4 ± 3.8	7.0 ± 3.5	
Δ TFEQ [suggestibility] (au) 12 weeks	−0.8 [−1.3; −0.3] **	−0.8 [−1.4; −0.3] ***,a	0.686
Δ TFEQ [suggestibility] (au) 52 weeks	−0.8 [−1.3; −0.2] **	−0.9 [−1.4; −0.4] ***,a	0.342
TFEQ [hunger] (au)	6.3 ± 3.7	5.6 ± 3.3	
Δ TFEQ [hunger] (au) 12 weeks	−1.3 [−1.8; −0.7] ***,a	−1.3 [−1.9; −0.7] ***,a	0.586
Δ TFEQ [hunger] (au) 52 weeks	−1.1 [−1.7; −0.5] ***,a	−1.4 [−2.0; −0.8] ***,a	0.074
SF36 [physical health] (au)	42 ± 10	43 ± 10	
Δ SF36 [physical health] (au) 12 weeks	1.5 [−0.2; 3.2]	1.4 [−0.3; 3.1]	0.773
Δ SF36 [physical health] (au) 52 weeks	0.2 [1.4; 1.8]	1.2 [−0.4; 2.8]	0.150
SF36 [mental health] (au)	47 ± 13	45 ± 15	
Δ SF36 [mental health] (au) 12 weeks	0.6 [−2.0; 3.2]	1.2 [−1.5; 3.8]	0.953
Δ SF36 [mental health] (au) 52 weeks	−0.4 [−3.0; 2.2]	−1.4 [−3.9; 1.2]	0.272
No medication (%)	8.0	8.2	
Δ no medication (%) 12 weeks	−1.6	0	0.652
Δ no medication (%) 52 weeks	−3.5	−0.1	0.179
Metformin (%)	81.6	77.0	
Δ Metformin (%) 12 weeks	0	−0.8	0.660
Δ Metformin (%) 52 weeks	−1.2	0.5	0.942
DPP4 inhibitors (%)	28.8	24.6	
Δ DPP4 inhibitors (%) 12 weeks	0.8	−0.8	0.314
Δ DPP4 inhibitors (%) 52 weeks	5.1	0.6	0.377
Sulfonylurea (%)	6.4	4.1	
Δ Sulfonylurea (%) 12 weeks	−2.4	−2.5	1.000
Δ Sulfonylurea (%) 52 weeks	2.5	0.4	0.920
Glinides (%)	0	0	
Δ Glinides (%) 12 weeks	0	0	NA
Δ Glinides (%) 52 weeks	2.7	0.9	0.622
Glitazone (%)	1.6	0.8	
Δ Glitazone (%) 12 weeks	−1.6	0	0.428
Δ Glitazone (%) 52 weeks	−0.5	−0.8	1.000
Glucosidase inhibitors (%)	0	0.8	
Δ Glucosidase inhibitors (%) 12 weeks	0	0	NA
Δ Glucosidase inhibitors (%) 52 weeks	0	0.1	1.000
GLP−1 receptor agonists (%)	12.0	8.2	
Δ GLP−1 receptor agonists (%) 12 weeks	−0.8	0.8	0.855
Δ GLP−1 receptor agonists (%) 52 weeks	0.4	0.8	1.000
Sodium-glucose co-transporter−2 (%)	0.8	0.8	
Δ Sodium-glucose co-transporter−2 (%) 12 weeks	0	0	NA
Δ Sodium-glucose co-transporter−2 (%) 52 weeks	0.1	0.1	1.000
Insulin (%)	19.2	19.7	
Δ Insulin (%) 12 weeks	−5.6	−0.8	0.290
Δ Insulin (%) 52 weeks	−3.9	−0.8	0.256

Data are shown as mean ± SD and mean [95% CI] or % as appropriate; *** $p < 0.001$ vs. baseline; ** $p < 0.01$ vs. baseline; Superscript letter a represents significance after Bonferroni correction for multiple testing ($p < 0.002$). Differences in changes after 12 and 52 weeks between both groups were analyzed using multivariable regression models adjusting baseline values. au, arbitrary units; BMI, body mass index; DBP, diastolic blood pressure; SBP, systolic blood pressure; SF36, short form-36 questionnaire; FBG, fasting blood glucose; HDL, high-density-lipoprotein; LDL, low-density-lipoprotein; TFEQ, three-factor eating questionnaire; DDP4, dipeptidyl peptidase 4; GLP-1, glucagon-like peptide-1. NA, not applicable.

When compared to the control group (12 weeks: −0.20 ± 0.80 standard deviation (SD); 52 weeks: −0.10 ± 0.90 SD), only the S-group (12 weeks: −0.97 ± 1.18 SD; 52 weeks: −0.81 ± 1.20 SD) demonstrated a significant difference in HbA1c after 52 weeks of follow-up ($p < 0.01$), while the M-group (−0.84 ± 1.14 SD; 52 weeks: −0.55 ± 1.31 SD) was not significantly different (Figure 3). Furthermore, a higher proportion of participants with a larger weight reduction was shown in the intervention groups after 12 and 52 weeks in comparison to the control group (all $p < 0.001$; Figure 2).

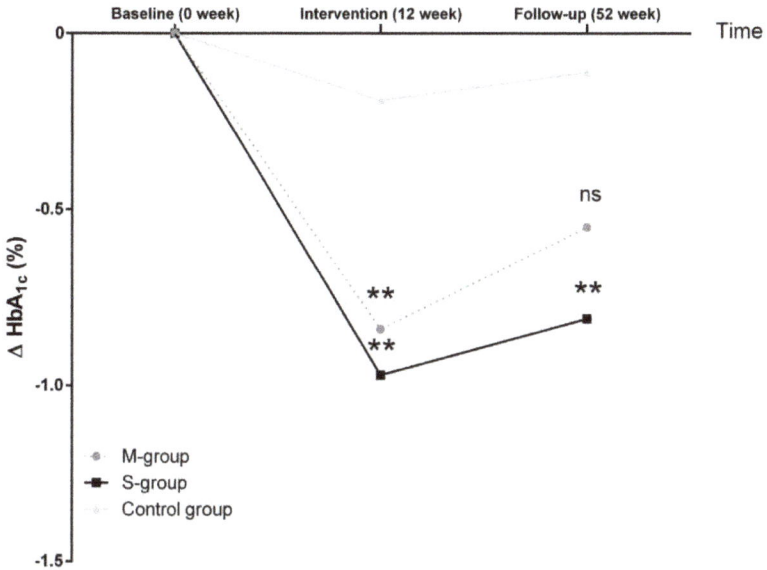

Figure 3. Change of glycemic control after 12 weeks of intervention and 52 weeks of follow-up. At baseline, M-, S- and control group were not significantly different, however, 12 weeks of diet intervention led to reductions in HbA1c in both intervention groups in comparison to the control group. Compared to controls, only the S-group showed a significant difference in HbA1c after 52 weeks of follow-up. Analyses of variance with repeated measures were performed to determine differences between groups; ns, not significant; ** $p < 0.01$ vs. controls.

4. Discussion

The results of the present study demonstrate that an individualized meal replacement therapy starting with intense low-carbohydrate formula diets and SMBG-accompanied reintervention of low-carbohydrate meals lead to clinically relevant improvements in HbA1c after 12 weeks of intervention in patients with poorly controlled long-standing type 2 diabetes. Particularly, patients of the more intense intervention group (S-group) showed long-term clinically relevant improvements after 52 weeks of follow-up as compared to the participants of the moderate intervention group (M-group), although this difference was not statistically significant. Furthermore, the overall dropout rate after allocation into both intervention groups was small (247:285; 13%) and not different (S-group = 12% and M-group = 14%). We hypothesize that the strict rules, the stringent and individual SMBG [17], and the complete replacement of all meals in the S-group during the first week contributed to a subtler change of behavior and higher motivation for the diet, which was shown to be necessary for long-term changes of behavior in high-risk individuals for type 2 diabetes in prior studies [19]. Furthermore, we assume that our personalized nutrition and treatment-approach with a more intense patient empowerment during the first week in the S-group contributed to a long-term difference in HbA1c after 52 weeks of follow-up. The recently published DIRECT study has demonstrated that a strict calorie restriction with only 825–853 kcal per day for 3–5 months contributes to significant improvements of HbA1c (−0.9%) and body weight, and in the further course to diabetes remission after 52 weeks of intervention [13]. However, the formula diet contained proteins and carbohydrates in a ratio of 1:2 [13]. We chose an opposite formula diet that was high in protein, but low in carbohydrates (ratio nearly 2:1) with individualized moderate-calorie supply (1300–1500 kcal/day), because we postulate that a higher amount of carbohydrates would stimulate an increase in insulin release and a decrease in fat burning [20]. Therefore, our strong carbohydrate reduction with an accompanied stepped food reintroduction should lead to long-term benefits like it was shown before in the DIRECT study [13]. Another explanation could be that the S-group was somewhat higher motivated to be physically active due to the complete change of nutrition and behavior, respectively. Previous studies have already demonstrated strong effects on HbA1c through very low-calorie liquid formula diets in small groups of patients with type 2 diabetes ($n < 30$) during an investigation period up to 26 weeks, especially after a short duration of diabetes (<4 years) [11,14,15]. This correlation between diabetes duration and changes of HbA1c after 12 or 52 weeks could be confirmed in our study by the whole intervention cohort ($r = 0.226$ (after 12 weeks) or 0.229 (after 52 weeks); both $p < 0.001$), independently of age.

Our approach of low-carbohydrate meal replacement is based on the recommendations for diets in type 2 diabetes, as well as recently published reviews and meta-analyses [21,22]. Although, a healthy diet is crucial for type 2 diabetes, there still exists controversy in the field about the feasibility and mechanisms of these stringent types of dietary interventions and their long-term effects in HbA1c [23]. The effects on the glucose metabolism (e.g., anti-diabetic medication was adjusted within the first week) occur immediately after beginning the meal replacement therapy [12] and before a significant weight loss takes place. The observed effects are comparable with those after bariatric surgery [7]. Possible explanation approaches in this context could be altered levels of incretin secretion [24], improved mitochondrial oxidative function [25], energy restriction [10], the sudden negative energy balance [14], or a combination of all these points. Furthermore, a reduced carbohydrate intake [26] or a reduced number of carbohydrate-containing meals might trigger the fast effects on the glucose metabolism. This would be in line with observations that two meals per day are better than six [27] for type 2 diabetes patients, especially in terms of body weight, insulin resistance/sensitivity, and beta cell function [10]. The results of the PREDIMED study, in which two high-fat/lower-carbohydrate Mediterranean diets were compared to a fat-reduced diet regarding the incidence of type 2 diabetes [28] or cardiovascular events [29], as well as changes of body weight and waist circumference [30], support our findings that carbohydrate-reduced diets are beneficial for patients with type 2 diabetes.

The improvements in glycemic control in both intervention groups in the present study were followed by strong reductions in body weight (Figure 2). In a recently published meta-analysis, it was shown that very low-calorie (<800 kcal per day) or low-energy liquid-formula (>800 kcal per day) diets can induce large reductions of body weight (ranging from 8.9 to 15.0 kg) in obese people (BMI: 35.5–42.6 kg/m^2) with and without type 2 diabetes [31]. The slight difference in body weight reduction in our trial can be explained by a higher calorie consumption per day ($\approx$1300–1500 kcal per day) when compared to the studies of the meta-analysis. Furthermore, our results are comparable to the findings of Steven et al. [11], who works with a very low-calorie and moderate-carbohydrate composition (43% carbohydrate, 34% protein, and 19.5% fat; 2.6 MJ/day [624 kcal/day]). They found that a very low-calorie diet over eight weeks can contribute to a meaningful weight reduction of $\approx$14 kg, which was still comparably high, even after 26 weeks ($\approx$13 kg) in individuals with type 2 diabetes. In regard to the aforementioned findings, we could demonstrate similar results of weight reduction with $\approx$7 kg after 12 and 52 weeks of intervention. In contrast to Steven et al., we designed an individualized low-carbohydrate and moderate-calorie diet intervention (31% carbohydrate), accompanied with SMBG as it might be more feasible for patients with type 2 diabetes, characterized with eating and motivation impairments [32]. The improvements, apart from the meal restriction, could be therefore also explained by improved education regarding nutrition, physical activity, and blood glucose control.

A recently published review supports our approach, as it states that a rather moderate weight loss is more sufficient for the transition from metabolically unhealthy obesity to metabolically healthy obesity with a lower risk for adverse outcomes in the long run than a large amount of weight loss in a short period [33]. We chose this calorie goal per day in order to reduce the rate for dropouts and increase the participants therapy adherence. Lifestyle interventions are always criticized in terms of their long-term effectiveness, and one possible hypothesis says that the major problem is that patients fail to adhere to the altered lifestyle prescriptions [34]. In contrast to many other long-term lifestyle intervention programs [35], the relatively high number of completers after 12 (83%) and 52 (72%) weeks supports our study design and approach. Potential reasons for nonadherence comprise: age, perception and duration of disease, polytherapy, social and psychological factors, costs, dislike for foods included in meal plans, education and a lack of understanding of the long-term benefits of treatment, adverse outcomes (e.g., weight gain or hypoglycemia), as well as negative treatment perceptions [36]. In this context, new innovative methods are needed to assist those patients. In light of these problems, we designed the study with almost no barriers for the participants (e.g., 1:1 personal support or no additional costs) and provided every participant with a personalized meal replacement and supported them in their SMBG.

Further improvements were achieved in the cardiometabolic parameters of fasting blood glucose, as well as systolic and diastolic blood pressure. These results are confirmative regarding other studies with low-calorie diets in patients with a short- and long-duration type 2 diabetes and moderate [14] or poor glycemic control [10,15]. Our results are also confirmed by a recently published review in terms of improvements of the cardiovascular risk profile in patients with type 2 diabetes showing a significant decrease in systolic and diastolic blood pressure as well as fasting blood glucose after low-calorie diets [37].

A further positive effect following the intervention was the improvement of eating behavior in the intervention groups. The simple and structured formula diet reduced feelings of hunger and increased the control regarding eating-associated actions. In patients with type 2 diabetes, a disordered eating behavior can be present and it is associated with poor quality of life [38]. When compared to individuals with the metabolic syndrome, type 2 diabetes participants of the present intervention groups showed a pronounced feeling of hunger and a weaker control over their suggestibility for food [39]. Another study supports our findings showing meaningful improvements in eating behavior after a three-month mindful eating intervention in non-insulin requiring patients with type 2 diabetes in a small cohort ($n < 30$) [40].

A previously published pilot study [12] revealed how a formula diet affects blood glucose control and weight, and how insulin is reduced or discontinued. However, it was also shown that participants sometimes found it difficult to maintain the stringent diet during the first week. Therefore, we were interested in whether a moderate approach also leads to success. The underlying idea was that the replacement of all three meals in the first week would lead to some kind of "reset". In combination with concomitant blood glucose self-monitoring in the following weeks, an individualized diet should be gradually rebuilt. However, because of the similarity of the intervention design, we expected that the moderate diet regimen would lead to a significant improvement as well. We, therefore, included the comparison with a control group that received standard treatment.

The strengths of the present study comprise: (i) a relatively large number of patients studied per group who had poor controlled type 2 diabetes and a long type 2 diabetes duration; (ii) a longer study period compared to previous studies with formula diets (52 weeks vs. ≤ 26 weeks); as well as (iii) a randomized trial design with two intervention groups and one observational control group. Furthermore, the (iv) chosen real-world setting with a combination of formula diet, SMBG, and dietary education could be easily implemented into present health care programs. Likewise, another study with a real-world approach could demonstrate that even the partial use of a formula diet with one pack of formula diet instead of one of three daily low-caloric meals for 24 weeks was much more effective in reducing body weight and improving coronary risk factors than a conventional diet with a reduced energy intake in obese type 2 diabetic patients [41].

A limitation of our study is that we did not use food diaries to control for decreased calorie consumption or incorrect food compositions (e.g., the amount of carbohydrate in the diet, glycemic index, fat or protein intake) after the acute meal replacement phase from week 13 to week 52. However, the 52-week follow-up revealed that participants of both intervention groups showed no difference in maintaining the formula diet and following the dietary intervention until the study end (S-group 65%; M-group 63%). Also, more profound and quantitative diagnostics, such as isotope measurements, could have been done to control for food-related study compliance. On the other side, interventional studies with formula diets and similar results in a real-world setting [31] support our therapeutic approach in patients with poorly controlled type 2 diabetes.

Another factor, which should be considered, is the adjusted glucose-lowering medication dose in response to glycemic improvements due to the meal replacement intervention. It is conceivable that the impact of our formula diet on the HbA1c reduction is underestimated due to this adjustment. Another limitation of our real-world study is that the participants of the control group were not randomly assigned. In one of our previously published studies (NCT02066831), we found dramatic negative effects on HbA1c and dropout rate (26%) for the participants of the control group [16]. This approach, without a randomized control group with standard care, was also conducted in other benchmark studies for formula diet trials, like the Counterbalance Study (CS) [14] and the Counterpoint Study (CP) [15]. Both of the studies with small sample sizes (n = 11–29) reduced HbA1c (CS: -1.4% and CP: -1.1% to -0.6%) similar, as it was shown in our study after eight weeks of intervention. Furthermore, when comparing the present study results with findings from other landmark studies (DIRECT and TeLiPro study [17,21]), one can see that an assignment to the control group with standard care is accompanied with serious and disadvantageous effects, such as high dropout rates or even an increase in HbA1c. These findings support our approach and study design.

In sum, individualized low-carbohydrate diets can produce clinically-relevant reductions in HbA1c after 12 weeks of intervention. Furthermore, body weight, fasting blood glucose, quality of life, eating behavior, and other cardiometabolic risk factors improved, although not all of the parameters showed statistically significant improvements. Moreover, the initiation of a weight loss program with one week of full meal replacement (three meals per day) resulted in a clinically relevant long-term HbA1c reduction, when compared to an observational control group that had standard care. Our practicable and real-world setting-based approach led to relevant long-term improvements that were comparable with procedures of bariatric surgery without adverse events or negative side-effects. These results support the therapeutic concept of low-carbohydrate diets by formula diets in patients with poorly controlled type 2 diabetes.

Supplementary Materials: The following are available online at http://www.mdpi.com/2072-6643/10/8/1022/s1. Table S1. Baseline characteristics of the drop-outs. Table S2. Baseline antidiabetic drugs.

Author Contributions: M.R. and K.K. wrote the manuscript, researched and collected data. M.R. and K.K. performed the statistical analysis. S.M. had the idea, initiated the study and revised the manuscript. K.N. and B.G. researched data and contributed to the manuscript. S.M. is the guarantor of this work and, as such, had full access to all the data in the study and take responsibility for the integrity of the data and the accuracy of the data analysis.

Funding: The study was financially supported by the Almased-Wellness-GmbH and the Gesellschaft von Freunden und Förderern der Heinrich-Heine-Universität Düsseldorf e.V. The funder had no influence on study design, data collection, data analysis, manuscript preparation and/or publication decisions.

Acknowledgments: We thank our study nurse Bettina Prete (West-German Centre of Diabetes and Health) for her excellent work.

Conflicts of Interest: K. Kempf and S. Martin received consultant fees from the Almased-Wellness-GmbH. M. Röhling, B. Gärtner and K. Niedermeier declare that there is no conflict of interest regarding the publication of this article.

References

1. Dunkley, A.J.; Bodicoat, D.H.; Greaves, C.J.; Russell, C.; Yates, T.; Davies, M.J.; Khunti, K. Diabetes prevention in the real world: Effectiveness of pragmatic lifestyle interventions for the prevention of type 2 diabetes and of the impact of adherence to guideline recommendations: A systematic review and meta-analysis. *Diabetes Care* **2014**, *37*, 922–933. [CrossRef] [PubMed]
2. Rise, M.B.; Pellerud, A.; Rygg, L.O.; Steinsbekk, A. Making and maintaining lifestyle changes after participating in group based type 2 diabetes self-management educations: A qualitative study. *PLoS ONE* **2013**, *8*, e64009. [CrossRef] [PubMed]
3. Giorgino, F.; Home, P.D.; Tuomilehto, J. Glucose Control and Vascular Outcomes in Type 2 Diabetes: Is the Picture Clear? *Diabetes Care* **2016**, *39* (Suppl. S2), S187–S195. [CrossRef] [PubMed]
4. U.K. Prospective Diabetes Study Group. U.K. prospective diabetes study 16. Overview of 6 years' therapy of type II diabetes: A progressive disease. U.K. Prospective Diabetes Study Group. *Diabetes* **1995**, *44*, 1249–1258. [CrossRef]
5. Yki-Jarvinen, H.; Ryysy, L.; Kauppila, M.; Kujansuu, E.; Lahti, J.; Marjanen, T.; Niskanen, L.; Rajala, S.; Salo, S.; Seppala, P.; et al. Effect of obesity on the response to insulin therapy in noninsulin-dependent diabetes mellitus. *J. Clin. Endocrinol. Metab.* **1997**, *82*, 4037–4043. [CrossRef] [PubMed]
6. Gloy, V.L.; Briel, M.; Bhatt, D.L.; Kashyap, S.R.; Schauer, P.R.; Mingrone, G.; Bucher, H.C.; Nordmann, A.J. Bariatric surgery versus non-surgical treatment for obesity: A systematic review and meta-analysis of randomised controlled trials. *BMJ* **2013**, *347*, f5934. [CrossRef] [PubMed]
7. Ackerman, N.B. Observations on the improvements in carbohydrate metabolism in diabetic and other morbidly obese patients after jejunoileal bypass. *Surg. Gynecol. Obstet.* **1981**, *152*, 581–586. [PubMed]
8. Backman, O.; Stockeld, D.; Rasmussen, F.; Naslund, E.; Marsk, R. Alcohol and substance abuse, depression and suicide attempts after Roux-en-Y gastric bypass surgery. *Br. J. Surg.* **2016**, *103*, 1336–1342. [CrossRef] [PubMed]
9. Colquitt, J.L.; Pickett, K.; Loveman, E.; Frampton, G.K. Surgery for weight loss in adults. *Cochrane Database Syst. Rev.* **2014**, *8*, Cd003641. [CrossRef] [PubMed]
10. Jackness, C.; Karmally, W.; Febres, G.; Conwell, I.M.; Ahmed, L.; Bessler, M.; McMahon, D.J.; Korner, J. Very low-calorie diet mimics the early beneficial effect of Roux-en-Y gastric bypass on insulin sensitivity and beta-cell Function in type 2 diabetic patients. *Diabetes* **2013**, *62*, 3027–3032. [CrossRef] [PubMed]
11. Steven, S.; Hollingsworth, K.G.; Al-Mrabeh, A.; Avery, L.; Aribisala, B.; Caslake, M.; Taylor, R. Very Low-Calorie Diet and 6 Months of Weight Stability in Type 2 Diabetes: Pathophysiological Changes in Responders and Nonresponders. *Diabetes Care* **2016**, *39*, 808–815. [CrossRef] [PubMed]
12. Kempf, K.; Schloot, N.C.; Gartner, B.; Keil, R.; Schadewaldt, P.; Martin, S. Meal replacement reduces insulin requirement, HbA1c and weight long-term in type 2 diabetes patients with >100 U insulin per day. *J. Hum. Nutr. Diet.* **2014**, *27* (Suppl. S2), 21–27. [CrossRef] [PubMed]
13. Lean, M.E.; Leslie, W.S.; Barnes, A.C.; Brosnahan, N.; Thom, G.; McCombie, L.; Peters, C.; Zhyzhneuskaya, S.; Al-Mrabeh, A.; Hollingsworth, K.G.; et al. Primary care-led weight management for remission of type 2 diabetes (DiRECT): An open-label, cluster-randomised trial. *Lancet* **2017**. [CrossRef]
14. Lim, E.L.; Hollingsworth, K.G.; Aribisala, B.S.; Chen, M.J.; Mathers, J.C.; Taylor, R. Reversal of type 2 diabetes: Normalisation of beta cell function in association with decreased pancreas and liver triacylglycerol. *Diabetologia* **2011**, *54*, 2506–2514. [CrossRef] [PubMed]
15. Steven, S.; Taylor, R. Restoring normoglycaemia by use of a very low calorie diet in long- and short-duration Type 2 diabetes. *Diabet. Med.* **2015**, *32*, 1149–1155. [CrossRef] [PubMed]
16. Kempf, K.; Altpeter, B.; Berger, J.; Reuss, O.; Fuchs, M.; Schneider, M.; Gartner, B.; Niedermeier, K.; Martin, S. Efficacy of the Telemedical Lifestyle intervention Program TeLiPro in Advanced Stages of Type 2 Diabetes: A Randomized Controlled Trial. *Diabetes Care* **2017**, *40*, 863–871. [CrossRef] [PubMed]
17. Kempf, K.; Kruse, J.; Martin, S. ROSSO-in-praxi follow-up: Long-term effects of self-monitoring of blood glucose on weight, hemoglobin A1c, and quality of life in patients with type 2 diabetes mellitus. *Diabetes Technol. Ther.* **2012**, *14*, 59–64. [CrossRef] [PubMed]
18. Thomas, D.E.; Elliott, E.J.; Naughton, G.A. Exercise for type 2 diabetes mellitus. *Cochrane Database Syst. Rev.* **2006**, *3*, Cd002968. [CrossRef] [PubMed]

19. den Braver, N.R.; de Vet, E.; Duijzer, G.; Ter Beek, J.; Jansen, S.C.; Hiddink, G.J.; Feskens, E.J.M.; Haveman-Nies, A. Determinants of lifestyle behavior change to prevent type 2 diabetes in high-risk individuals. *Int. J. Behav. Nutr. Phys. Act.* **2017**, *14*, 78. [CrossRef] [PubMed]
20. Gower, B.A.; Goss, A.M. A lower-carbohydrate, higher-fat diet reduces abdominal and intermuscular fat and increases insulin sensitivity in adults at risk of type 2 diabetes. *J. Nutr.* **2015**, *145*, 177s–183s. [CrossRef] [PubMed]
21. Qian, F.; Korat, A.A.; Malik, V.; Hu, F.B. Metabolic Effects of Monounsaturated Fatty Acid-Enriched Diets Compared With Carbohydrate or Polyunsaturated Fatty Acid-Enriched Diets in Patients with Type 2 Diabetes: A Systematic Review and Meta-analysis of Randomized Controlled Trials. *Diabetes Care* **2016**, *39*, 1448–1457. [CrossRef] [PubMed]
22. Snorgaard, O.; Poulsen, G.M.; Andersen, H.K.; Astrup, A. Systematic review and meta-analysis of dietary carbohydrate restriction in patients with type 2 diabetes. *BMJ Open Diabetes Res. Care* **2017**, *5*, e000354. [CrossRef] [PubMed]
23. Wheeler, M.L.; Dunbar, S.A.; Jaacks, L.M.; Karmally, W.; Mayer-Davis, E.J.; Wylie-Rosett, J.; Yancy, W.S., Jr. Macronutrients, food groups, and eating patterns in the management of diabetes: A systematic review of the literature, 2010. *Diabetes Care* **2012**, *35*, 434–445. [CrossRef] [PubMed]
24. Rubino, F.; Forgione, A.; Cummings, D.E.; Vix, M.; Gnuli, D.; Mingrone, G.; Castagneto, M.; Marescaux, J. The mechanism of diabetes control after gastrointestinal bypass surgery reveals a role of the proximal small intestine in the pathophysiology of type 2 diabetes. *Ann. Surg.* **2006**, *244*, 741–749. [CrossRef] [PubMed]
25. Urbanova, M.; Mraz, M.; Durovcova, V.; Trachta, P.; Klouckova, J.; Kavalkova, P.; Haluzikova, D.; Lacinova, Z.; Hansikova, H.; Wenchich, L.; et al. The effect of very-low-calorie diet on mitochondrial dysfunction in subcutaneous adipose tissue and peripheral monocytes of obese subjects with type 2 diabetes mellitus. *Physiol. Res.* **2017**, *66*, 811–822. [PubMed]
26. Esposito, K.; Maiorino, M.I.; Ciotola, M.; Di Palo, C.; Scognamiglio, P.; Gicchino, M.; Petrizzo, M.; Saccomanno, F.; Beneduce, F.; Ceriello, A.; et al. Effects of a Mediterranean-style diet on the need for antihyperglycemic drug therapy in patients with newly diagnosed type 2 diabetes: A randomized trial. *Ann. Intern. Med.* **2009**, *151*, 306–314. [CrossRef] [PubMed]
27. Kahleova, H.; Belinova, L.; Malinska, H.; Oliyarnyk, O.; Trnovska, J.; Skop, V.; Kazdova, L.; Dezortova, M.; Hajek, M.; Tura, A.; et al. Eating two larger meals a day (breakfast and lunch) is more effective than six smaller meals in a reduced-energy regimen for patients with type 2 diabetes: A randomised crossover study. *Diabetologia* **2014**, *57*, 1552–1560. [CrossRef] [PubMed]
28. Salas-Salvado, J.; Bullo, M.; Babio, N.; Martinez-Gonzalez, M.A.; Ibarrola-Jurado, N.; Basora, J.; Estruch, R.; Covas, M.I.; Corella, D.; Aros, F.; et al. Reduction in the incidence of type 2 diabetes with the Mediterranean diet: Results of the PREDIMED-Reus nutrition intervention randomized trial. *Diabetes Care* **2011**, *34*, 14–19. [CrossRef] [PubMed]
29. Estruch, R.; Ros, E.; Salas-Salvado, J.; Covas, M.I.; Corella, D.; Aros, F.; Gomez-Gracia, E.; Ruiz-Gutierrez, V.; Fiol, M.; Lapetra, J.; et al. Primary prevention of cardiovascular disease with a Mediterranean diet. *N. Engl. J. Med.* **2013**, *368*, 1279–1290. [CrossRef] [PubMed]
30. Estruch, R.; Martinez-Gonzalez, M.A.; Corella, D.; Salas-Salvado, J.; Fito, M.; Chiva-Blanch, G.; Fiol, M.; Gomez-Gracia, E.; Aros, F.; Lapetra, J.; et al. Effect of a high-fat Mediterranean diet on bodyweight and waist circumference: A prespecified secondary outcomes analysis of the PREDIMED randomised controlled trial. *Lancet Diabetes Endocrinol.* **2016**, *4*, 666–676. [CrossRef]
31. Leslie, W.S.; Taylor, R.; Harris, L.; Lean, M.E. Weight losses with low-energy formula diets in obese patients with and without type 2 diabetes: Systematic review and meta-analysis. *Int. J. Obes. (Lond.)* **2017**, *41*, 96–101. [CrossRef] [PubMed]
32. Rehackova, L.; Araujo-Soares, V.; Adamson, A.J.; Steven, S.; Taylor, R.; Sniehotta, F.F. Acceptability of a very-low-energy diet in Type 2 diabetes: Patient experiences and behaviour regulation. *Diabet. Med.* **2017**. [CrossRef] [PubMed]
33. Stefan, N.; Haring, H.U.; Schulze, M.B. Metabolically healthy obesity: The low-hanging fruit in obesity treatment? *Lancet Diabetes Endocrinol.* **2017**. [CrossRef]
34. Banasik, J.L.; Walker, M.K.; Randall, J.M.; Netjes, R.B.; Foutz, M.S. Low-calorie diet induced weight loss may alter regulatory hormones and contribute to rebound visceral adiposity in obese persons with a family history of type-2 diabetes. *J. Am. Assoc. Nurse Pract.* **2013**, *25*, 440–448. [CrossRef] [PubMed]

35. Garcia-Perez, L.E.; Alvarez, M.; Dilla, T.; Gil-Guillen, V.; Orozco-Beltran, D. Adherence to therapies in patients with type 2 diabetes. *Diabetes Ther.* **2013**, *4*, 175–194. [CrossRef] [PubMed]
36. Shultz, J.A.; Sprague, M.A.; Branen, L.J.; Lambeth, S. A comparison of views of individuals with type 2 diabetes mellitus and diabetes educators about barriers to diet and exercise. *J. Health Commun.* **2001**, *6*, 99–115. [CrossRef] [PubMed]
37. Sellahewa, L.; Khan, C.; Lakkunarajah, S.; Idris, I. A Systematic Review of Evidence on the Use of Very Low Calorie Diets in People with Diabetes. *Curr. Diabetes Rev.* **2017**, *13*, 35–46. [CrossRef] [PubMed]
38. Cerrelli, F.; Manini, R.; Forlani, G.; Baraldi, L.; Melchionda, N.; Marchesini, G. Eating behavior affects quality of life in type 2 diabetes mellitus. *Eat. Weight Disord.* **2005**, *10*, 251–257. [CrossRef] [PubMed]
39. Carbonneau, E.; Royer, M.M.; Richard, C.; Couture, P.; Desroches, S.; Lemieux, S.; Lamarche, B. Effects of the Mediterranean Diet before and after Weight Loss on Eating Behavioral Traits in Men with Metabolic Syndrome. *Nutrients* **2017**, *9*, 305. [CrossRef] [PubMed]
40. Miller, C.K.; Kristeller, J.L.; Headings, A.; Nagaraja, H. Comparison of a mindful eating intervention to a diabetes self-management intervention among adults with type 2 diabetes: A randomized controlled trial. *Health Educ. Behav.* **2014**, *41*, 145–154. [CrossRef] [PubMed]
41. Shirai, K.; Saiki, A.; Oikawa, S.; Teramoto, T.; Yamada, N.; Ishibashi, S.; Tada, N.; Miyazaki, S.; Inoue, I.; Murano, S.; et al. The effects of partial use of formula diet on weight reduction and metabolic variables in obese type 2 diabetic patients-multicenter trial. *Obes. Res. Clin. Pract.* **2013**, *7*, e43–e54. [CrossRef] [PubMed]

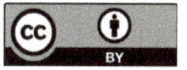

© 2018 by the authors. Licensee MDPI, Basel, Switzerland. This article is an open access article distributed under the terms and conditions of the Creative Commons Attribution (CC BY) license (http://creativecommons.org/licenses/by/4.0/).

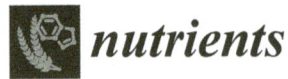

Review

Personalized Nutrition Approach in Food Allergy: Is It Prime Time Yet?

Enza D'Auria [1,*], Mariette Abrahams [2], Gian Vincenzo Zuccotti [1] and Carina Venter [3]

1. Department of Pediatrics, Children's Hospital V. Buzzi, University of Milan, Milan 20154, Italy; gianvincenzo.zuccotti@unimi.it
2. Faculty of Social Sciences, University of Bradford, Bradford BD7 1DP, UK; mariette@marietteabrahams.com
3. Section of Allergy and Immunology, Children's Hospital Colorado, University of Colorado, Aurora, CO 80045, USA; carina.venter@childrenscolorado.org
* Correspondence: enza.dauria@unimi.it

Received: 27 December 2018; Accepted: 5 February 2019; Published: 9 February 2019

Abstract: The prevalence of food allergy appears to be steadily increasing in infants and young children. One of the major challenges of modern clinical nutrition is the implementation of individualized nutritional recommendations. The management of food allergy (FA) has seen major changes in recent years. While strict allergen avoidance is still the key treatment principle, it is increasingly clear that the avoidance diet should be tailored according to the patient FA phenotype. Furthermore, new insights into the gut microbiome and immune system explain the rising interest in tolerance induction and immunomodulation by microbiota-targeted dietary intervention. This review article focuses on the nutritional management of IgE mediated food allergy, mainly focusing on different aspects of the avoidance diet. A personalized approach to managing the food allergic individual is becoming more feasible as we are learning more about diagnostic modalities and allergic phenotypes. However, some unmet needs should be addressed to fully attain this goal.

Keywords: food allergy; avoidance diet; nutrition; personalized nutrition; phenotype; microbiome

---

1. Introduction

The true prevalence of food allergy is still unclear: a systematic review of challenge proven food allergy (FA) prevalence in Europe estimates a very low prevalence of FA of 1% [1] compared to single center studies reporting challenge proven prevalence figures of up to 10%. The latest paper on the prevalence of food allergies in children in the USA reports the number of reported FA of 7.6% in children [2] and 10.8% in adults [3].

A small number of foods, such as milk, egg, peanut, tree nuts, wheat, soy, fish, and shellfish, are responsible of most of IgE mediated allergic reactions [4,5]. These reactions are induced by allergenic proteins in the foods and are characterized by rapid onset (usually <2 h). These foods can provoke severe reactions, especially tree nut and peanuts [5,6]. Clinical reactivity to carbohydrates in mammalian meat is an exception—symptoms can be delayed for as long as 6 h [7].

The cornerstone of the management of FA still relies on avoiding the culprit food, since accidental ingestion of the offending food may lead to symptoms including serious and potentially life-threatening reactions, like anaphylaxis [8].

The management of food allergies has seen major transformations in the last decade. It is increasingly clear that the avoidance diet should be tailored according to the patient FA phenotype [9]. Better characterization of FA phenotypes could help to personalize the dietary management of FA by the degree of avoidance required.

Furthermore, there is a greater focus seen on tolerance induction and immunomodulation by microbiota-targeted dietary intervention to allow for greater control of allergies. In the era of precision medicine, the field of precision nutrition involves tailored nutritional recommendations to the individual. To plan personalized nutrition advice for patients with a food allergy, many factors including clinical history, type of allergen, sensitization profiles, threshold level, dietary habits, food preferences, physical activity, microbiome and genotype should all be considered.

In the field of food allergy, some of these factors are better-defined thanks to new diagnostic molecular technologies [10]. Allergen-component resolved diagnostics (CRD) allows differentiating between a true food allergy from pollen-food syndrome or clinically irrelevant sensitization. CRD may predict the risk or severity of allergic reactions to specific food by identifying IgE to epitopes within an allergen source. However, many other components necessary for dietary guidance are poorly understood and need further investigation to be incorporated into clinical practice.

In this review, we will focus on the nutritional management of IgE mediated food allergy, the avoidance diet, state of the art tools/therapies, and the remaining knowledge gap.

2. Making an Accurate Diagnosis: The First Step Required to Develop an Avoidance Diet

The first step in the diagnosis of a FA is to distinguish IgE-mediated from non–IgE-mediated reactions. Most IgE caused reactions occur rapidly (minutes up to 2 h after ingestion) with the rare exception [11]. Anaphylaxis is the most serious allergic reaction; it is rapid in onset, life-threatening, and potentially fatal [12]. Different geographical locations show some differences in food allergen triggers for anaphylaxis. A recent one from Spain suggested milk and eggs allergies are more severe than nuts in their population [13].

Unlike IgE mediated, non IgE-mediated reactions are typically delayed from hours to weeks after ingestion of the culprit food(s) [11].

A thourough clinical history is central in diagnosing FA. Components of this history should ideally include food recalls, as well as timing, characteristics, and severity of symptoms. If the history suggests an IgE mediated food allergy, skin prick tests (SPT) or food-specific IgE blood tests can be used to confirm allergy diagnosis [5,14]. A positive test result does not confirm an IgE-mediated allergic reaction, whereas a negative test, with rare exception, eliminates it [15].

In addition to the SPT and specific IgE tests, oral food challenges (OFC) and CRD are important tools for allergy diagnosis. OFC remains the gold standard to confirm clinical reactivity, in most cases [16,17]. Component-resolved diagnostics helps further define specific allergens and reduces misdiagnosis due to cross-reactivity [18,19]. The usefulness of these tools can be explained through the classic example—wheat allergy. Wheat allergy is often over diagnosed, due to the low specificity of wheat IgE testing [20,21]. A patient with a grass pollen allergy may have elevated "wheat IgE levels" while being wheat tolerant [22]. Therefore, both CRD and OFCs should be implemented in children with an SPT or IgE positive wheat allergy. CRD increases the accuracy of wheat allergy diagnosis by identifying the presence of specific IgE to omega-5 gliadin, the antibody highly specific to wheat allergy [23]. Currently, oral provocation with wheat is the reference test for the diagnosis of wheat/cereal allergy as it definitely shows if a child will tolerate wheat.

Additionally, profiling the specific IgE repertoire by CRD may help identify falsely diagnosed allergies in highly polysensitized patients. This can be explained with the case of patients with allergen extract positive but negative genuine components. In children with multiple sensitization to tree nuts, including hazelnut, positive IgE extract but negative IgE genuine component are markers of a probable cross-sensitization with grass pollen. These patients are very likely to be tolerant to hazelnut in vivo [24]. CRD has become a useful tool for diagnosing FA, though the use of these tests varies from country to country.; This technique has some limitations that should be considered. For instance, the allergens are in a recombinant form and not always show the same IgE reactivity that natural allergens. This is even more relevant in food allergy testing as the allergens used in the reagents are processed. Indeed, the oral food challenge (OFC) is the only effective method to confirm the FA diagnosis, although the other preliminary diagnostic techniques could support the diagnosis.

3. Risk Assessment and Individual Threshold Level

In general, for IgE mediated-food allergy it is very important to identify patients who are likely to have severe reactions from patients with mild to moderate ones. Unfortunately, as allergy severity is multifactorial, this is difficult. Possible contributors to severe reactions are allergen bioavailability, patient habits (e.g., Exercise [25]), and history of anaphylaxis—although many people who have a history of only mild symptoms can develop anaphylaxis. Allergen-specific IgE levels and CRD may assist in risk assessment as sensitization to some allergenic molecules is more likely to be related to systemic rather than local reactions.

For instance, high levels of casein IgE has been shown to correlate with severe reactions, due to accidental exposure, in cow's milk allergic children [26]. Similarly, an association between specific IgE to omega-5 gliadin component and severity of reactions during wheat challenge has been reported [21,27]. In peanut allergic children, Eller and Bindslev–Jensen documented that symptom severity elicited during challenge correlated significantly with the levels of Ara h 2 ($r(s) = 0.60$, $P < 0.0001$) [28]. However, patients with very low or undetectable sIgE may still experience severe allergic reactions [25,29].

The OFC allows us to ascertain information about individual threshold level can guide the necessary level of food avoidance.

For instance, the challenge food for baked milk contains 1.3 g CM protein (equivalent to 40 mL CM), and children who react during their CM OFC should avoid it completely due to their severe phenotype [30].

Lieberman et al. showed that 66% of the patients with egg allergy undergoing baked egg OFC tolerated baked egg and that most of the reactions were mild and treated with antihistamine alone, regardless of sIgE and/or SPT. [31].

In our opinion, performing OFC with baked milk or egg in a controlled-setting has the potential to greatly improve children's quality of life [32].

4. Avoidance Diet: Towards Personalized Nutrition Advice

Managing food allergies and avoiding food allergic reactions involves an individualized approach to food allergen avoidance while providing sufficient nutrition [33].

An avoidance diet is a complex undertaking that requires education about label reading, cooking, preventing cross-contamination, and communicating information to family, caregivers, friends, and restaurant personnel [34,35]. See Table 1

Table 1. Nutritional management according to risk assessment: What are the challenges?

Challenges of the Nutritional Management According to Risk Assessment
- local availability of food
- lack of understanding about foods to be avoided
- unexpected allergens in foods
- prepacked foods with inadequate allergen labeling
- defining "baked" milk and egg
- identify the "eliciting dose"
- risks of over restrictive diet
- potential long-term effects on health and quality of life

The standard information that should be provided to all patients includes advice on food labels and relevant labeling laws, hidden allergens, and suitable replacement foods [36]. However, avoidance advice should be individualized considering individual tolerances, cross-reactivity, and specific allergens that drive the reaction. Allergies to novel allergens such as alpha-gal will also require individualized avoidance advice.

Individualized Allergen Avoidance

4.0.1. Milk and Egg

It is known that a large proportion of children with cow's milk and egg allergies will be tolerant to baked milk and egg irrespective of the age or population studied [37]. Baked milk or egg-containing foods typically refer to muffins, but other forms such as cookies, waffles, and pancakes have also been suggested. Baked cheese (pizza) has also been suggested for baked milk challenges [38–43]. No established guidelines to determine when to challenge have been established, so testing depends on combination of history, sIgE, and skin test results. There is limited consensus about the exact time and temperature of baking/cooking that is required, the need for a wheat/starch matrix, and where the challenge/food reintroduction should be conducted, e.g., hospital/in-office vs. at home [44–46]. It is, however, important to realize that some children who react to baked milk or baked egg may experience severe symptoms, requiring epinephrine. [31,32,46]. Risk factors for severe reactions to baked foods need further clarification but may include asthma requiring preventative treatment, multiple IgE mediated food allergies, and a history of anaphylaxis. [45,47]. Baked milk and egg-containing foods are successfully introduced at home in most children's diets post a negative challenge with good compliance; positively affecting the child's food and texture repertoire [48]. However, as it is unclear if continued and regular consumption of baked milk and egg-containing foods will speed up tolerance to uncooked milk or egg [49,50], families should not be pressured about frequent intake unnecessarily.

4.0.2. Peanut, Tree Nuts, Seeds

Previously, patients with peanut or tree nut allergies were advised to avoid all nuts, due to the risk of cross-reactivity or possible cross-contact/contamination. However, recent studies indicate that clinical cross-reactivity may be as low as 30% [51]. For instance, walnuts and pecans are highly cross-reactive with each other, but not with peanuts, hazelnuts or almonds Sensitization or clinical allergy may develop after a period of unnecessarily exclusion [52]. The British Society for Allergy and Clinical Immunology (BSACI) guidelines were the first food allergy management guidelines to recommend active inclusion of tolerated nuts in diets of individuals with peanut or tree nut allergy [53,54]. Peanuts are legumes, but allergy to other legumes is generally uncommon among those with peanut allergy, though this does depend on geography and local diet [55,56]. Lupine, pea, and soybean show some apparent cross-reactivity for patients who are highly allergic to peanut, although it is very difficult to separate cross-reactivity from de novo sensitization. The risk of cross-reaction may be higher for lupin than for other beans, particularly in Europe [57–59]. In the case of lupine allergy, patients need to be informed about foods containing lupin which may include pies, certain breads, and pastries.

Seeds are being used more often in commercial and gourmet foods—most commonly flaxseed, sesame, sunflower, poppy, pumpkin, and mustard seeds [60]. Sesame and mustard seeds are among the 14 most prevalent allergens in the EU, but not in the US [61]. In Europe, prevalence data indicates sesame and mustard seed allergies are geographically disproportionate: high in some areas (France and Spain), much lower in others (Germany and the Nordic countries) and unknown in Eastern Europe [62]. Mustard and sesame seeds are often hidden in commercial foods, making scrutiny of labels required at all times. Sesame seed allergy is not commonly seen outside of Israel and Europe [63]. In addition to scrutiny of labels, children with sesame allergy should always avoid sesame oil as it is cold/expeller pressed [64].

4.0.3. Fruit and Vegetable Allergies

Allergies to fruit and vegetables, in particular, require individualized advice as symptoms range from milder symptoms triggered by pollen-food syndrome (PFS, secondary IgE mediated food allergy) to more severe symptoms triggered by lipid transfer protein syndrome (LTP, primary IgE mediated food allergy) [65]. It is important to differentiate between these two presentations of fruit and vegetable allergies as that will direct the dietary advice given. With PFS, cooked, canned, baked, microwaved fruit and vegetables are allowed, whereas fruit/vegetable should be completely avoided in the case of LTP allergies. The degree to which cross-reactive fruit and vegetables (including soy and nuts) should be avoided requires careful diagnostic evaluation as blanket avoidance advice is not advocated [66–68].

4.0.4. Fish and Shellfish Allergy

It is important to distinguish between fish and shellfish (crustacean and mollusks) allergies. Fish and shellfish allergies may co-exist [69] but the main allergens differ, and cross-reactivity between fish and shellfish is unlikely. The main allergen in fish is β parvalbumin; in the case of shellfish, the major allergen is tropomyosin [70]. Additionally, allergy to a certain fish or shellfish does not imply allergies to all species in that particular group [71,72]. Subjects who suffer from fish allergy have only about a 50% probability of being cross-reactive to another fish species. This is significantly lower than those with shellfish allergies, who have up to a 75% chance of cross-reactivity [15]. In addition to the allergens derived from fish themselves, fish contaminants, such as the parasite Anisakis, can also cause allergic reactions, meaning Anisakis allergy can be falsely diagnosed as a fish allergy. In particular, Anisakis allergy correlated to prevalence of parasitic infection in fish—for example, in Spain and Southern Italy, there is a higher prevalence of Anisakis allergy due to moderately frequent Anisakis infection. These allergic patients develop IgE against tropomyosin from Anisakis. As always, sensitization depends in part on the consumption pattern of fish (cooked, undercooked or raw) and the infection pattern of fish in the local region [73].

4.0.5. Alpha-Galactosidase

Alpha galactosidase (Alpha-gal) allergy is characterized by delayed (4 to 6 h after the ingestion) hypersensitivity reactions to mammalian meats and is mediated by IgE antibodies to the oligosaccharide galactose-alpha 1,3-galactose. It requires avoidance of mammalian meats and their organ meat. Some individuals also need to avoid ice-cream, milk, and milk products but the degree of avoidance and foods being avoided should be discussed with the allergist. This decision can be made based on past history of reactions or tolerance [74,75]. Where the history is unclear, or the food has not been eaten in the past, an oral food challenge can be conducted [76].

5. Nutritional Impact of Food Allergies: Growth and Nutrient Intake

There is rising concern that children with FA have an insufficient nutrient intake or nutrient imbalance leading to adverse health implications. Data published over the past few years indicates that children with food allergies (IgE, non-IgE, and mixed presentations of IgE and non-IgE) show growth impairment, both in weight and length. They are often underweight [77], and in the case of chronic malnutrition, they become stunted, e.g., a child who is too short for his/her age [78,79]. However, excessive weight gain has also been reported in children with food allergies, but poorly researched [77,80,81]. A recent international survey conducted by Meyer et al. [82] included 430 patients from twelve allergy centers world-wide. The pooled data indicated that 6% were underweight, 9% stunted, 5% undernourished, and 3–5% were overweight. In this study, growth impairments varied by allergy profile. Children with cow's milk allergy (CMA) had a lower weight for age z-score, as a result of acute malnutrition or "wasting"; children with mixed IgE and non-IgE mediated FA were stunted, and children with only non-IgE FA were underweight with lower body mass index (BMI). Very different growth patterns were observed between children from different countries. Atopic comorbidities did not affect growth.

Avoidance diets required for FA management place children at risk for potential inadequate nutrition. In this regard, a number of studies have investigated the nutritional adequacy of elimination diets. However, most of them have been conducted in young children aged six months to four years. Children with food allergies (IgE, non-IgE, and mixed presentations of IgE and non-IgE) are also at higher risk of insufficient intake of protein, calories, vitamins, and minerals [83–87]. The micronutrients implicated are iodine, calcium, and vitamin D, especially in children with CMA [83,88,89]. However, it has been shown that children with cow's milk allergies or multiple food allergies are able to achieve similar mean intakes of nutrients as healthy children when receiving nutrition counselling and substitution of nutritionally equivalent foods [78,83,90–92].

Limited data exist on dietary intake in teenagers and adults with food allergies, with contrasting results [93,94]. One study reports, higher intakes of calcium, iron, folate, and vitamin E have been demonstrated in participants >20 years with food allergy [44]. Conversely, lower intakes of calcium and phosphorous have been reported in young adults with CMA, with one study reporting that 27% were at risk of osteoporosis [48]. Maslin et al. showed no significant difference between these two groups and control groups with the intake of calcium. Iron, copper, zinc, selenium, and iodine were below the Recommended National Intakes (RNI) for both groups and their controls [94]. There are currently no data on BMI status on adults with IgE mediated food allergy. These factors need to be considered when providing nutrition advice to children and adults with food allergies. Although information on healthy eating is important, consideration to vitamin and mineral supplementation in hypoallergenic formulas in the case of children should be given [84,95]. Nutritional counselling and monitoring growth and development are crucial in the management of FA, as the avoidance diet may affect the well-being of FA patients (see Table 2).

Table 2. Effect of avoidance diet on patients.

Effect of Avoidance Diet
- poor growth
- micronutrient deficiencies
- altered taste perception
- long term effects on food preferences and choices
- reduced quality of life

6. Food Behaviour and Preferences

In children with FA, the development of their food habits and preferences takes place in the context of their chronic condition. Since parents have the main responsibility for the dietary management of their child's food allergies [96], their parenting style and the way they interact with the child during feedings both have an effect on a child's food habits [97]. A child's food allergies add a burden to parents [98]. Food refusal has also been shown to occur in toddlers with food allergies [99] and more specifically eosinophilic gastrointestinal disease [100]. Additionally, a study on children aged 5 to 14 years in France showed that children who have outgrown their food allergies are more reluctant to try new foods than their siblings [101]. Food neophobia and refusal could result from unnecessarily high dietary restrictions that parents place on their children due to increased anxiety and fear of an allergic reaction [102]. The long-term effects of avoidance diet on food behavior and preferences needs further investigation.

Food choice behavioral problems have been documented in older children or adults with food allergies. Teenagers with food allergies, strive to eat the same foods as their peers, often leading to risk taking behavior. However, they reported reluctance to try new foods when away from home. In contrast to the non-food allergic teens, those with food allergies felt that parental control over food intake was to protect them [103].

Adults with FA felt that their allergies limited them from the pleasure of eating and they often found it difficult to find safe foods. They also felt that the need to be constantly organized to have safe foods available was a burden [104].

7. Microbiota-Diet and Genetic Factors: A Complex and Still Unknown Interplay

FA is thought to be the result of a disruption of mucosal immunological tolerance, due to dietary factors, gut microbiota, and interactions between them [105]. Different bacterial taxa may be associated with different food allergy subphenotyes. Differences in gut microbiome have been observed in subjects with tree-nut allergy in respect to those with cow's milk allergy [106,107]. The observed differences may however be influenced by age, population, sex and diet. Furthermore, recent data indicate that for cow's milk allergy, the microbiome differs between those children who are sensitized vs. not sensitized [108], those with clinical allergy vs. those with no allergy [109], and those who develop tolerance vs. those who do not [110]. Overall, these findings suggest the possibility to manipulate the gut microbiota with preventive or therapeutic purposes.

Data in pediatric studies indicate that certain pre and probiotics tested may address dysbiosis [111] and may even induce tolerance development [112]. More clinical trials regarding the use of pre and probiotics in the management of food allergies are needed before clinical recommendations can be made. These studies should also consider genetic background and age in their design. Another important issue to be considered is that the gut microbiome composition and diversity can be modulated by host genetic profiling [113]. A host's genetic composition is able to modulate their gut microbiota, which is another paramount area of study [114].

Whether diet diversity may improve dysbiosis and microbial diversity in those with food allergies remains to be seen [115].

Further studies need to investigate the complex interplay between the host genetic components and environmental factors, including the microbiota and diet, in the pathogenesis and expression of food allergy that is still largely unknown.

8. The Technology Revolution in FA Management

Increasingly, personalized devices to aid in allergen detection have been invented, and the industry has grown rapidly over the last decade [116]. These technologies have resulted both from increased demand for transparency of product information and scientific advancements. [117]. The rapid drop in the price of personalised nutrition devices has resulted in mass accessibility [118]. Deciphering food labels is a difficult task and for those with allergies, a daily chore that if done incorrectly, can lead to negative and possibly fatal outcomes [119,120].

New digital technologies have started to appear on the market that attempts to address the daily challenges families face when choosing products for a child with allergies. For a full review of technologies involved in portable allergy products, we refer readers to the comprehensive article by Ross, G.M.S [121]. There have been a number of technology services advising about potential risks related to food composition. For concerned consumers, having instant access to information can remove the guesswork and can potentially save time. However, there are no validated, personalized systems for testing individual meals for specific food source products. It is also noteworthy that sometimes component recipes change and accuracy as well of lack of clinical validation of these products are issues frequently raised.

With such rapid advances in the scientific and technology industry, it is, however, important to have comprehensive communication between consumer advocates, the food industry, and the clinicians to help improve avoidance of allergens by technical fixes, while being fully aware of the limitations and current lack of validation of these products in a variety of matrices or in foods with multiple ingredients (see Figure 1). What is clear, is that management of allergies will require the intervention of a specialist multidisciplinary team with registered dietitians playing a key role in supporting families while staying abreast of new technologies [122].

Some examples of products currently available on the market, outlining their pros, cons and future considerations, are listed below (Table 3).

Table 3. Personalized nutrition offering for Food allergies.

Currently Available Resources or Tools	Description	Pros	Cons	Future directions
Apps	Smartwithfood™, Spoonguru™, Foodmaestro™, Whisk™. These apps are available free to consumers. Through barcode scanning, image recognition, natural language processing and machine learning technology, consumers can obtain instant information whether a product contains allergens.	• These app scanners provide quick results that are easy to understand and can always be on hand. • They can provide peace of mind as a second line. • The platforms rely on food manufacturers to provide accurate product information in terms of their recipes.	• The app only reports on a limited number of allergens. • The app is not a medical device and, therefore, cannot replace a medical professional's advice; consumers should always ask questions and always check the food label.	• Apps should increase the number of allergens they have information about. • New products could ideally be developed based on the popularity of scanned products.
Food scanners	Scanners such as Tellspec™, Scioscan™ and Nima™ are handheld, mobile devices that use hyperspectral or imaging technology to analyse nutritional information and detect allergens.	• These scanners are small, provide quick results that are easy to understand. • They can provide peace of mind as a second line. • These products may provide some reassurance once standard allergen avoidance advice has been followed but should NOT be used instead of advice provided by the allergist or dietitian.	• Costs can be prohibitive. • It is not a medical device and, therefore, consultation with a healthcare professional is still required. • Concerns have been raised about the accuracy in detecting allergens (Popping et al., 2017). Scanners work best with homogenous solid products. For example, testing may be highly inaccurate in foods with multiple ingredients or high-fat matrices. • It is not clear who holds the data on these products.	• These tools need to be clinically validated. • These tools need to comply with medical devices regulation
Wearable devices	Such as Allergy Amulet™ is a device that is worn as a necklace and works by inserting strips into food, available in 2019.	• A mobile and attractive device that provides instant results. • These products may provide some reassurance once standard allergen avoidance advice has been followed.	• It is not a medical device • It is important the consumers read labels and ask about ingredients to the dietitian. • Have not been validated for accuracy	• Needs to be clinically validated. • In the future, potentially sensors or implants could detect from a nanoparticle of food.
CRISPR	Is the new technology which enables DNA of food (and humans) to be edited. This means that new foods and products can be developed where the culprit allergen's DNA has been edited without the devastating effects.	Consumers with allergies will have a wider variety of foods to eat	• Technology is still expensive. • Some allergens can be removed. • It is not clear how differentiating appropriately altered foods from native food sources. For some allergenic sources, such as wheat, the genetic complexity of the crop is unlikely to allow simple genetic knockout of allergenic genes.	• Current lack of understanding of the long-term impact of eating gene-edited foods. • Extensive public education will be required.

53

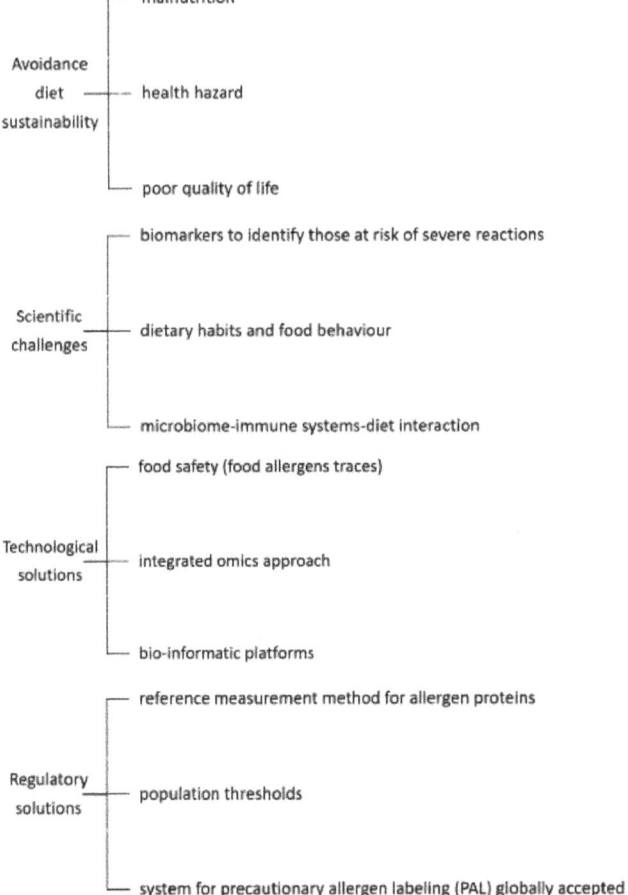

Figure 1. Nutrition approach: unmet needs.

9. Conclusions

A personalized approach to managing the food allergic individual is becoming more feasible as we are learning more about diagnostic modalities and allergic phenotypes. The availability of specialized foods and technology are increasing which also enables the clinicians to provide personalized advice. A multidisciplinary team approach, including a dietitian, is crucial to provide individualized recommendations to patients.

Author Contributions: E.D. and C.V contributed to the conception and design of the review, drafting the review; M.A. contributed in the review drafting; G.V.Z. and C.V. contributed to revise the manuscript. All the authors approved the manuscript for publication.

Funding: This research received no external funding

Acknowledgments: We would like to acknowledge Miriam Ben Abdallah for editing the paper.

Conflicts of Interest: The authors declare no conflict of interests.

References

1. Nwaru, B.I.; Hickstein, L.; Panesar, S.S.; Muraro, A.; Werfel, T.; Cardona, V.; Dubois, A.E.; Halken, S.; Hoffmann-Sommergruber, K.; Poulsen, L.K.; et al. EAACI Food Allergy and Anaphylaxis Guidelines Group. The epidemiology of food allergy in Europe: A systematic review and meta-analysis. *Allergy* **2014**, *69*, 62–75. [CrossRef]
2. Gupta, R.S.; Warren, C.M.; Smith, B.M.; Blumenstock, J.A.; Jiang, J.; Davis, M.M.; Nadeau, K.C. The Public Health Impact of Parent-Reported Childhood Food Allergies in the United States. *Pediatrics* **2018**, *142*, e20181235. [CrossRef] [PubMed]
3. Osborne, N.J.; Koplin, J.J.; Martin, P.E.; Gurrin, L.C.; Lowe, A.J.; Matheson, M.C.; Ponsonby, A.L.; Wake, M.; Tang, M.L.; Dharmage, S.C.; et al. HealthNuts Investigators. Prevalence of challenge-proven IgE-mediated food allergy using population-based sampling and predetermined challenge criteria in infants. *J. Allergy ClinImmunol.* **2011**, *127*, e1–e2. [CrossRef] [PubMed]
4. Chafen, J.J.; Newberry, S.J.; Riedl, M.A.; Bravata, D.M.; Maglione, M.; Suttorp, M.J.; Sundaram, V.; Paige, N.M.; Towfigh, A.; Hulley, B.J.; et al. Diagnosing and managing common food allergies: A systematic review. *JAMA* **2010**, *303*, 1848–1856. [CrossRef] [PubMed]
5. Boyce, J.A.; Assa'ad, A.; Burks, A.W.; Jones, S.M.; Sampson, H.A.; Wood, R.A.; Plaut, M.; Cooper, S.F.; Fenton, M.J.; Arshad, S.H.; et al. NIAID-sponsored expert panel. Guidelines for the diagnosis and management of food allergy in the United States: Report of the NIAID-sponsored expert panel. *J. Allergy ClinImmunol.* **2010**, *126*, S1–S58. [CrossRef] [PubMed]
6. Gupta, R.S.; Springston, E.E.; Warrier, M.R.; Smith, B.; Kumar, R.; Pongracic, J.; Holl, J.L. The prevalence, severity, and distribution of childhood food allergy in the United States. *Pediatrics* **2011**, *128*, e9–e17. [CrossRef] [PubMed]
7. Commins, S.P.; Satinover, S.M.; Hosen, J.; Mozena, J.; Borish, L.; Lewis, B.D.; Woodfolk, J.A.; Platts-Mills, T.A.E. Delayed anaphylaxis, angioedema, or urticaria after consumption of red meat in patients with IgE antibodies specific for galactose-alpha-1,3-galactose. *J. Allergy ClinImmunol.* **2009**, *123*, 426–433. [CrossRef] [PubMed]
8. Sova, C.; Feuling, M.B.; Baumler, M.; Gleason, L.; Tam, J.S.; Zafra, H.; Goday, P.S. Systematic review of nutrient intake and growth in children with multiple IgE-mediated food allergies. *Nutr. Clin. Pract.* **2013**, *28*, 669–675. [CrossRef] [PubMed]
9. Deschildre, A.; Lejeune, S.; Cap, M.; Flammarion, S.; Jouannic, L.; Amat, F.; Just, J. Food allergy phenotypes: The key to personalized therapy. *ClinExp Allergy* **2017**, *47*, 1125–1137. [CrossRef] [PubMed]
10. Matricardi, P.M.; Kleine-tebbe, J.; Hoffmann, H.J.; Valenta, R.; Hilger, C.; Hofmaier, S.; Aalberse, R.C.; Agache, I.; Asero, R.; Ballmer-Weber, B.; et al. EAACI Molecular Allergology User's Guide. *Pediatr. Allergy Immunol.* **2016**, *27*, 1–250. [CrossRef]
11. Sampson, H.A.; Aceves, S.; Bock, S.A.; James, J.; Jones, S.; Lang, D.; Nadeau, K.; Nowak-Wegrzyn, A.; Oppenheimer, J.; Perry, T.T.; et al. Food allergy: A practice parameter update-2014. *J. Allergy Clin. Immunol.* **2014**, *134*, 1016–1025. [CrossRef] [PubMed]
12. Muraro, A.; Roberts, G.; Worm, M.; Bilo, M.B.; Brockow, K.; Fernandez-Rivas, M.; Santos, A.F.; Zolkipli, Z.Q.; Bellou, A.; Bindslev-Jensen, C.; et al. Anaphylaxis: Guidelines from the European Academy of Allergy and Clinical Immunology. *Allergy* **2014**, *69*, 1026–1045. [CrossRef] [PubMed]
13. Benedé, S.; Garrido-Arandia, M.; Martín-Pedraza, L.; Bueno, C.; Díaz-Perales, A.; Villalba, M. Multifactorial modulation of food-induced anaphylaxis. *Front. Immunol.* **2017**, *8*, 552. [CrossRef]
14. Centre for Clinical Practice at NICE (UK). *Food Allergy in Children and Young People: Diagnosis and Assessment of Food Allergy in Children and Young People in Primary Care and Community Settings*; National Institute for Health and Clinical Excellence: London, UK, 2011.
15. Sicherer, S.H.; Sampson, H.A. Food allergy. *J. Allergy Clin. Immunol.* **2010**, *125*, S116–S125. [CrossRef] [PubMed]
16. Petersen, T.H.; Mortz, C.G.; Bindslev-jensen, C.; Eller, E. Cow's milk allergic children-Can component-resolved diagnostics predict duration and severity? *Pediatr. Allergy Immunol.* **2018**, *29*, 194–199. [CrossRef] [PubMed]
17. Sicherer, S.H.; Sampson, H.A. Food allergy: A review and update on epidemiology, pathogenesis, diagnosis, prevention, and management. *J. Allergy ClinImmunol.* **2018**, *141*, 41–58. [CrossRef] [PubMed]

18. D'auria, E.; Mameli, C.; Piras, C.; Cococcioni, L.; Urbani, A.; Zuccotti, G.V.; Roncada, P. Precision medicine in cow's milk allergy: Proteomics perspectives from allergens to patients. *J. Proteomics* **2018**, *188*, 173–180. [CrossRef]
19. Mirnezami, R.; Nicholson, J.; Darzi, A. Preparing for precision medicine. *N. Engl. J. Med.* **2012**, *366*, 489–491. [CrossRef]
20. Venter, C.; Maslin, K.; Arshad, S.H.; Patil, V.; Grundy, J.; Glasbey, G.; Twiselton, R.; Dean, T. Very low prevalence of IgE mediated wheat allergy and high levels of cross-sensitisation between grass and wheat in a UK birth cohort. *Clin. Transl. Allergy* **2016**, *6*, 22. [CrossRef]
21. Nilsson, N.; Sjölander, S.; Baar, A.; Berthold, M.; Pahr, S.; Vrtala, S.; Valenta, R.; Morita, E.; Hedlin, G.; Borres, M.P.; et al. Wheat allergy in children evaluated with challenge and IgE antibodies to wheat components. *Pediatr. Allergy Immunol.* **2015**, *26*, 119–125. [CrossRef]
22. Constantin, C.; Quirce, S.; Poorafshar, M.; Touraev, A.; Niggemann, B.; Mari, A.; Ebner, C.; Akerström, H.; Heberle-Bors, E.; Nystrand, M.; et al. Micro-arrayed wheat seed and grass pollen allergens for component-resolved diagnosis. *Allergy* **2009**, *64*, 1030–1037. [CrossRef] [PubMed]
23. Palosuo, K.; Varjonen, E.; Kekki, O.M.; Klemola, T.; Kalkkinen, N.; Alenius, H.; Reunala, T. Wheat omega-5 gliadin is a major allergen in children with immediate allergy to ingested wheat. *J. Allergy ClinImmunol.* **2001**, *108*, 634–638. [CrossRef] [PubMed]
24. Beyer, K.; Grabenhenrich, L.; Härtl, M.; Beder, A.; Kalb, B.; Ziegert, M.; Finger, A.; Harandi, N.; Schlags, R.; Gappa, M.; et al. Predictive values of component-specific IgE for the outcome of peanut and hazelnut food challenges in children. *Allergy* **2015**, *70*, 90–98. [CrossRef] [PubMed]
25. Turner, P.J.; Baumert, J.L.; Beyer, K.; Boyle, R.J.; Chan, C.H.; Clark, A.T.; Crevel, R.W.; DunnGalvin, A.; Fernández-Rivas, M.; Gowland, M.H.; et al. Can we identify patients at risk of life-threatening allergic reactions to food? *Allergy* **2016**, *71*, 1241–1255. [CrossRef] [PubMed]
26. Boyano-martínez, T.; García-ara, C.; Pedrosa, M.; Díaz-pena, J.M.; Quirce, S. Accidental allergic reactions in children allergic to cow's milk proteins. *J. Allergy ClinImmunol.* **2009**, *123*, 883–888. [CrossRef] [PubMed]
27. Ito, K.; Futamura, M.; Borres, M.P.; Takaoka, Y.; Dahlstrom, J.; Sakamoto, T.; Tanaka, A.; Kohno, K.; Matsuo, H.; Morita, E. IgE antibodies to omega-5 gliadin associate with immediate symptoms on oral wheat challenge in Japanese children. *Allergy* **2008**, *63*, 1536–1542. [CrossRef] [PubMed]
28. Eller, E.; Bindslev-jensen, C. Clinical value of component-resolved diagnostics in peanut-allergic patients. *Allergy* **2013**, *68*, 190–194. [CrossRef]
29. Perry, T.T.; Matsui, E.C.; Conover-walker, M.K.; Wood, R.A. The relationship of allergen-specific IgE levels and oral food challenge outcome. *J. Allergy ClinImmunol.* **2004**, *114*, 144–149. [CrossRef]
30. Yanagida, N.; Okada, Y.; Sato, S.; Ebisawa, M. New approach for food allergy management using low-dose oral food challenges and low-dose oral immunotherapies. *Allergol. Int.* **2016**, *65*, 135–140. [CrossRef]
31. Lieberman, J.A.; Huang, F.R.; Sampson, H.A.; Nowak-węgrzyn, A. Outcomes of 100 consecutive open, baked-egg oral food challenges in the allergy office. *J. Allergy ClinImmunol.* **2012**, *129*, 1682–1684. [CrossRef]
32. Nowak-Wegrzyn, A.; Bloom, K.A.; Sicherer, S.H.; Shreffler, W.G.; Noone, S.; Wanich, N.; Sampson, H.A. Tolerance to extensively heated milk in children with cow's milk allergy. *J. Allergy ClinImmunol.* **2008**, *122*, 342–347. [CrossRef] [PubMed]
33. Venter, C.; Groetch, M.; Netting, M.; Meyer, R. A patient-specific approach to develop an exclusion diet to manage food allergy in infants and children. *Clin. Exp. Allergy* **2018**, *48*, 121–137. [CrossRef] [PubMed]
34. Kim, J.S.; Sicherer, S.H. Living with food allergy: Allergen avoidance. *Pediatr. Clin. North Am* **2011**, *58*, 459–470. [CrossRef] [PubMed]
35. Muñoz-furlong, A. Daily coping strategies for patients and their families. *Pediatrics* **2003**, *111*, 1654–1661. [PubMed]
36. Venter, C.; Meyer, R. Session 1: Allergic disease: The challenges of managing food hypersensitivity. *Proc. Nutr. Soc.* **2010**, *69*, 11–24. [CrossRef] [PubMed]
37. Savage, J.; Sicherer, S.; Wood, R. The natural history of food allergy. *J. Allergy Clin. Immunol. Pract.* **2016**, *4*, 196–203. [CrossRef] [PubMed]
38. Leonard, S.A.; Caubet, J.C.; Kim, J.S.; Groetch, M.; Nowak-Wegrzyn, A. Baked milk- and egg-containing diet in the management of milk and egg allergy. *J. Allergy Clin. Immunol. Pract.* **2015**, *3*, 13–23. [CrossRef] [PubMed]

39. Leonard, S.A.; Nowak-Wegrzyn, A.H. Baked milk and egg diets for milk and egg allergy management. *Immunol. Allergy Clin. North Am* **2016**, *36*, 147–159. [CrossRef]
40. Leonard, S.A.; Sampson, H.A.; Sicherer, S.H.; Noone, S.; Moshier, E.L.; Godbold, J.; Nowak-Wegrzyn, A. Dietary baked egg accelerates resolution of egg allergy in children. *J. Allergy Clin. Immunol.* **2012**, *130*, 473–480. [CrossRef]
41. MiceliSopo, S.; Greco, M.; Cuomo, B.; Bianchi, A.; Liotti, L.; Monaco, S.; DelloIacono, I. Matrix effect on baked egg tolerance in children with IgE-mediated hen's egg allergy. *Pediatr. Allergy Immunol.* **2016**, *27*, 465–470. [CrossRef]
42. MiceliSopo, S.; Greco, M.; Monaco, S.; Bianchi, A.; Cuomo, B.; Liotti, L.; Iacono, I.D. Matrix effect on baked milk tolerance in children with IgE cow milk allergy. *Allergol. Immunopathol.* **2016**, *44*, 517–523. [CrossRef] [PubMed]
43. Kim, J.S.; Nowak-Wegrzyn, A.; Sicherer, S.H.; Noone, S.; Moshier, E.L.; Sampson, H.A. Dietary baked milk accelerates the resolution of cow's milk allergy in children. *J. Allergy Clin. Immunol.* **2011**, *128*, 125–131. [CrossRef] [PubMed]
44. Dupont, C. How to reintroduce cow's milk? *Pediatr. Allergy Immunol.* **2013**, *24*, 627–632. [CrossRef] [PubMed]
45. Luyt, D.; Ball, H.; Makwana, N.; Green, M.R.; Bravin, K.; Nasser, S.M.; Clark, A.T. Standards of Care Committee (SOCC) of the British Society for Allergy and Clinical Immunology (BSACI). BSACI guideline for the diagnosis and management of cow's milk allergy. *Clin. Exp. Allergy* **2014**, *44*, 642–672. [CrossRef] [PubMed]
46. Athanasopoulou, P.; Deligianni, E.; Dean, T.; Dewey, A.; Venter, C. Use of baked milk challenges and milk ladders in clinical practice: A worldwide survey of healthcare professionals. *Clin. Exp. Allergy* **2017**, *47*, 430–434. [CrossRef] [PubMed]
47. Mehr, S.; Turner, P.J.; Joshi, P.; Wong, M.; Campbell, D.E. Safety and clinical predictors of reacting to extensively heated cow's milk challenge in cow's milk-allergic children. *Ann. Allergy Asthma. Immunol.* **2014**, *113*, 425–429. [CrossRef] [PubMed]
48. Lee, E.; Mehr, S.; Turner, P.J.; Joshi, P.; Campbell, D.E. Adherence to extensively heated egg and cow's milk after successful oral food challenge. *J. Allergy Clin. Immunol. Pract.* **2015**, *3*, 125–127. [CrossRef]
49. Netting, M.; Gold, M.; Quinn, P.; El-Merhibi, A.; Penttila, I.; Makrides, M. Randomised controlled trial of a baked egg intervention in young children allergic to raw egg but not baked egg. *World Allergy Organ. J.* **2017**, *10*, 22. [CrossRef]
50. Lambert, R.; Grimshaw, K.E.C.; Ellis, B.; Jaitly, J.; Roberts, G. Evidence that eating baked egg or milk influences egg or milk allergy resolution: A systematic review. *Clin. Exp. Allergy* **2017**, *47*, 829–837. [CrossRef]
51. Couch, C.; Franxman, T.; Greenhawt, M. Characteristics of tree nut challenges in tree nut allergic and tree nut sensitized individuals. *Ann. Allergy Asthma. Immunol.* **2017**, *118*, 591–596. [CrossRef]
52. Elizur, A.; Bollyky, J.B.; Block, W.M. Elimination diet and the development of multiple tree-nut allergies. *Pediatr. Res.* **2017**, *82*, 671. [CrossRef]
53. Stiefel, G.; Anagnostou, K.; Boyle, R.K.; Brathwaite, N.; Ewan, P.; Fox, A.T.; Huber, P.; Luyt, D.; Till, S.J.; Venter, C. BSACI guideline for the diagnosis and management of peanut and tree nut allergy. *Clin. Exp. Allergy* **2017**, *47*, 719–739. [CrossRef] [PubMed]
54. Eigenmann, P.A.; Lack, G.; Mazon, A.; Nieto, A.; Haddad, D.; Brough, H.A.; Caubet, J.C. Managing nut allergy: A remaining clinical challenge. *J. Allergy Clin. Immunol. Pract.* **2017**, *5*, 296–300. [CrossRef]
55. Pascual, C.Y.; Fernandez-Crespo, J.; Sanchez-Pastor, S.; Padial, M.A.; Diaz-Pena, J.M.; Martin-Munoz, F.; Martin-Esteban, M. Allergy to lentils in Mediterranean pediatric patients. *J. Allergy Clin. Immunol.* **1999**, *103*, 154–158. [CrossRef]
56. Martinez San Ireneo, M.; Ibanez, M.D.; Sanchez, J.J.; Carnes, J.; Fernandez-Caldas, E. Clinical features of legume allergy in children from a Mediterranean area. *Ann. Allergy Asthma. Immunol.* **2008**, *101*, 179–184. [CrossRef]
57. Moneret-Vautrin, D.A.; Guerin, L.; Kanny, G.; Flabbee, J.; Fremont, S.; Morisset, M. Cross-allergenicity of peanut and lupine: The risk of lupine allergy in patients allergic to peanuts. *J. Allergy Clin. Immunol.* **1999**, *104*, 883–888. [CrossRef]

58. Fiocchi, A.; Sarratud, P.; Terracciano, L.; Vacca, E.; Bernardini, R.; Fuggetta, D.; Ballabio, C.; Duranti, M.; Magni, C.; Restani, P. Assessment of the tolerance to lupine-enriched pasta in peanut-allergic children. *Clin. Exp. Allergy* **2009**, *39*, 1045–1051. [CrossRef] [PubMed]
59. Peeters, K.A.; Koppelman, S.J.; Penninks, A.H.; Lebens, A.; Bruijnzeel-Koomen, C.A.; Hefle, S.L.; Taylor, S.L.; van Hoffen, E.; Knulst, A.C. Clinical relevance of sensitization to lupine in peanut-sensitized adults. *Allergy* **2009**, *64*, 549–555. [CrossRef]
60. Patel, A.; Bahna, S.L. Hypersensitivities to sesame and other common edible seeds. *Allergy* **2016**, *71*, 1405–1413. [CrossRef] [PubMed]
61. Allen, K.J.; Turner, P.J.; Pawankar, R.; Taylor, S.; Sicherer, S.; Lack, G.; Rosario, N.; Ebisawa, M.; Wong, G.; Mills, E.N.C; et al. Precautionary labelling of foods for allergen content: Are we ready for a global framework? *World Allergy Organ. J.* **2014**, *7*, 10. [CrossRef]
62. Moonesinghe, H.; Kilburn, S.; Mackenzie, H.; Venter, C.; Lee, K.; Dean, T. The prevalence of "novel" food allergens worldwide: a systematic review. *Clin. Transl. Allergy* **2015**, *5*, 9. [CrossRef]
63. Adatia, A.; Clarke, A.E.; Yanishevsky, Y.; Ben-Shoshan, M. Sesame allergy: Current perspectives. *J. Asthma. Allergy* **2017**, *10*, 141–151. [CrossRef] [PubMed]
64. Efsa Panel on Dietetic Products NaA. Scientific Opinion on Dietary Reference Values for fats, including saturated fatty acids, polyunsaturated fatty acids, monounsaturated fatty acids, trans fatty acids, and cholesterol. *EFSA J.* **2010**, *8*, 1461–1568.
65. Fernandez-Rivas, M. Fruit and vegetable allergy. *Chem. Immunol. Allergy* **2015**, *101*, 162–170. [PubMed]
66. Goikoetxea, M.J.; D'Amelio, C.M.; Martinez-Aranguren, R.; Gamboa, P.; Garcia, B.E.; Gomez, F.; Fernandez, J.; Bartra, J.; Parra, A.; Alvarado, M.I.; et al. Is microarray analysis really useful and sufficient to diagnose nut allergy in the mediterranean area? *J. Investig. Allergol. Clin. Immunol.* **2016**, *26*, 31–39. [PubMed]
67. Gomez, F.; Aranda, A.; Campo, P.; Diaz-Perales, A.; Blanca-Lopez, N.; Perkins, J.; Garrido, M.; Blanca, M.; Mayorga, C.; Torres, M.J. High prevalence of lipid transfer protein sensitization in apple allergic patients with systemic symptoms. *PLoS One* **2014**, *9*, e107304. [CrossRef] [PubMed]
68. Haroun-Diaz, E.; Azofra, J.; Gonzalez-Mancebo, E.; de Las Heras, M.; Pastor-Vargas, C.; Esteban, V.; Villalba, M.; Diaz-Perales, A.; Cuesta-Herranz, J.I. Nut allergy in two different areas of Spain: Differences in clinical and molecular pattern. *Nutrients* **2017**, *9*, 909. [CrossRef]
69. Moonesinghe, H.; Mackenzie, H.; Venter, C.; Kilburn, S.; Turner, P.; Weir, K.; Dean, T. Prevalence of fish and shellfish allergy: A systematic review. *Ann. Allergy Asthma. Immunol.* **2016**, *117*, 264–272. [CrossRef]
70. Faber, M.A.; Pascal, M.; El Kharbouchi, O.; Sabato, V.; Hagendorens, M.M.; Decuyper, I.; Bridts, C.H.; Ebo, D.G. Shellfish allergens: Tropomyosin and beyond. *Allergy* **2017**, *72*, 842–848. [CrossRef]
71. Sharp, M.F.; Lopata, A.L. Fish allergy: In review. *Clin. Rev. Allergy Immunol.* **2014**, *46*, 258–271. [CrossRef]
72. Stephen, J.N.; Sharp, M.F.; Ruethers, T.; Taki, A.; Campbell, D.E.; Lopata, A.L. Allergenicity of bony and cartilaginous fish—Molecular and immunological properties. *Clin. Exp. Allergy* **2017**, *47*, 300–312. [CrossRef] [PubMed]
73. Lopata, A.L.; Lehrer, S.B. New insights into seafood allergy. *Curr. Opin. Allergy Clin. Immunol.* **2009**, *9*, 270–277. [CrossRef] [PubMed]
74. Scott, P. Commins invited commentary: Alpha-gal allergy: Tip of the iceberg to a pivotal immune response. *Curr. Allergy Asthma. Rep.* **2016**, *16*, 61.
75. Mullins, R.J.; James, H.; Platts-Mills, T.A.; Commins, S. Relationship between red meat allergy and sensitization to gelatin and galactose-α-1,3-galactose. *J. Allergy Clin. Immunol.* **2012**, *129*, 1334–1342. [CrossRef] [PubMed]
76. Steinke, J.W.; Platts-Mills, T.A.; Commins, S.P. The alpha-gal story: Lessons learned from connecting the dots. *J. Allergy Clin. Immunol.* **2015**, *135*, 589–596. [CrossRef] [PubMed]
77. Meyer, R.; De Koker, C.; Dziubak, R.; Skrapac, A.K.; Godwin, H.; Reeve, K.; Chebar-Lozinsky, A.; Shah, N. A practical approach to vitamin and mineral supplementation in food allergic children. *Clin. Transl. Allergy* **2015**, *5*, 11. [CrossRef] [PubMed]
78. Flammarion, S.; Santos, C.; Guimber, D.; Jouannic, L.; Thumerelle, C.; Gottrand, F.; Deschildre, A. Diet and nutritional status of children with food allergies. *Pediatr. Allergy Immunol.* **2011**, *22*, 161–165. [CrossRef]
79. Vieira, M.C.; Morais, M.B.; Spolidoro, J.V.; Toporovski, M.S.; Cardoso, A.L.; Araujo, G.T.; Nudelman, V.; Fonseca, M.C. A survey on clinical presentation and nutritional status of infants with suspected cow' milk allergy. *BMC Pediatr.* **2010**, *10*, 25. [CrossRef]

80. Fleischer, D.M.; Conover-Walker, M.K.; Christie, L.; Burks, A.W.; Wood, R.A. Peanut allergy: Recurrence and its management. *J. Allergy Clin. Immunol.* **2004**, *114*, 1195–1201. [CrossRef]
81. De Swert, L.F.A.; Gadisseur, R.; Sjolander, S.; Raes, M.; Leus, J.; Van Hoeyveld, E. Secondary soy allergy in children with birch pollen allergy may cause both chronic and acute symptoms. *Pediat. Allerg. Imm.UK* **2012**, *23*, 118–124. [CrossRef]
82. Meyer, R.M.; Vieira, M.C.; Chong, K.W.; Chatchatee, P.; Vlieg-Boerstra, B.J.; Groetch, M.; Dominguez-Ortega, G.; Heath, S.; Lang, S.; Archibald-Durham, L.; et al. International survey on growth indices and impacting factors in children with food allergies. *J. Hum. Nutr. Diet.* **2018**, in press. [CrossRef] [PubMed]
83. Christie, L.; Hine, R.J.; Parker, J.G.; Burks, W. Food allergies in children affect nutrient intake and growth. *J. Am. Diet. Assoc.* **2002**, *102*, 1648–1651. [CrossRef]
84. Meyer, R.; De Koker, C.; Dziubak, R.; Godwin, H.; Dominguez-Ortega, G.; Shah, N. Dietary elimination of children with food protein induced gastrointestinal allergy—Micronutrient adequacy with and without a hypoallergenic formula? *Clin. Transl. Allergy* **2014**, *4*, 31. [CrossRef] [PubMed]
85. Toyran, M.; Kaymak, M.; Vezir, E.; Harmanci, K.; Kaya, A.; Ginis, T.; Kose, G.; Kocabas, C.N. Trace element levels in children with atopic dermatitis. *J. Investig. Allergol. Clin. Immunol.* **2012**, *22*, 341–344. [PubMed]
86. Noimark, L.; Cox, H.E. Nutritional problems related to food allergy in childhood. *Pediatr. Allergy Immunol.* **2008**, *19*, 188–195. [CrossRef] [PubMed]
87. Ojuawo, A.; Lindley, K.J.; Milla, P.J. Serum zinc, selenium and copper concentration in children with allergic colitis. *East. Afr. Med. J.* **1996**, *73*, 236–238. [PubMed]
88. Foong, R.X.; Meyer, R.; Dziubak, R.; Lozinsky, A.C.; Godwin, H.; Reeve, K.; Hussain, S.T.; Nourzaie, R.; Shah, N. Establishing the prevalence of low vitamin D in non-immunoglobulin-E mediated gastrointestinal food allergic children in a tertiary centre. *World Allergy Organ. J.* **2017**, *10*, 4. [CrossRef]
89. Thomassen, R.A.; Kvammen, J.A.; Eskerud, M.B.; Juliusson, P.B.; Henriksen, C.; Rugtveit, J. Iodine status and growth in 0-2-year-old infants with cow's milk protein allergy. *J. Pediatr. Gastroenterol. Nutr.* **2016**, *64*, 806–811. [CrossRef]
90. D'Auria, E.; Fabiano, V.; Bertoli, S.; Bedogni, G.; Bosetti, A.; Pendezza, E.; Sartorio, M.U.A.; Leone, A.; Spadafranca, A.; Borsani, B.; et al. Growth Pattern, resting energy expenditure, and nutrient intake of children with food allergies. *Nutrients* **2019**, *11*, 212. [CrossRef]
91. Seppo, L.; Korpela, R.; Lönnerdal, B.; Metsäniitty, L.; Juntunen-Backman, K.; Klemola, T.; Paganus, A.; Vanto, T. A follow-up study of nutrient intake, nutritional status, and growth in infants with cow milk allergy fed either a soy formula or an extensively hydrolyzed whey formula. *Am. J. Clin. Nutr.* **2005**, *82*, 140–145. [CrossRef]
92. BerniCanani, R.; Leone, L.; D'auria, E.; Riva, E.; Nocerino, R.; Ruotolo, S.; Terrin, G.; Cosenza, L.; Di Costanzo, M.; Passariello, A.; et al. The effects of dietary counseling on children with food allergy: A prospective, multicenter intervention study. *J. Acad. Nutr. Diet.* **2014**, *114*, 1432–1439. [CrossRef] [PubMed]
93. Goldberg, M.R.; Nachshon, L.; Sinai, T.; Epstein-Rigbi, N.; Oren, Y.; Eisenberg, E.; Katz, Y.; Elizur, A. Risk factors for reduced bone mineral density measurements in milk-allergic patients. *Pediatr. Allergy Immunol.* **2018**, *29*, 850–856. [CrossRef] [PubMed]
94. Maslin, K.; Venter, C.; Mackenzie, H.; Vlieg-boerstra, B.; Dean, T.; Sommer, I. Comparison of nutrient intake in adolescents and adults with and without food allergies. *J. Hum. Nutr. Diet.* **2018**, *31*, 209–217. [CrossRef] [PubMed]
95. Giovannini, M.; D'auria, E.; Caffarelli, C.; Verduci, E.; Barberi, S.; Indinnimeo, L.; Iacono, I.D.; Martelli, A.; Riva, E.; Bernardini, R. Nutritional management and follow up of infants and children with food allergy: Italian Society of Pediatric Nutrition/Italian Society of Pediatric Allergy and Immunology Task Force Position Statement. *Ital. J. Pediatr.* **2014**, *40*, 1. [CrossRef] [PubMed]
96. Mandell, D.; Curtis, R.; Gold, M.; Hardie, S. Anaphylaxis: How do you live with it? *Health. Soc. Work* **2005**, *30*, 325–335. [CrossRef]
97. Sommer, I.; Chisholm, V.; Mackenzie, H.; Venter, C.; Dean, T. Relationship between maternal and child behaviors in pediatric food allergy–an exploratory study. *Ann. Allergy. Asthma. Immunol.* **2016**, *116*, 78–80. [CrossRef]
98. Komulainen, K. Parental burden in families with a young food-allergic child. *Child. Care Pract.* **2010**, *16*, 287–302. [CrossRef]

99. Fortunato, J.E.; Scheimann, A.O. Protein-energy malnutrition and feeding refusal secondary to food allergies. *Clin. Pediatr.* **2008**, *47*, 496–499. [CrossRef]
100. Mukkada, V.A.; Haas, A.; Maune, N.C.; Capocelli, K.E.; Henry, M.; Gilman, N.; Petersburg, S.; Moore, W.; Lovell, M.A.; Fleischer, D.M.; et al. Feeding dysfunction in children with eosinophilic gastrointestinal diseases. *Pediatrics* **2010**, *126*, e672–e677. [CrossRef]
101. Rigal, N.; Reiter, F.; Morice, C.; De boissieu, D.; Dupont, C. Food allergy in the child: An exploratory study on the impact of the elimination diet on food neophobia. *Arch. Pediatr.* **2005**, *12*, 1714–1720. [CrossRef]
102. Ng, I.E.; Turner, P.J.; Kemp, A.S.; Campbell, D.E. Parental perceptions and dietary adherence in children with seafood allergy. *Pediatr. Allergy Immunol.* **2011**, *22*, 720–728. [CrossRef] [PubMed]
103. Sommer, I.; Mackenzie, H.; Venter, C.; Dean, T. An exploratory investigation of food choice behavior of teenagers with and without food allergies. *Ann. Allergy Asthma Immunol.* **2014**, *112*, 446–452. [CrossRef] [PubMed]
104. Sommer, I.; Mackenzie, H.; Venter, C.; Dean, T. Factors influencing food choices of food-allergic consumers: Findings from focus groups. *Allergy* **2012**, *67*, 1319–1322. [CrossRef]
105. Berin, M.C.; Sampson, H.A. Mucosal immunology of food allergy. *Curr. Biol.* **2013**, *23*, 389–400. [CrossRef]
106. Hua, X.; Goedert, J.J.; Pu, A.; Yu, G.; Shi, J. Allergy associations with the adult fecal microbiota: Analysis of the American Gut Project. *E. Bio. Med.* **2016**, *3*, 172–179. [CrossRef] [PubMed]
107. Berni, C.R.; Sangwan, N.; Stefka, A.T.; Nocerino, R.; Paparo, L.; Aitoro, R.; Calignano, A.; Khan, A.A.; Gilbert, J.A.; Nagler, C.R. Lactobacillus rhamnosus GG-supplemented formula expands butyrate-producing bacterial strains in food allergic infants. *ISME J.* **2016**, *10*, 742–750. [CrossRef] [PubMed]
108. Azad, M.B.; Konya, T.; Guttman, D.S.; Field, C.J.; Sears, M.R.; HayGlass, K.T.; Mandhane, P.J.; Turvey, S.E.; Subbarao, P.; Becker, A.B.; et al. CHILD Study Investigators. Infant gut microbiota and food sensitization: Associations in the first year of life. *Clin. Exp. Allergy* **2015**, *45*, 632–643. [CrossRef] [PubMed]
109. Dong, P.; Feng, J.J.; Yan, D.Y.; Lyu, Y.J.; Xu, X. Early-life gut microbiome and cow's milk allergy—A prospective case—Control 6-month follow-up study. *Saudi. J. BiolSci.* **2018**, *25*, 875–880. [CrossRef]
110. Bunyavanich, S.; Shen, N.; Grishin, A.; Wood, R.; Burks, W.; Dawson, P.; Jones, S.M.; Leung, D.Y.M.; Sampson, H.; Sicherer, S. Early-life gut microbiome composition and milk allergy resolution. *J. Allergy ClinImmunol.* **2016**, *138*, 1122–1130. [CrossRef]
111. Candy, D.C.A.; Van Ampting, M.T.J.; Oude Nijhuis, M.M.; Wopereis, H.; Butt, A.M.; Peroni, D.G.; Vandenplas, Y.; Fox, A.T.; Shah, N.; West, C.E.; et al. A synbiotic-containing amino-acid-based formula improves gut microbiota in non-IgE-mediated allergic infants. *Pediatr. Res.* **2018**, *83*, 677–686. [CrossRef]
112. BerniCanani, R.; Nocerino, R.; Terrin, G.; Coruzzo, A.; Cosenza, L.; Leone, L.; Troncone, R. Effect of Lactobacillus GG on tolerance acquisition in infants with cow's milk allergy: A randomized trial. *J. Allergy ClinImmunol.* **2012**, *129*, 580–582. [CrossRef] [PubMed]
113. Ridaura, V.K.; Faith, J.J.; Rey, F.E.; Cheng, J.; Alexis, E.; Kau, A.L.; Griffin, N.W.; Lombard, V.; Henrissat, B.; Bain, J.R.; et al. Cultured gut microbiota from twins discordant for obesity modulate adiposity and metabolic phenotypes in mice. *Science* **2014**, *341*, 1241214. [CrossRef] [PubMed]
114. Bonder, M.J.; Kurilshikov, A.; Tigchelaar, E.F.; Mujagic, Z.; Imhann, F.; Vila, A.V.; Deelen, P.; Vatanen, T.; Schirmer, M.; Smeekens, S.P.; et al. The effect of host genetics on the gut microbiome. *Nat. Genet.* **2016**, *48*, 1407–1412. [CrossRef] [PubMed]
115. Claesson, M.J.; Jeffery, I.B.; Conde, S.; Power, S.E.; O'Connor, E.M.; Cusack, S.; Harris, H.M.; Coakley, M.; Lakshminarayanan, B.; O'Sullivan, O.; et al. Gut microbiota composition correlates with diet and health in the elderly. *Nature* **2012**, *488*, 178–184. [CrossRef] [PubMed]
116. Ronteltap, A.; Van trijp, H.; Berezowska, A.; Goossens, J. Nutrigenomics-based personalised nutritional advice: In search of a business model? *Genes Nutr.* **2013**, *8*, 153–163. [CrossRef] [PubMed]
117. Ordovas, J.M.; Ferguson, L.R.; Tai, E.S.; Mathers, J.C. Personalised nutrition and health. *BMJ* **2018**, *361*, 2173. [CrossRef] [PubMed]
118. Van ommen, B.; Van den broek, T.; De hoogh, I.; van Erk, M.; van Someren, E.; Rouhani-Rankouhi, T.; Anthony, J.C.; Hogenelst, K.; Pasman, W.; Boorsma, A.; et al. Systems biology of personalized nutrition. *Nutr. Rev.* **2017**, *75*, 579–599. [CrossRef]
119. Miller, L.M.; Cassady, D.L. The effects of nutrition knowledge on food label use. A review of the literature. *Appetite* **2015**, *92*, 207–216. [CrossRef]

120. Bahri, R.; Custovic, A.; Korosec, P.; Tsoumani, M.; Barron, M.; Wu, J.; Sayers, R.; Weimann, A.; Ruiz-Garcia, M.; Patel, N.; et al. Mast cell activation test in the diagnosis of allergic disease and anaphylaxis. *J. Allergy ClinImmunol.* **2018**, *142*, 485–496. [CrossRef]
121. Ross, G.M.S.; Bremer, M.G.E.G.; Nielen, M.W.F. Consumer-friendly food allergen detection: Moving towards smartphone-based immunoassays. *Anal. Bioanal.Chem.* **2018**, *410*, 5353–5371. [CrossRef]
122. Abrahams, M.; Frewer, L.J.; Bryant, E.; Stewart-Knox, B. Perceptions and experiences of early-adopting registered dietitians in integrating nutrigenomics into practice. *Br. Food J.* **2018**, *120*, 763–776. [CrossRef]

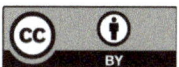 © 2019 by the authors. Licensee MDPI, Basel, Switzerland. This article is an open access article distributed under the terms and conditions of the Creative Commons Attribution (CC BY) license (http://creativecommons.org/licenses/by/4.0/).

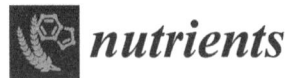

Article

The Differences in Postprandial Serum Concentrations of Peptides That Regulate Satiety/Hunger and Metabolism after Various Meal Intake, in Men with Normal vs. Excessive BMI

Edyta Adamska-Patruno [1,*], Lucyna Ostrowska [2], Joanna Goscik [1], Joanna Fiedorczuk [1], Monika Moroz [1], Adam Kretowski [1,3] and Maria Gorska [3]

1. Clinical Research Centre, Medical University of Bialystok, MC Sklodowskiej 24A, 15-276 Bialystok, Poland; joanna.goscik@umb.edu.pl (J.G.); j.fiedorczuk@wp.pl (J.F.); monika_bakun@wp.pl (M.M.); adamkretowski@wp.pl (A.K.)
2. Department of Dietetics and Clinical Nutrition, Medical University of Bialystok, Mieszka I-go 4B, 15-054 Bialystok, Poland; lucyna.ostrowska@umb.edu.pl
3. Department of Endocrinology, Diabetology and Internal Medicine, Medical University of Bialystok, MC Sklodowskiej 24A, 15-276 Bialystok, Poland; mgorska@wp.pl
* Correspondence: edyta.adamska@wp.pl; Tel.: +48-85-8318153

Received: 25 January 2019; Accepted: 22 February 2019; Published: 26 February 2019

Abstract: The energy balance regulation may differ in lean and obese people. The purposes of our study were to evaluate the hormonal response to meals with varying macronutrient content, and the differences depending on body weight. Methods. The crossover study included 46 men, 21–58 years old, normal-weight and overweight/obese. Every subject participated in two meal-challenge-tests with high-carbohydrate (HC), and normo-carbohydrate (NC) or high-fat (HF) meals. Fasting and postprandial blood was collected for a further 240 min, to determine adiponectin, leptin and total ghrelin concentrations. Results. In normal-weight individuals after HC-meal we observed at 60min higher adiponectin concentrations (12,554 ± 1531 vs. 8691 ± 1070 ng/mL, $p = 0.01$) and significantly ($p < 0.05$) lower total ghrelin concentrations during the first 120 min, than after HF-meal intake. Fasting and postprandial leptin levels were significantly ($p < 0.05$) higher in overweigh/obese men. Leptin concentrations in normal-weight men were higher (2.72 ± 0.8 vs. 1.56 ± 0.4 ng/mL, $p = 0.01$) 180 min after HC-meal than after NC-meal intake. Conclusions. Our results suggest that in normal-body weight men we can expect more beneficial leptin, adiponectin, and total ghrelin response after HC-meal intake, whereas, in overweight/obese men, the HC-meal intake may exacerbate the feeling of hunger, and satiety may be induced more by meals with lower carbohydrate content.

Keywords: obesity; postprandial adiponectin; postprandial leptin; postprandial total ghrelin; high-carbohydrate meal; high-fat meal

1. Introduction

Obesity is a chronic disease resulting from excess fat accumulation. Currently, adipose tissue is recognized as a major endocrine organ and many hormones, growth factors, and cytokines are synthesized and secreted into the circulation by the cells of subcutaneous and visceral adipose tissue. These factors (called adipokines) show auto-, endo-, and paracrine activity and regulate energy homeostasis and insulin sensitivity, inflammatory processes, glucose and lipid metabolism, blood pressure, blood coagulation and proliferation, cell differentiation, as well as apoptosis processes [1–3]. The central nervous system receives peripheral signals through numerous receptors, especially from the gastrointestinal tract and adipose tissue, in response to the current energy status and in response to changes in the body energy status [4].

Energy balance regulation also has a short-term component and includes metabolic and hormonal changes induced by food consumption. Current studies suggest that ghrelin and leptin and their interactions seem to play a key role in appetite regulation. The increase of leptin hypothalamic expression results in a decrease in ghrelin and adiponectin concentrations [5].

The main ghrelin activity is associated with hunger stimulation and stimulation of growth hormone secretion; it also influences energy homeostasis [4]. The highest ghrelin concentrations are observed before a meal intake. During starvation, ghrelin concentrations increase, and they are reduced 60 to 120 min after meal intake [6]. Ghrelin concentrations depend also on the diet energy value, and a postprandial decrease of ghrelin levels is proportional to the meal energy value [7]. Furthermore, ghrelin concentrations depend on the content of essential nutrients in the diet—proteins, fats and carbohydrates—but their influence is not thoroughly known. It seems that after high-carbohydrate and high-protein meals, ghrelin concentrations may be significantly reduced, compared to the high-fat meals [8].

Adiponectin synthesis is stimulated by insulin, insulin-like growth factor and peroxisome proliferator-activated receptor gamma (PPARγ-receptor antagonist [9]. Decreased adiponectin synthesis and secretion are observed in both high-energy [10] and high-fat diets [11]. Decreased adiponectin concentrations in peripheral blood are also observed with increased body mass index (BMI), and it increases with body weight reduction [12].

Taking into consideration the functions of leptin, ghrelin, and adiponectin, in obese individuals we would expect higher concentrations of ghrelin and adiponectin and lower leptin levels, but the tendencies are reversed [12]. Moreover, in obesity, the metabolic and hormonal response in the postprandial state may differ from the changes observed in subjects with normal body weight [13–17]. The mechanisms of these phenomena are not completely known. People spend most of the day in the postprandial state; therefore, meals that induce the longest possible satiety and an advantageous metabolic response are important in both the prevention and treatment of obesity.

The aim of our study was to evaluate the hormonal changes after meals of varying carbohydrate and fat content, in men with normal body weight and in men who are overweight/obese (in cross-over study design).

2. Materials and Methods

This study is a part of our larger project, which is registered at www.clinicaltrials.gov as NCT03792685, and all methods have been previously described in details [13,14,17–21].

2.1. Ethics

The study protocol was approved by the local Ethics Committee (Medical University of Bialystok, Poland, R-I-002/35/2009). All aspects of the study were performed in accordance with the ethical standards set forth in the Declaration of Helsinki of 1975, revised in 2013. Written informed consent was obtained from all participants prior to inclusion in the study.

2.2. Study Participants

The study included 46 men, 23 with normal body weight (N) and 23 who were overweight/obese (O/O), ranging in age between 21 and 58 years old. Excluded from the study were any subjects suffering from glucose metabolism disorders, endocrine disorders, liver or renal failure, digestive system diseases, or any other diseases that could influence the study results (including people with history of any gastroenterological and bariatric surgeries) as well as individuals who were receiving pharmaceutical treatment (or any other products with unknown impact on metabolism). Only men were enrolled, since the factors to be analyzed may be characteristic of sexual dimorphism. The study population characteristics are presented in Table 1.

Table 1. The study population characteristic.

		Normal-weight Men	Overweight/Obese Men	*p*-Value
Group I	*n*	11	12	
	Age (years)	33 ± 2	40 ± 2	0.01
	BMI	23.8 ± 0.5	31.4 ± 1.5	0.0002
	Body fat content (%)	17.9 ± 1.0	28.6 ± 1.7	0.00003
Group II	*n*	12	11	
	Age (years)	33 ± 3	36 ± 3	0.24
	BMI	23.9 ± 0.2	33.7 ± 2.2	0.000001
	Body fat content (%)	18.6 ± 1.5	31.9 ± 2.7	0.0002

The results are presented as mean values ± SE.

2.3. Study Procedures

Based on BMI, the men were divided into two groups (N and O/O). Subsequently, participants were randomly assigned to one of two sub-groups: Group I comprised 11 men with normal body weight (N1) and 12 overweight/obese men (O/O1), while Group II comprised 12 men with normal body weight (N2) and 11 overweight/obese men (O/O2). The crossover method was used to carry out the study. Subjects from Group I received a standardized high-carbohydrate (HC) meal (Nutridrink Fat Free, Nutricia, Poland) and an isocaloric (450 kcal) normo-carbohydrate (NC) meal (Cubitan, Nutricia, Poland). Similarly, men from Group II received the same standardized HC-meal (Nutridrink Fat Free, Nutricia, Poland) and an isocaloric (450 kcal) HF-meal (Calogen, Nutricia, Poland). Subjects received meals in random order, at 1–2 weeks intervals. Subjects were asked to avoid coffee, alcohol, and excessive physical activity at least on the day before each test and to maintain their regular lifestyle throughout the study. The meal contents are presented in Table 2.

Table 2. The energy and macronutrients composition of meals.

	High-carbohydrate Meal	Normo-carbohydrate Meal	High-fat Meal
Energy (kcal)	450	450	450
Carbohydrate (g)	100.5	51.1	4.0
Carbohydrate (% of total energy)	89.3	45.1	4.0
Fat (g)	0	12.6	47.5
Fat (% of total energy)	0	25.2	96
Protein (g)	12	36	0
Protein (% of total energy)	10.7	29.7	0
Fiber (g)	0	0.1	0

Subjects arrived at the laboratory between 8:00 and 8:30 in the morning, after at least 12-h fasting, Each participant's height and weight measurements and body composition analysis (using the bioimpedance method, InBody 220, Biospace, Korea) were carried out. A peripheral venous catheter was placed in the elbow crook and before receiving the standardized meal, venous blood was collected to determine the fasting adiponectin, leptin, and total ghrelin concentrations. Then the subjects received a randomly assigned meal (at room temperature), with a recommendation to consume it within 10 min. Venous blood was drawn 30, 60, 120, 180, and 240 min after meal consumption to determine postprandial adiponectin, ghrelin, and leptin levels. The blood preparation and laboratory procedures were in accordance with the recommendations of the laboratory kits. The concentrations were determined using the following methods: total adiponectin—radioimmunoassay (Human Adiponectin RIA, Millipore, USA); leptin—immunoenzymatic method (Human Leptin ELISA, BioVendor, Czech Republic); total ghrelin—radioimmunometric method (Ghrelin (total) RIA, Millipore, USA). Biochemical analyses were performed at the Laboratory of the Department of Endocrinology, Diabetology and Internal Medicine, Medical University of Bialystok, Poland.

Statistical analysis. Descriptive statistics, including mean and its standard error (SE), were calculated for all numerical features representing concentrations of interest, which underwent further, consecutive steps of the analysis. The aim of the study was to evaluate whether postprandial hormonal responses differ significantly when the types of meals and patients' characteristic were used as a grouping factor. We stated two main null hypotheses: (1) the type of meal has no influence on postprandial metabolic response in normal body weight and overweight/obese men (the Is of participants were analyzed separately), (2) there is no statistically significant difference in postprandial hormonal response to a particular meal in normal body weight and overweight/obese men (the meal types were analyzed separately). The first hypothesis was verified for the following pairs of meals: HC vs. NC in Group I, and HC vs. HF in Group II. The procedure was conducted twice—for normal body weight and overweight/obese subjects—and, since both meals were given to the same individuals, the lack of independence was taken into consideration, resulting in the choice of statistical tests. Either one-way ANOVA (analysis of variance) or Wilcoxon signed-rank test (both for paired samples) was carried out, depending on fulfillment of the condition of the normality of the variables' distribution, analyzed with the Shapiro–Wilk test. The second hypothesis was verified for the investigated meal types: HC, NC, and HF. The goal was to investigate whether there are any statistically significant differences in postprandial hormonal response between normal body weight and overweight/obese men. To test the stated hypothesis we used the one-way ANOVA or Wilcoxon rank-sum test (both for unpaired samples)—dependently on the fulfillment of the condition of normality of the variables' distribution and the homogeneity of variances. The homogeneity of variances was verified with the Levene test. To address the issue of multiple hypothesis testing, the false discovery rate p-value adjustment method was used [22]. For all calculations, the alpha level was set at 0.05. The areas under the curve (AUCs) were calculated using a trapezoidal method and underwent the same analysis schema, like the rest of the features.

3. Results

The fasting and postprandial differences in adiponectin concentrations between normal body weight and overweight/obese individuals were not significant (Figure 1A,B). However, in subjects with normal body weight, we noted significantly higher ($p = 0.01$) adiponectin concentrations 60 min after the HC-meal than after the HF-meal intake (Figure 1B), while in overweight/obese men, we observed significantly higher ($p = 0.03$) adiponectin levels 120 min after the HF-meal than after the HC-meal intake.

In normal body weight participants, we observed significantly higher ($p = 0.01$) leptin concentrations 180 min after HC-meal than after NC-meal intake (Figure 2A). In overweight/obese men, although leptin concentrations before the HC-meal were significantly higher (8.44 ± 1.68 vs. 7.07 ± 1.51 ng/mL, $p = 0.01$), postprandially we did not observe any significant differences. The AUC for postprandial leptin levels was significantly higher after the HC-meal intake than after the NC-meal (670 ± 220 vs. 391 ± 103, $p = 0.04$) in the N group. When we compared the postprandial leptin levels between the HC and HF-meals, we found that men with normal body weight showed a tendency, which was on the margin of significance ($p = 0.05$), to higher leptin concentrations 240 min after the HC-meal intake (Figure 2B). In overweight/obese subjects, we did not observe any significant differences in postprandial leptin concentrations dependent on meal type. Leptin levels in O/O men were significantly higher than in N subjects, at fasting state and during the further 4 h of all of the meal challenge tests (Figure 2A,B).

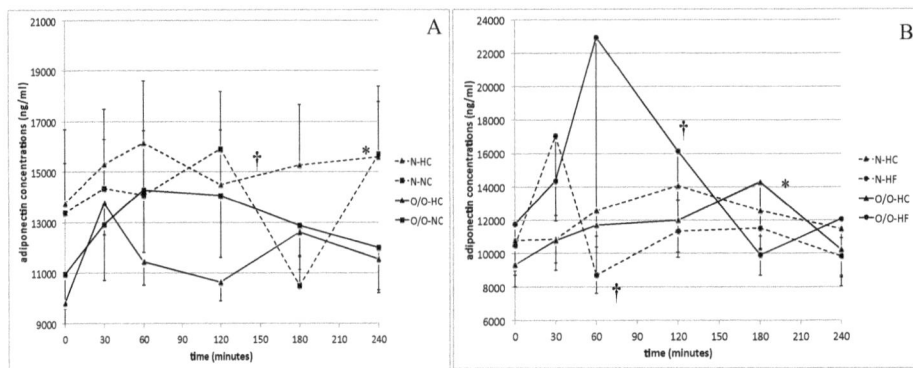

Figure 1. (**A**) Adiponectin concentrations (ng/mL) in men with normal body weight (N, the broken line) and overweight/obese people (O/O, the solid line) in fasting state (time 0 min) and after consumption (time 30–240 min) of a high carbohydrate meal (HC) and a normal carbohydrate meal (NC). The results are presented as mean values ± SE. * The comparison between study groups N and O/O, $p < 0.05$. † The comparison between meals HC and NC, $p < 0.05$. (**B**) Adiponectin concentrations (ng/mL) in men with normal body weight (N, the broken line) and overweight/obese people (O/O, the solid line) in fasting state (time 0 min) and after consumption (time 30–240 min) of a high carbohydrate meal (HC) and a high fat meal (HF). The results are presented as mean values ± SE. * The comparison between study groups N and O/O, $p < 0.05$. † The comparison between meals HC and HF, $p < 0.05$.

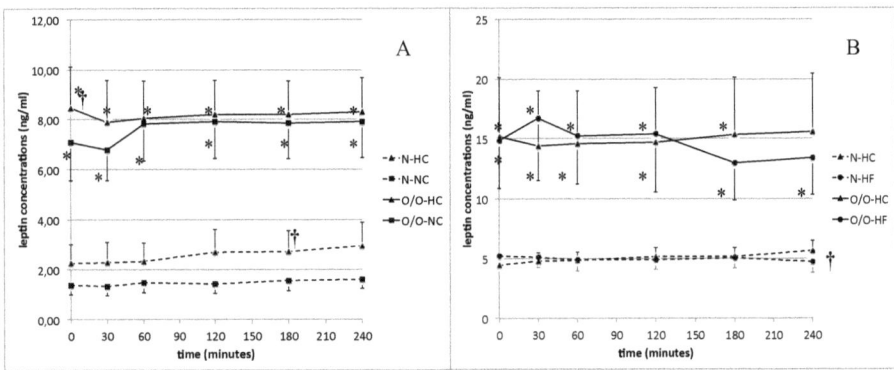

Figure 2. (**A**) Leptin concentrations (ng/mL) in men with normal body weight (N, the broken line) and overweight/obese people (O/O, the solid line) in fasting state (time 0 min) and after consumption (time 30–240 min) of a high carbohydrate meal (HC) and a normal carbohydrate meal (NC). The results are presented as mean values ± SE. * The comparison between study groups N and O/O, $p < 0.05$. † The comparison between meals HC and NC, $p < 0.05$. (**B**) Leptin concentrations (ng/mL) in men with normal body weight (N, the broken line) and overweight/obese people (O/O, the solid line) in fasting state (time 0 min) and after consumption (time 30–240 min) of a high carbohydrate meal (HC) and a high fat meal (HF). The results are presented as mean values ± SE. * The comparison between study groups N and O/O *$p < 0.05$. † The comparison between meals HC and HF $p < 0.05$.

The total ghrelin concentration analysis in Group I showed that there were not any significant differences dependent on meal type in N and O/O men (Figure 3A). However, in Group II, we found that in N subjects the total ghrelin concentrations were significantly lower after the HC-meal intake than after the HF-meal intake (Figure 3B). Lower values were observed at fasting state (744 ± 79 vs. 884 ± 105 ng/mL; $p = 0.02$) and during the first 120 min of the test (30 min: 701 ± 56 vs. 929 ± 101 ng/mL, $p = 0.0005$; 60 min: 637 ± 57 vs. 787 ± 82 ng/mL, $p = 0.0005$; 120 min: 673 ± 64 vs. 804 ± 93 ng/mL,

$p = 0.03$). At 240 min the total ghrelin levels were significantly higher after the HC-meal intake than after the HF-meal (860 ± 92 vs. 748 ± 79 ng/mL, $p = 0.03$). In addition, the AUC for postprandial ghrelin levels was significantly lower after the HC-meal intake than after the HF-meal (174,263 ± 15,962 vs. 202,764 ± 24,214, $p = 0.007$) in N men. In O/O individuals we did not find any significant differences between total ghrelin concentrations after the HC-meal and the HF-meal intake, except at 240 min of the test, when total ghrelin concentrations were significantly lower after the HF-meal consumption (774 ± 77 vs. 586 ± 52 ng/mL, $p = 0.003$) (Figure 3B). In Group I, we did not notice any differences in total ghrelin concentrations between N men and O/O men (Figure 3A). In Group II (Figure 3B) 30 min after the HF-meal intake 30 we observed lower total ghrelin levels in O/O men than in N individuals.

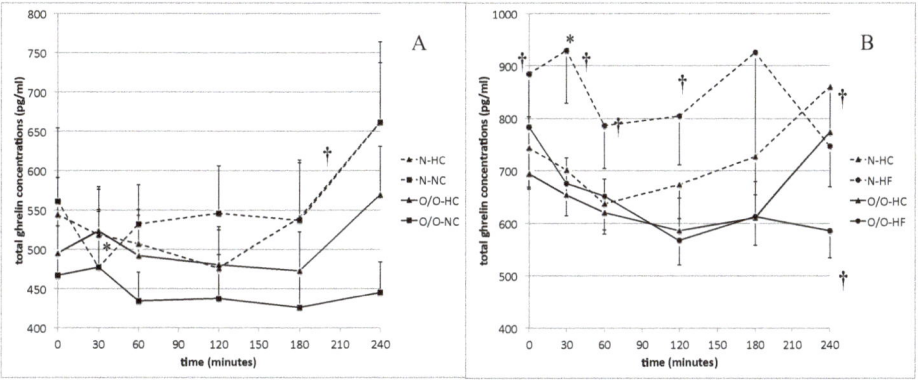

Figure 3. (**A**) Total ghrelin concentrations (ng/mL) in men with normal body weight (N, the broken line) and overweight/obese people (O/O, the solid line) in fasting state (time 0 min) and after consumption (time 30–240 min) of a high carbohydrate meal (HC) and a normal carbohydrate meal (NC). The results are presented as mean values ± SE. * The comparison between study groups N and O/O, $p < 0.05$. † The comparison between meals HC and NC, $p < 0.05$. (**B**) Total ghrelin concentrations (ng/mL) in men with normal body weight (N, the broken line) and overweight/obese people (O/O, the solid line) in fasting state (time 0 min) and after consumption (time 30–240 min) of a high carbohydrate meal (HC) and a high fat meal (HF). The results are presented as mean values ± SE. * The comparison between study groups N and O/O, $p < 0.05$. † The comparison between meals HC and HF, $p < 0.05$.

4. Discussion

The conducted experiment revealed the differences in postprandial adiponectin, leptin and total ghrelin response dependently on the macronutrients meal composition, and also dependently on the body weight. In normal-weight individuals after an HC-meal, we observed higher adiponectin and lower total ghrelin concentrations, than after an HF-meal intake. After the HC-meal intake, we noted also higher leptin concentrations than after NC-meal intake, in normal body weight men. However, higher fasting and postprandial leptin levels we observed in overweight/obese individuals. Investigated hormones and adipokines are involved in energy homeostasis regulation, and play a crucial role in body fat accumulation.

Pathological amounts of adipose tissue lead to cardiovascular diseases, lipid disorders, and type 2 diabetes, which are significant medical problems [3,23–25]. Due to the dynamic nature of obesity [26], it is necessary to broaden our knowledge about the physiological mechanisms involved in energy balance regulation. Hunger and satiety are regulated by the central nervous system's receipt of central and peripheral signals [27–29], which are influenced by environmental factors, including diet [29,30]. In our study, we have observed that the postprandial levels of investigated factors depend on the meal content and may differ in N and O/O men. In N men we noted higher adiponectin levels after the HC-meal intake than after the HF-meal; while in O/O subjects, adiponectin concentrations were significantly higher after the HF-meal intake than after the HC-meal. Our results contrast with those of some other studies, which showed that serum levels of adiponectin are very stable and are not acutely affected by oral glucose or fat load [31,32], but these differences between findings may result from the different nutritional composition of the standardized meals.

We did not observe any significant differences in fasting adiponectin concentrations between N subjects and O/O subjects, although it is generally accepted that people with obesity are characterized by lower adiponectin concentrations [33,34]. However, it was also shown that adiponectin levels in obese and metabolically healthy individuals are comparable with adiponectin concentrations in normal body weight individuals [35], what may explain the lack of significant differences in fasting adiponectin concentrations in our observations.

Another hormone secreted primarily by adipose tissue that is involved in the regulation of body energy homeostasis is leptin. In O/O men, we noted significantly higher leptin concentrations at fasting state and throughout the meal challenge tests. The higher levels in the postprandial period in O/O men were undoubtedly the result of higher baseline values, which may be a consequence of positive energy balance and leptin resistance development [36]. In the context of hunger and satiety regulation, more important are the postprandial changes in leptin levels. In Group I, we have noted significantly higher postprandial leptin concentrations only after the HC-meal in N subjects. We did not observe this effect in O/O men, even if the baseline leptin levels before the HC-meal intake were significantly higher. Our results are inconsistent with the results of Marzullo et al. [15], who showed a slight increase in leptin concentrations in subjects with obesity for 2 h after the HC-meal consumption, whereas, in individuals with normal body weight, authors noted lower leptin concentrations than their baseline values. However, other researchers [16] noticed a greater increase in leptin concentrations after the HC-meal in women with normal body weight, compared to women who were obese, in whom leptin concentrations started to increase just 4 h after HC-meal intake, which is in line with our results. It is worth emphasizing that, in the cited study, the authors considered the HC-meal a meal in which carbohydrates covered 53% of the meal energy, which corresponds better to our NC-meal composition.

After the HF-meal the observations from our study differ from the results obtained by some other researchers, who observed an increase in leptin concentrations after the HF-meal in subjects with normal body mass, whereas in obese individuals they noted a significant decrease in leptin concentrations [37]. However, our results seem to be comparable to the results of studies conducted by Marzullo et al. [15], who showed that postprandial leptin levels in subjects with normal body weight, after HF-meal intake, remained unchanged for 2 h into the test, while in obese individuals postprandial leptin concentrations decreased. The other authors showed that, after a mixed meal intake, leptin concentrations in people with normal body weight were reduced, and an increase was noted from 2 to 8 h after the meal intake [38]. Kim S. et al. [39] noted reduced leptin levels in women after a meal in which carbohydrates accounted for 60% of the energy. Other authors [40] have demonstrated that in obese individuals leptin levels are reduced for the first 2 h after a mixed meal intake, and it returns to baseline values after the next 6 to 12 h. In men with normal body weight, we have noted an increase in postprandial leptin levels only after meals that contained carbohydrates (the difference 240 min after meal intake was on the margin of significance), and this observation seems to be consistent with the results of Monteleone et al. [41] and Romon et al. [42], who showed that in people with normal body weight and BMI ≤ 27 kg/m^2, leptin concentrations after an HC-meal were higher than after consumption of the HF-meals, while leptin levels decreased. Other researchers have shown that after a high-fat meal intake, leptin concentrations were reduced for the first 2 h but then a significant increase was noticed, with a maximum concentration 8 h after meal intake [43]. A study by Raben et al. [44] showed that the decrease in leptin levels is more pronounced after the HC-meal than after the HF-meal, whereas a greater increase in leptin concentrations in relation to fasting values was observed only at 195 min after the HC-meal intake.

Taken together, the results of these studies are inconsistent and it seems that comparisons of leptin concentrations between studies make sense only with similar study protocols and similar nutrient contents of tested meals, but also with comparable study groups, since leptin concentrations are also determined by sexual dimorphism [45].

Besides leptin, which shows anorexigenic activity (decreasing appetite) [46], also ghrelin plays an important role, and both hormones together participate in the regulation of hunger and satiety [47]. Ghrelin is a gastrointestinal hormone with a well-documented orexigenic effect [48]. In our study, despite the apparently higher mean fasting total ghrelin concentrations in subjects with normal body weight than in overweight/obese men, these differences were not statistically significant, probably due to a too-small study sample, which was a major limitation of our study. Other researchers [49] have shown that people with normal body weight tend to have higher ghrelin concentrations. Moreover, in our study we did not notice any important differences in total ghrelin levels between subjects with normal body weight and overweight/obese subjects, except one time-point, which was 30 min after HF-meal intake, when in the overweight/obese men the total ghrelin level decreased, while surprisingly in the normal body weight men it increased. Our results are in line with the study by Heinonen M. et al. [50], who in subjects with obesity and metabolic syndrome, did not observe any decrease in ghrelin levels after HC-meal intake, compared to subjects with normal body weight. An experiment conducted by Zwirska-Korczala et al. [49] showed a more pronounced decrease in ghrelin concentrations after mixed meals in normal body weight subjects than in obese participants, but the study group consisted exclusively of women and different changes depending on sex cannot be excluded. Moreover, the investigated meals differed in essential nutrient content from the meals used in our study, and the test lasted for 120 min.

When we compared the HC-meals with the HF-meals, we found that we could expect a more beneficial response in lean subjects after the HC-meal intake, while after the HF-meal the total ghrelin levels tended to be even higher than at fasting state, and started to decrease at 60 min of the test. The differences were statistically significant also at baseline before meal intake, in the same study group, probably due to the daily variations of total ghrelin levels. Importantly, in overweight/obese men from Group II, we have noted that ghrelin levels decreased postprandially after both meals, but the decrease was more pronounced after the HF-meal intake than after the HC-meal consumption. These results differ from those obtained by Marzullo et al. [15], who showed that the decrease in ghrelin levels after an HF-meal is more pronounced in subjects with normal body weight than in subjects with obesity. It seems that the difference in results can be caused by different compositions of the tested meals, which contained a lower percentage of fat than meals in our study.

The major limitations of our study are the small sample size and the fact that we could not create one study group, in which all volunteers would receive all of the three investigated meals. The main reason is that the presented study is a part of our larger project, with very long and laborious protocol procedures, what limited the final number of volunteers who would agree to participate in the all of the meal challenge tests, with various meals intake. Therefore, it was needed to divide participants into two groups (Group I and Group II), if we aimed to compare the postprandial responses to different meals in the same individuals, following a crossover study design. The other limitations include enrolling only the male participants and the liquid form of meals. These limitations were actually intended and allowed us to reduce the impact of possible confounding factors, such as the influences of sex hormones and sex differences; or to decrease the time of meal digestion and absorption, to not discourage volunteers with a long time spent at each visit etc. However, limitations mentioned above could affect our results, and therefore, our observations regarding the differences in personal postprandial hormonal response dependently on BMI and meal content need further investigation.

5. Conclusions

In conclusion, our study showed that postprandial concentrations and/or changes in concentrations of adiponectin, leptin, and total ghrelin may differ depending on current body energy status, as well as on meal macronutrients content. Our findings suggest that in men with normal body weight we can expect a more beneficial hormonal response after an HC-meal intake, whereas in overweight/obese men, more beneficial effects we have observed after meals with lower carbohydrate and higher fat content. Thus, the practical implications of our study may be the recommendation for overweight/obese people to limit the consumption of high-carbohydrate meals, in exchange for meals in which less than 50% of the energy value comes from carbohydrates.

Author Contributions: Conceptualization, E.A.-P., L.O., A.K. and M.G.; methodology, E.A.-P., L.O., A.K. and M.G.; statistical analysis, J.G.; investigation and data curation, E.A.-P., J.F. and M.M.; writing—original draft preparation, E.A.-P. and L.O.; writing—review and editing, A.K. and M.G.; visualization, E.A.-P., J.F. and M.M.; supervision, A.K. and M.G.

Funding: This study was founded by the Polish Ministry of Science and Higher Education (4774/B/P01/2009/37).

Acknowledgments: The authors would like to thank the Study Team of the Clinical Research Centre and Department of Endocrinology, Diabetology and Internal Medicine of Medical University of Bialystok for technical support. This study was supported by grants from the Medical University of Bialystok, Poland.

Conflicts of Interest: The authors declare no conflict of interest.

References

1. Frühbeck, G.; Gómez-Ambrosi, J.; Muruzábal, F.J.; Burrell, M.A. The adipocyte: A model for integration of endocrine and metabolic signaling in energy metabolism regulation. *Am. J. Physiol. Endocrinol. Metab.* **2001**, *280*, E827–E847. [CrossRef] [PubMed]
2. Rabe, K.; Lehrke, M.; Parhofer, K.G.; Broedl, U.C. Adipokines and insulin resistance. *Mol. Med.* **2008**, *14*, 741–751. [CrossRef] [PubMed]
3. Mattu, H.S.; Randeva, H.S. Role of adipokines in cardiovascular disease. *J. Endocrinol.* **2013**, *216*, T17–T36. [CrossRef] [PubMed]
4. Gil-Campos, M.; Aguilera, C.M.; Cañete, R.; Gil, A. Ghrelin: A hormone regulating food intake and energy homeostasis. *Br. J. Nutr.* **2016**, *96*, 201–226. [CrossRef]
5. Ueno, N.; Dube, M.G.; Inui, A.; Kalra, P.S.; Kalra, S.P. Leptin modulates orexigenic effects of ghrelin and attenuates adiponectin and insulin levels and selectively the dark-phase feeding as revealed by central leptin gene therapy. *Endocrinology* **2004**, *145*, 4176–4184. [CrossRef] [PubMed]
6. Cummings, D.E.; Purnell, J.Q.; Frayo, R.S.; Schmidova, K.; Wisse, B.E.; Weigle, D.S. A preprandial rise in plasma ghrelin levels suggests a role in meal initiation in humans. *Diabetes* **2001**, *50*, 1714–1719. [CrossRef] [PubMed]
7. Leidy, H.J.; Williams, N.I. Meal energy content is related to features of meal-related ghrelin profiles across a typical day of eating in non-obese premenopausal women. *Horm. Metab. Res.* **2006**, *38*, 317–322. [CrossRef] [PubMed]
8. Williams, D.L.; Cummings, D.E. Regulation of ghrelin in physiologic and pathophysiologic states. *J. Nutr.* **2005**, *135*, 1320–1325. [CrossRef] [PubMed]
9. Kadowaki, T.; Yamauchi, T. Adiponectin and adiponectin receptors. *Endocr. Rev.* **2005**, *26*, 439–451. [CrossRef] [PubMed]
10. Saltiel, A.R. You are what you secrete. *Nat. Med.* **2001**, *7*, 887–888. [CrossRef] [PubMed]
11. Yamauchi, T.; Kamon, J.; Waki, H.; Terauchi, Y.; Kubota, N.; Hara, K.; Mori, Y.; Ide, T.; Murakami, K.; Tsuboyama-Kasaoka, N.; et al. The fat-derived hormone adiponectin reverses insulin resistance associated with both lipoatrophy and obesity. *Nat. Med.* **2001**, *7*, 941–946. [CrossRef] [PubMed]
12. Yang, W.S.; Lee, W.J.; Funahashi, T.; Tanaka, S.; Matsuzawa, Y.; Chao, C.L.; Chen, C.L.; Tai, T.Y.; Chuang, L.M. Weight reduction increases plasma levels of an adipose-derived anti-inflammatory protein, adiponectin. *J. Clin. Endocrinol. Metab.* **2001**, *86*, 3815–3819. [CrossRef] [PubMed]
13. Adamska, E.; Ostrowska, L.; Gościk, J.; Waszczeniuk, M.; Krętowski, A.; Górska, M. Intake of Meals Containing High Levels of Carbohydrates or High Levels of Unsaturated Fatty Acids Induces Postprandial Dysmetabolism in Young Overweight/Obese Men. *Biomed. Res. Int.* **2015**, *2015*. [CrossRef] [PubMed]
14. Adamska-Patruno, E.; Ostrowska, L.; Goscik, J.; Pietraszewska, B.; Kretowski, A.; Gorska, M. The relationship between the leptin/ghrelin ratio and meals with various macronutrient contents in men with different nutritional status: A randomized crossover study. *Nutr. J.* **2018**, *17*, 118. [CrossRef] [PubMed]

15. Marzullo, P.; Caumo, A.; Savia, G.; Verti, B.; Walker, G.E.; Maestrini, S.; Tagliaferri, A.; Di Blasio, A.M.; Liuzzi, A. Predictors of postabsorptive ghrelin secretion after intake of different macronutrients. *J. Clin. Endocrinol. Metab.* **2006**, *91*, 4124–4130. [CrossRef] [PubMed]
16. Romon, M.; Lebel, P.; Fruchart, J.C.; Dallongeville, J. Postprandial leptin response to carbohydrate and fat meals in obese women. *J. Am. Coll. Nutr.* **2003**, *22*, 247–251. [CrossRef] [PubMed]
17. Adamska-Patruno, E.; Ostrowska, L.; Golonko, A.; Pietraszewska, B.; Goscik, J.; Kretowski, A.; Gorska, M. Evaluation of Energy Expenditure and Oxidation of Energy Substrates in Adult Males after Intake of Meals with Varying Fat and Carbohydrate Content. *Nutrients* **2018**, *10*, 5. [CrossRef] [PubMed]
18. Adamska, E.; Waszczeniuk, M.; Gościk, J.; Golonko, A.; Wilk, J.; Pliszka, J.; Maliszewska, K.; Lipińska, D.; Milewski, R.; Wasilewska, A.; et al. The usefulness of glycated hemoglobin A1c (HbA1c) for identifying dysglycemic states in individuals without previously diagnosed diabetes. *Adv. Med. Sci.* **2012**, *57*, 296–301. [CrossRef] [PubMed]
19. Adamska, E.; Kretowski, A.; Goscik, J.; Citko, A.; Bauer, W.; Waszczeniuk, M.; Maliszewska, K.; Paczkowska-Abdulsalam, M.; Niemira, M.; Szczerbinski, L.; et al. The type 2 diabetes susceptibility TCF7L2 gene variants affect postprandial glucose and fat utilization in non-diabetic subjects. *Diabetes Metab.* **2018**, *44*, 379–382. [CrossRef] [PubMed]
20. Kretowski, A.; Adamska, E.; Maliszewska, K.; Wawrusiewicz-Kurylonek, N.; Citko, A.; Goscik, J.; Bauer, W.; Wilk, J.; Golonko, A.; Waszczeniuk, M.; et al. The rs340874 PROX1 type 2 diabetes mellitus risk variant is associated with visceral fat accumulation and alterations in postprandial glucose and lipid metabolism. *Genes. Nutr.* **2015**, *10*, 454. [CrossRef] [PubMed]
21. Ostrowska, L.; Witczak, K.; Adamska, E. Effect of nutrition and atherogenic index on the occurrence and intensity of insulin resistance. *Pol. Arch. Med. Wewn.* **2013**, *123*, 289–296. [CrossRef] [PubMed]
22. Benjamini, Y.; Hochberg, Y. Controlling the false discovery rate: A practical and powerful approach to multiple testing. *J. R. Statist. Soc. Ser. B* **1995**, *57*, 289–300. [CrossRef]
23. Trayhurn, P.; Wood, I.S. Adipokines: Inflammation and the pleiotropic role of white adipose tissue. *Br. J. Nutr.* **2004**, *92*, 347–355. [CrossRef] [PubMed]
24. Lakka, H.M.; Laaksonen, D.E.; Lakka, T.A.; Niskanen, L.K.; Kumpusalo, E.; Tuomilehto, J.; Salonen, J.T. The metabolic syndrome and total and cardiovascular disease mortality in middle-aged men. *JAMA* **2002**, *288*, 2709–2716. [CrossRef] [PubMed]
25. Mottillo, S.; Filion, K.B.; Genest, J.; Joseph, L.; Pilote, L.; Poirier, P.; Rinfret, S.; Schiffrin, E.L.; Eisenberg, M.J. The metabolic syndrome and cardiovascular risk a systematic review and meta-analysis. *J. Am. Coll. Cardiol.* **2001**, *56*, 1113–1132. [CrossRef] [PubMed]
26. Kelly, T.; Yang, W.; Chen, C.S.; Reynolds, K.; He, J. Global burden of obesity in 2005 and projections to 2030. *Int. J. Obes.* **2008**, *32*, 1431–1437. [CrossRef] [PubMed]
27. Gross, P.M. Circumventricular organ capillaries. *Prog. Brain. Res.* **1992**, *91*, 219–233. [PubMed]
28. Briggs, D.I.; Andrews, Z.B. Metabolic status regulates ghrelin function on energy homeostasis. *Neuroendocrinology* **2001**, *93*, 48–57. [CrossRef] [PubMed]
29. Anubhuti Arora, S. Role of neuropeptides in appetite regulation and obesity–A review. *Neuropeptides* **2006**, *40*, 375–401. [CrossRef] [PubMed]
30. Crowell, M.D.; Decker, G.A.; Levy, R.; Jeffrey, R.; Talley, N.J. Gut-brain neuropeptides in the regulation of ingestive behaviors and obesity. *Am. J. Gastroenterol.* **2006**, *101*, 2848–2856. [CrossRef] [PubMed]
31. Peake, P.W.; Kriketos, A.D.; Denyer, G.S.; Campbell, L.V.; Charlesworth, J.A. The postprandial response of adiponectin to a high-fat meal in normal and insulin-resistant subjects. *Int. J. Obes. Relat. Metab. Disord.* **2003**, *27*, 657–662. [CrossRef] [PubMed]
32. Heliövaara, M.K.; Strandberg, T.E.; Karonen, S.L.; Ebeling, P. Association of serum adiponectin concentration to lipid and glucose metabolism in healthy humans. *Horm. Metab. Res.* **2006**, *38*, 336–340. [CrossRef] [PubMed]
33. Haluzík, M.; Parízková, J.; Haluzík, M.M. Adiponectin and its role in the obesity-induced insulin resistance and related complications. *Physiol. Res.* **2004**, *53*, 123–129. [PubMed]
34. Lubkowska, A.; Radecka, A.; Bryczkowska, I.; Rotter, I.; Laszczyńska, M.; Dudzińska, W. Serum Adiponectin and Leptin Concentrations in Relation to Body Fat Distribution, Hematological Indices and Lipid Profile in Humans. *Int. J. Environ. Res. Public Health* **2015**, *12*, 11528–11548. [CrossRef] [PubMed]

35. Aguilar-Salinas, C.A.; García, E.G.; Robles, L.; Riaño, D.; Ruiz-Gomez, D.G.; García-Ulloa, A.C.; Melgarejo, M.A.; Zamora, M.; Guillen-Pineda, L.E.; Mehta, R.; et al. High adiponectin concentrations are associated with the metabolically healthy obese phenotype. *J. Clin. Endocrinol. Metab.* **2008**, *93*, 4075–4079. [CrossRef] [PubMed]
36. Kolaczynski, J.W.; Ohannesian, J.P.; Considine, R.V.; Marco, C.C.; Caro, J.F. Response of leptin to short-term and prolonged overfeeding in humans. *J. Clin. Endocrinol. Metab.* **1996**, *81*, 4162–4165. [PubMed]
37. Imbeault, P.; Doucet, E.; Mauriège, P.; St-Pierre, S.; Couillard, C.; Alméras, N.; Després, J.P.; Tremblay, A. Difference in leptin response to a high-fat meal between lean and obese men. *Clin. Sci.* **2001**, *101*, 359–365. [CrossRef] [PubMed]
38. Joannic, J.L.; Oppert, J.M.; Lahlou, N.; Basdevant, A.; Auboiron, S.; Raison, J.; Bornet, F.; Guy-Grand, B. Plasma leptin and hunger ratings in healthy humans. *Appetite* **1998**, *30*, 129–138. [CrossRef] [PubMed]
39. Kim, S.J.; Lee, H.; Choue, R. Short-term effects of ratio of energy nutrients on appetite-related hormones in female college students. *Clin. Nutr. Res.* **2012**, *1*, 58–65. [CrossRef] [PubMed]
40. Pratley, R.E.; Nicolson, M.; Bogardus, C.; Ravussin, E. Plasma leptin responses to fasting in Pima Indians. *Am. J. Physiol.* **1997**, *273*, E644–E649. [CrossRef] [PubMed]
41. Monteleone, P.; Bencivenga, R.; Longobardi, N.; Serritella, C.; Maj, M. Differential responses of circulating ghrelin to high-fat or high-carbohydrate meal in healthy women. *J. Clin. Endocrinol. Metab.* **2003**, *88*, 5510–5514. [CrossRef] [PubMed]
42. Romon, M.; Lebel, P.; Velly, C.; Marecaux, N.; Fruchart, J.C.; Dallongeville, J. Leptin response to carbohydrate or fat meal and association with subsequent satiety and energy intake. *Am. J. Physiol.* **1999**, *277*, E855–E861. [CrossRef] [PubMed]
43. Dallongeville, J.; Hecquet, B.; Lebel, P.; Edmé, J.L.; Le Fur, C.; Fruchart, J.C.; Auwerx, J.; Romon, M. Short term response of circulating leptin to feeding and fasting in man: Influence of circadian cycle. *Int. J. Obes. Relat. Metab. Disord.* **1998**, *22*, 728–733. [CrossRef] [PubMed]
44. Raben, A.; Agerholm-Larsen, L.; Flint, A.; Holst, J.J.; Astrup, A. Meals with similar energy densities but rich in protein, fat, carbohydrate, or alcohol have different effects on energy expenditure and substrate metabolism but not on appetite and energy intake. *Am. J. Clin. Nutr.* **2003**, *77*, 91–100. [CrossRef] [PubMed]
45. Montague, C.T.; Prins, J.B.; Sanders, L.; Digby, J.E.; O'Rahilly, S. Depot- and sex-specific differences in human leptin mRNA expression: Implications for the control of regional fat distribution. *Diabetes* **1997**, *46*, 342–347. [CrossRef] [PubMed]
46. Belgardt, B.F.; Brüning, J.C. CNS leptin and insulin action in the control of energy homeostasis. *Ann. N. Y. Acad. Sci.* **2010**, *1212*, 97–113. [CrossRef] [PubMed]
47. Konturek, P.C.; Konturek, J.W.; Cześnikiewicz-Guzik, M.; Brzozowski, T.; Sito, E.; Konturek, S.J. Neuro-hormonal control of food intake: Basic mechanisms and clinical implications. *J. Physiol. Pharmacol.* **2005**, *56*, 5–25. [PubMed]
48. Huda, M.S.; Dovey, T.; Wong, S.P.; English, P.J.; Halford, J.; McCulloch, P.; Cleator, J.; Martin, B.; Cashen, J.; Hayden, K.; et al. Ghrelin restores 'lean-type' hunger and energy expenditure profiles in morbidly obese subjects but has no effect on postgastrectomy subjects. *Int. J. Obes.* **2009**, *33*, 317–325. [CrossRef] [PubMed]
49. Zwirska-Korczala, K.; Konturek, S.J.; Sodowski, M.; Wylezol, M.; Kuka, D.; Sowa, P.; Adamczyk-Sowa, M.; Kukla, M.; Berdowska, A.; Rehfeld, J.F.; et al. Basal and postprandial plasma levels of PYY, ghrelin, cholecystokinin, gastrin and insulin in women with moderate and morbid obesity and metabolic syndrome. *J. Physiol. Pharmacol.* **2007**, *58*, 13–35. [PubMed]
50. Heinonen, M.V.; Karhunen, L.J.; Chabot, E.D.; Toppinen, L.K.; Juntunen, K.S.; Laaksonen, D.E.; Siloaho, M.; Liukkonen, K.H.; Herzig, K.H.; Niskanen, L.K.; et al. Plasma ghrelin levels after two high-carbohydrate meals producing different insulin responses in patients with metabolic syndrome. *Regul. Pept.* **2007**, *138*, 118–125. [CrossRef] [PubMed]

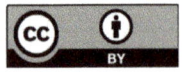

© 2019 by the authors. Licensee MDPI, Basel, Switzerland. This article is an open access article distributed under the terms and conditions of the Creative Commons Attribution (CC BY) license (http://creativecommons.org/licenses/by/4.0/).

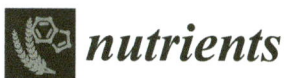

Article

Pretreatment Fasting Glucose and Insulin as Determinants of Weight Loss on Diets Varying in Macronutrients and Dietary Fibers—The POUNDS LOST Study

Mads F. Hjorth [1,*], George A. Bray [2], Yishai Zohar [3], Lorien Urban [3], Derek C. Miketinas [2,4], Donald A. Williamson [2], Donna H. Ryan [2], Jennifer Rood [2], Catherine M. Champagne [2], Frank M. Sacks [5] and Arne Astrup [1]

1. Department of Nutrition, Exercise and Sports, Faculty of Sciences, University of Copenhagen, Rolighedsvej 26, 1958 Frederiksberg, Denmark; ast@nexs.ku.dk
2. Pennington Biomedical Research Center of the Louisiana State University System, Baton Rouge, LA 70803, USA; George.Bray@pbrc.edu (G.A.B.); Derek.Miketinas@pbrc.edu (D.C.M.); WilliaDA@pbrc.edu (D.A.W.); ryandh@pbrc.edu (D.H.R.); Jennifer.Rood@pbrc.edu (J.R.); Catherine.Champagne@pbrc.edu (C.M.C.)
3. Gelesis, Boston, MA 02116, USA; yzohar@gelesis.com (Y.Z.); lurban@gelesis.com (L.U.)
4. School of Nutrition and Food Sciences, Texas Woman's University, Denton, TX 76204, USA
5. Nutrition Department, Harvard T.H Chan School of Public Health and Department of Medicine, Harvard Medical School, Boston, MA 02115, USA; fsacks@hsph.harvard.edu
* Correspondence: madsfiil@nexs.ku.dk; Tel.: +45-353-32489

Received: 28 January 2019; Accepted: 6 March 2019; Published: 11 March 2019

Abstract: Efforts to identify a preferable diet for weight management based on macronutrient composition have largely failed, but recent evidence suggests that satiety effects of carbohydrates may depend on the individual's insulin-mediated cellular glucose uptake. Therefore, using data from the POUNDS LOST trial, pre-treatment fasting plasma glucose (FPG), fasting insulin (FI), and homeostatic model assessment of insulin resistance (HOMA-IR) were studied as prognostic markers of long-term weight loss in four diets differing in carbohydrate, fat, and protein content, while assessing the role of dietary fiber intake. Subjects with FPG <100 mg/dL lost 2.6 (95% CI 0.9;4.4, $p = 0.003$) kg more on the low-fat/high-protein ($n = 132$) compared to the low-fat/average-protein diet ($n = 136$). Subjects with HOMA-IR ≥ 4 lost 3.6 (95% CI 0.2;7.1, $p = 0.038$) kg more body weight on the high-fat/high-protein ($n = 35$) compared to high-fat/average-protein diet ($n = 33$). Regardless of the randomized diet, subjects with prediabetes and FI below the median lost 5.6 kg (95% CI 0.6;10.6, $p = 0.030$) more when consuming ≥ 35 g ($n = 15$) compared to <35 g dietary fiber/10 MJ ($n = 16$). Overall, subjects with normal glycemia lost most on the low-fat/high-protein diet, subjects with high HOMA-IR lost most on the high-fat/high protein diet, and subjects with prediabetes and low FI had particular benefit from dietary fiber in the diet.

Keywords: glucose; insulin; weight; diet; macronutrient composition; clinical nutrition

---

1. Introduction

During the past 30 years, there has been a great deal of controversy about the composition of the optimal diet for weight loss and maintenance. Some have defended the more conventional low-fat/high-carbohydrate diet [1,2], whereas others point to a restriction in carbohydrates as being more effective [3]. Numerous strategies for modifying carbohydrate intake have been proposed, from ketogenic very-low-carbohydrate diets [4] to diets with increased protein and a lowered glycemic index (GI) of the carbohydrates [5]. Efforts to identify a preferable diet for weight loss and weight loss maintenance based on macronutrient composition have largely failed [6], implying that no single diet is ideal for all participants with overweight and obesity [7]. On the other hand, dietary fiber is regarded as important for weight regulation [8], as diets including more fruits, vegetables and whole grains are associated with lower body weight in randomized dietary studies [9,10], as well as in observational studies [8].

The glucostatic hypothesis suggests that the central nervous system monitors blood glucose as part of the established appetite regulatory system. As eating progresses, glucose in the blood increases, leading to increased hypothalamic glucose utilization, ultimately causing the individual to become satiated and to stop eating [11]. Recently, the glucose uptake in the brain during a hyperglycemic clamp, simulating postprandial levels, was found to be reduced in individuals with obesity compared to normal weight subjects and even more so in patients with type 2 diabetes [12]. Furthermore, brain glucose uptake was positively correlated with fullness and satiety [12]. Collectively, this suggests that whether or not a carbohydrate-rich diet, which, in the case of high glycemic index foods, would result in rapid increases in blood glucose, should be recommended as diets for weight loss and weight loss maintenance depends on the degree to which glucose enters the brain. Carbohydrate-rich meals may, therefore, be satiating in insulin-sensitive individuals, but less so in more insulin-resistant individuals. Individuals with prediabetes or type 2 diabetes may instead depend more on dietary fiber intake to stimulate satiety and improve glycemic control [13], as well as other satiety hormones, such as CCK, GLP-1, and PYY, which are released mainly in response to fats and protein reaching the small intestine [8].

Based on stratified analysis of several studies summarized in a recent review [14], it was proposed that diets low in fat and high in protein will work best for individuals with normal fasting glucose and diets high in dietary fibers will work particularly well among subjects with impaired fasting glucose. The POUNDS LOST study offers the opportunity to test this hypothesis, since it randomized subjects to four diets varying in macronutrients with a minimum of 20 g of dietary fiber per day. In the main paper, there were no differences in weight loss between the randomized groups [15]. However, the potential role of pretreatment fasting plasma glucose (FPG) and fasting insulin (FI) on weight loss according to randomized diets and dietary fiber intake was not investigated, and is the subject of this paper.

The purpose of this study was to analyze data from the POUNDS LOST trial [15], to investigate whether FPG and FI are prognostic markers for long-term weight loss in four diets differing in carbohydrate, fat, and protein content, and assess the role of dietary fiber intake. We hypothesized that normoglycemic subjects would lose more weight on the low-fat/high-protein diet, that dietary fiber intake would be positively associated with weight loss particularly among subjects with prediabetes, and that those being most insulin resistance would lose more weight on the high-fat/high-protein diet.

2. Materials and Methods

In the original trial, 811 overweight adults were randomized to one of four energy-reduced diets (deficit of 750 kcal per day from baseline) varying in macronutrient composition for 24 months with the goals for all groups of having at least 20 g of dietary fiber per day while recommending carbohydrates with a low glycemic index. The nutrient goals for the four diet groups were: 20% fat, 15% protein, and 65% carbohydrates (low-fat/average-protein); 20% fat, 25% protein, and 55% carbohydrates (low-fat/high-protein); 40% fat, 15% protein, and 45% carbohydrates (high-fat/average-protein); and 40% fat, 25% protein, and 35% carbohydrates (high-fat/high-protein). At baseline, FPG and FI were measured from which homeostatic model assessment of insulin resistance (HOMA-IR) was calculated, and participants were asked to complete a 5-day diet record. Body weight was measured at baseline and after 24 months of intervention. After 6 and 24 months, 24-h dietary recalls were collected during telephone interviews on 3 nonconsecutive days in a random sample of 50% of the participants. The proportion of attended counseling sessions for weight loss during the 24 months was calculated as sessions attended divided by sessions offered and split into high and low attendance using the median value (0.44). Among others, the presence of diabetes was a criterion for exclusion. Detailed information about the study has been published [15]. The study was approved by the human subjects committee and by the data and safety monitoring board. All participants gave written informed consent. The study was registered on clinicaltrials.gov with the identifier: NCT00072995.

For this re-analysis, baseline FPG levels were used to stratify subjects as being normoglycemic (FPG < 100 mg/dL) or prediabetic (FPG ≥ 100 mg/dL, NOTE: no upper limit as diabetes was a criterion for exclusion) through the use of the FPG cutoffs published by the American Diabetes Association [16], as pre-treatment FPG was recently shown to determine weight loss and weight loss maintenance success to diets varying in macronutrient composition and fiber content [14]. Furthermore, median FI concentration among subjects with prediabetic having dietary records (13.8 µIU/mL) was used to dichotomize subjects into low and high FI in accordance with previous procedures in which cut-offs ranging between 10.5 and 13 µIU/mL were used [17]. Similarly, median HOMA-IR value among subjects with prediabetic having dietary records (4.0) was used to dichotomize subjects into low and high HOMA-IR. Subjects were included in the current study if they had a baseline measure of FPG and FI as well as a 24-month measurement of body weight. Dietary fiber intake during the 24 months was calculated as mean intake at 6 and 24 months expressed as g/10 MJ (~2400 kcal). If the 24-h recall was missing at either 6 or 24 months, the other constituted the mean value. Furthermore, changes in dietary fiber intake (g/10 MJ) were calculated using the mean intake during the intervention by subtracting the baseline fiber intake.

Descriptive characteristics of the study population (completers only) are presented as mean ± SD or as proportions (%) and differences between glycemic groups was tested using one-way ANOVA or Pearson's chi-squared test. Differences in weight change between FPG and FI groups (and the combination of the two using an interaction term) were analyzed by means of linear mixed models. The linear mixed models comprised fixed effects including age, gender, and baseline BMI and site as random effect. Results are shown as 24-month mean weight change from baseline with 95% confidence interval (CI). Differences in weight change from baseline between diets were compared within each blood marker group through the use of pairwise comparisons with post hoc t-tests. The 24-month weight change according to self-reported dietary fiber intake (during the intervention and as changes from baseline to intervention) in the overall population, as well as in selected groups based on FPG and FI groups (and the combination of the two) were reported as Pearson correlation coefficients and partial correlation coefficients adjusting for age, gender, and baseline BMI. Finally, the difference in 24-month weight loss between participants consuming ≥35 g fiber/10 MJ and <35 g fiber/10 MJ during the intervention was compared using t-tests. The level of significance was set at $P < 0.05$, with no adjustment for multiple testing, and statistical analyses were conducted using STATA/SE 14.1 (Houston, TX, USA).

3. Results

The 639 subjects used for these analyses included participants who were 61% women, were 52 ± 9 years of age and had a BMI of 32.7 ± 3.8 kg/m². Differences in age, BMI, weight and gender distribution ($p ≤ 0.008$), but not in completion rate ($p = 0.81$), were observed between the FPG/FI subgroups (Table 1). In addition, among the 317 subjects having valid dietary records, total energy intake, dietary fat and fiber intake ($p ≤ 0.035$), but not carbohydrate and protein intake ($p ≥ 0.22$), varied slightly between FPG/FI subgroups at baseline (Table 1).

Table 1. Baseline characteristics of the completing study populations stratified by fasting glucose and insulin.

	FPG < 100 mg/dL & FI < 13.8 μIU/mL	FPG < 100 mg/dL & FI ≥ 13.8 μIU/mL	FPG ≥100 mg/dL & FI < 13.8 μIU/mL	FPG ≥ 100 mg/dL & FI ≥ 13.8 μIU/mL	p-Value
All (n = 639)	386	136	50	67	
Completion (%)	78.6	79.5	82.0	82.7	0.81
Age	50.9 ± 9.4 [a]	52.3 ± 8.4 [ab]	55.0 ± 6.9 [b]	53.1 ± 9.7 [ab]	0.008
Sex, % females	68.9	53.7	46.0	43.3	<0.001
Body weight, kg	88.8 ± 14.6 [a]	100.0 ± 14.7 [bc]	95.3 ± 13.3 [c]	101.4 ± 14.4 [b]	<0.001
BMI, kg/m²	31.6 ± 3.7 [a]	34.5 ± 3.6 [c]	32.8 ± 3.8 [b]	34.7 ± 3.1 [c]	<0.001
Fasting glucose, mg/dL	88 (83;92)	92 (87;96)	106 (102;115)	108 (103;115)	
Fasting Insulin, μIU/mL	7.9 (6.1;10.5)	17.3 (15.4;21.8)	10.3 (8.3;11.9)	19.8 (16.7;26.2)	
HOMA-IR	1.7 (1.3;2.3) [a]	3.9 (3.5;4.7) [b]	2.8 (2.2;3.3) [c]	5.4 (4.6;7.1) [d]	<0.001
Diet record subgroup (n = 317)	179	75	31	32	
Age	52.3 ± 9.2	53.4 ± 8.6	55.1 ± 7.1	52.1 ± 8.8	0.38
Sex, % females	62.6	49.3	48.4	28.1	0.002
Body weight, kg	89.3 ± 15.8 [a]	100.9 ± 14.3 [b]	95.3 ± 14.2 [b]	101.5 ± 14.4 [b]	<0.001
BMI, kg/m²	31.4 ± 3.8 [a]	34.3 ± 3.4 [b]	32.6 ± 3.9 [a]	34.7 ± 2.7 [b]	<0.001
Fasting glucose, mg/dL	88 (83;92)	93 (87;96)	106 (103;110)	110 (106;119)	
Fasting Insulin, μIU/mL	8.1 (6.1;10.5)	17.2 (15.7;19.8)	10.3 (8.3;11.9)	19.1 (16.5;23.3)	
HOMA-IR	1.7 (1.3;2.3) [a]	3.9 (3.5;4.5) [b]	2.8 (2.2;3.3) [c]	5.3 (4.6;6.9) [d]	<0.001
Energy intake (kcal/day)	1976 ± 494 [a]	2126 ± 579 [b]	1856 ± 630 [a]	2301 ± 647 [b]	0.002
Carbohydrate (E%)	45.1 ± 7.7	44.7 ± 7.0	45.2 ± 8.4	41.9 ± 6.6	0.17
Fat (E%)	36.9 ± 6.0 [ab]	37.9 ± 5.4 [b]	35.4 ± 6.9 [a]	39.3 ± 5.6 [bc]	0.035
Protein (E%)	17.9 ± 3.4	17.4 ± 3.2	18.8 ± 3.8	17.6 ± 2.5	0.22
Fiber intake (g/day)	18.1 ± 7.3	16.9 ± 5.4	17.6 ± 5.4	17.9 ± 5.8	0.61
Fiber intake (g/10 MJ)	22.2 ± 7.7 [a]	19.5 ± 5.7 [b]	24.5 ± 10.1 [a]	19.1 ± 6.3 [b]	0.002

Abbreviations: BMI, Body mass index; E%, Energy percentage; FI, Fasting insulin; FPG, Fasting plasma glucose; HOMA-IR, Homeostatic model assessment of insulin resistance. Data are mean ± SD, median (IQR), and proportions. Tested by one-way ANOVA with different superscript letters within a row indicate significant differences ($p < 0.05$) or tested for overall difference by chi-square.

Overall, the low-fat/high-protein diet (n = 157) produced a 1.8 (95% CI 0.2;3.4, p = 0.03) kg greater weight loss compared to the low-fat/average-protein diet (n = 166) (Table 2). This difference was 2.6 (95% CI 0.9;4.4, p = 0.003) kg among subjects with normoglycemic and −1.4 (95% CI −5.3;2.4, p = 0.46) kg among subjects with prediabetes [mean difference: 4.1 kg (95% CI −0.1;8.3, p = 0.057)]. This indicates that glycemic status modulates the effect of a low-fat, high-protein diet on weight loss over 2 years. The diet appears more effective in those with normoglycemia than prediabetes. Further subdividing the normoglycemia group showed that this difference was 2.9 (95% CI 0.9;4.9, p = 0.005) kg among subjects with normoglycemia and low FI, and 2.1 (95% CI −1.4;5.6, p = 0.25) kg among subjects with normoglycemia and high FI [mean difference: 0.8 kg (95% CI −3.3;4.8, p = 0.71).

Furthermore, subjects with high HOMA-IR lost 3.6 (95% CI 0.2;7.1, p = 0.038) kg more body weight on the high-fat/high-protein diet compared to high-fat/average-protein diet, whereas this difference was −0.9 (95% CI −2.7;0.9, p = 0.32) kg among subjects with low HOMA-IR [mean difference: 4.5 (95% CI 0.7;8.4, p = 0.022)].

Independent of the type of diet, subjects attending at least 44 percent (median value) of the counseling sessions lost 5.6 (95% CI 4.5;6.6, p < 0.001) kg more compared to those attending fewer sessions (−6.9 vs. −1.3 kg). Among this subgroup with attendance above the median, subjects who had high HOMA-IR lost 4.8 kg (95% CI 0.01;9.6, p = 0.049) more body weight when randomized to the high-fat/high-protein diet compared to the high-fat/average-protein, whereas this difference was −1.1 (95% CI −3.5;1.2, p = 0.35) kg among subjects with low HOMA-IR [mean difference: 5.9 (95% CI 0.6;11.3, p = 0.029)] (Table S1).

The self-reported dietary fiber intake was 9.8 (95% CI 8.7;11.0, SD 10.4, n = 317, p < 0.001) g/10 MJ higher during the intervention compared to the baseline. The fiber intake mainly came from the carbohydrate-rich foods, so fiber intake was highest in the low-fat/average-protein diet and lowest in the high-fat/high-protein diet and intermediate in the two remaining diets (Table 3).

Table 2. Two-year weight change according to randomization and stratified on pretreatment FPG and FI ($n = 639$).

	LF-AP 65% Carb	LF-HP 55% Carb	Δ (LF-AP vs. LF-HP) Weight Change (kg)	HF-AP 45% Carb	HF-HP 34% Carb	Δ (HF-AP vs. HF-HP) Weight Change (kg)
All [1]	($n = 166$) −3.3 (−4.4; −2.1) a	($n = 157$) −5.0 (−6.2; −3.9) b	1.8 (0.2;3.4) *	($n = 148$) −4.0 (−5.2; −2.8) ab	($n = 168$) −4.0 (−5.1; −2.9) ab	−0.03 (−1.7;1.6)
FPG < 100 mg/dL	($n = 136$) −2.9 (−4.2; −1.7) a	($n = 132$) −5.6 (−6.8; −4.3) b	2.6 (0.9;4.4) *	($n = 119$) −4.2 (−5.5; −2.9) ab	($n = 135$) −3.9 (−5.1; −2.6) ab	−0.4 (−2.1;1.4)
FI < 13.8 μIU/mL	($n = 97$) −2.6 (−4.1; −1.2) a	($n = 105$) −5.5 (−6.9; −4.1) b	2.9 (0.9;4.9) *	($n = 80$) −4.5 (−6.1; −2.9) ab	($n = 104$) −3.6 (−5.0; −2.2) ab	−0.9 (−3.0;1.2)
FI ≥ 13.8 μIU/mL	($n = 39$) −3.7 (−5.9; −1.4)	($n = 27$) −5.7 (−8.5; −3.0)	2.1 (−1.4;5.6)	($n = 39$) −3.6 (−5.9; −1.3)	($n = 31$) −4.7 (−7.3; −2.2)	1.1 (−2.3;4.5)
FPG ≥ 100 mg/dL	($n = 30$) −4.6 (−7.2; −2.0)	($n = 25$) −3.2 (−6.0; −0.3)	−1.4 (−5.3;2.4)	($n = 29$) −2.4 (−5.1;0.2)	($n = 33$) −4.4 (−6.9; −2.0)	2.0 (−1.6;5.6)
FI < 13.8 μIU/mL	($n = 11$) −5.4 (9.7; −1.2)	($n = 9$) −2.2 (−6.9;2.5)	−3.2 (−9.6;3.1)	($n = 14$) −1.9 (−5.7;1.9)	($n = 16$) −3.6 (−7.1; −0.1)	1.7 (−3.4;6.9)
FI ≥ 13.8 μIU/mL	($n = 19$) −4.1 (−7.4; −0.9)	($n = 16$) −3.7 (−7.3; −0.2)	−0.4 (−5.2;4.4)	($n = 15$) −3.0 (−6.6;0.7)	($n = 17$) −5.3 (−8.7; −1.8)	2.3 (−2.7;7.3)
HOMA-IR < 4.0	($n = 131$) −3.4 (−4.6; −2.1) a	($n = 130$) −5.3 (−6.6; −4.1) b	2.0 (0.2;3.7) *	($n = 115$) −4.6 (−5.9; −3.3) ab	($n = 133$) −3.7 (−4.9; −2.5) ab	−0.9 (−2.7;0.9)
HOMA-IR > 4.0	($n = 35$) −2.8 (−5.2; −0.4) ab	($n = 27$) −4.5 (−7.2; −1.7) ab	1.7 (−1.9;5.3)	($n = 33$) −1.3 (−3.8;1.1) a	($n = 35$) −5.0 (−7.4; −2.5) b	3.6 (0.2;7.1) *

Abbreviations: AP, Average protein; FI, Fasting insulin; FPG, Fasting plasma glucose; HOMA-IR, Homeostatic model assessment of insulin resistance; HF, High fat; HP, High protein; LF, Low fat. Data are presented as estimated mean weight changes from baseline for each combination of the diet × FPG × FI strata interaction in the linear mixed models, which were also adjusted for age, sex, and BMI (fixed effects) as well as sites (random effect). Differences in weight change from baseline between diets were compared within each blood marker group through the use of pairwise comparisons with post hoc t tests. Different superscript letters within a row indicate significant differences ($p < 0.05$). * $p < 0.05$; [1] Not adjusted for any fixed effects.

Table 3. Self-reported dietary fiber intake in the four randomized groups.

	LF-AP 65% Carb	LF-HP 55% Carb	HF-AP 45% Carb	HF-HP 34% Carb
Fiber g/10 MJ (month 6)	$n = 80$ 36.6 ± 12.4 [a]	$n = 79$ 32.1 ± 10.8 [b]	$n = 68$ 32.1 ± 9.3 [b]	$n = 80$ 28.0 ± 9.9 [c]
Fiber g/10 MJ (month 24)	$n = 43$ 33.6 ± 12.8 [a]	$n = 46$ 29.1 ± 9.3 [ab]	$n = 41$ 28.6 ± 11.5 [b]	$n = 39$ 26.2 ± 10.2 [b]
Fiber g/10 MJ (month 6 and 24) [1]	$n = 83$ 35.4 ± 11.7 [a]	$n = 81$ 31.4 ± 9.6 [b]	$n = 72$ 30.9 ± 9.2 [b]	$n = 81$ 27.3 ± 8.6 [c]

Abbreviations: AP, Average protein; Carb, Carbohydrates; HF, High fat; HP, High protein; LF, Low fat. Data are mean ± SD and tested by one-way ANOVA with different superscript letters within a row indicate significant differences ($p < 0.05$). [1] Mean dietary fiber intake from month 6 and 24. If only one measurement was present this was used.

Overall, differences in dietary fiber intake between baseline and intervention, as well as fiber intake during the intervention, were negatively correlated with weight change ($r = -0.17$ to -0.23, $p \leq 0.002$). This negative correlation existed for most subgroups of FPG, FI, and HOMA-IR but was most pronounced among subjects with prediabetes and low FI ($r = -0.45$ to -0.47, $p \leq 0.011$) (Table 4). This correlation remained significant ($r = -0.40$, $p = 0.047$) after additionally adjusting for fat, protein and carbohydrate intake during the intervention.

Subjects consuming ≥35 g dietary fiber/10 MJ during the intervention lost 2.4 kg (95% CI 0.6;4.1, $p = 0.008$) more compared to those consuming <35 g dietary fiber/10 MJ. This difference existed for most subgroups of FPG, FI, and HOMA_IR, but was most pronounced among subjects with prediabetes and low FI [5.6 kg (95% CI 0.6;10.6, $p = 0.030$)] (Table 4 and Figure 1).

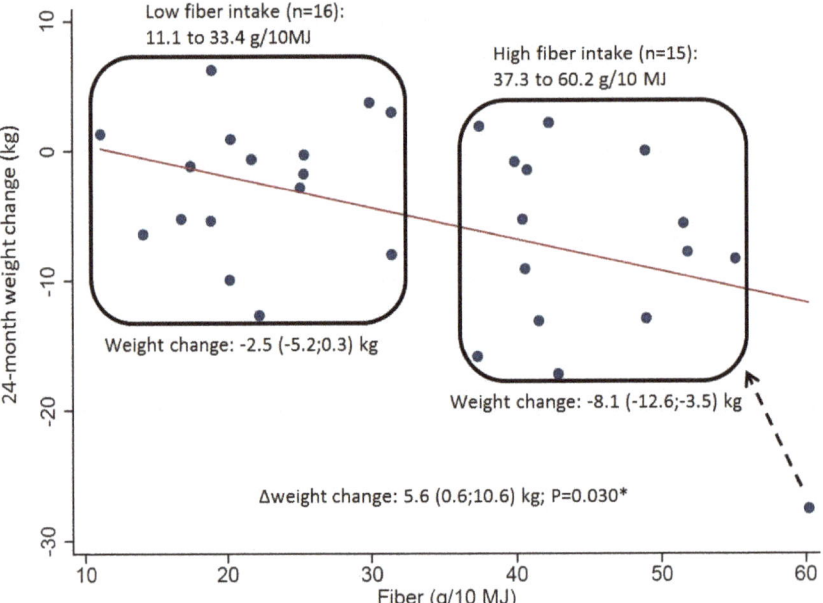

Figure 1. Dietary fiber intake as a function of weight change among subjects with prediabetes and low fasting insulin. Values for fiber intake is reported as range and weight change is reported as mean (95%CI). *Analyzed using *t*-test. When excluding the one subject with self-reported fiber intake of 60 g/10 MJ the *p*-value was $p = 0.057$.

Table 4. Correlations between self-reported dietary fiber intake (g/10 MJ) and 24-month weight change (24-month − baseline) as well as weight change in groups of dietary fiber intake according to baseline glycemic and insulinemic status.

	n	Correlations [1] (Change in Fiber Intake [2])	Correlations [1] (Fiber Intake during Intervention [3])	n	Weight Change (kg) [<35 g Fiber/10 MJ [3]]	n	Weight Change (kg) [≥35 g Fiber/10 MJ [3]]	Δ Weight Change (kg) [3]
All	317	−0.23 */−0.22 *	−0.17 */−0.18 *	210	−4.1 (−5.1;3.1)	107	−6.5 (−8.0; −4.9)	2.4 (0.6;4.1) *
FPG (mg/dL)								
<100	254	−0.21 */−0.21 *	−0.15 */−0.15 *	170	−4.0 (−5.1; −2.9)	84	−6.3 (−8.1; −4.5)	2.3 (0.3;4.3) *
≥100	63	−0.31 */−0.27 *	−0.25 */−0.27 *	40	−4.5 (−6.9; −2.0)	23	−7.1 (−10.2; −4.0)	2.7 (−1.3;6.6)
FI								
<13.8	210	−0.28 */−0.28 *	−0.23 */−0.22 *	138	−3.3 (−4.3; −2.3)	72	−6.0 (−7.7; −4.3)	2.7 (0.8;4.5) *
≥13.8	107	−0.15/−0.15	−0.12/−0.12	72	−5.6 (−7.8; −3.5)	35	−7.5 (−10.7; −4.3)	1.9 (−1.9;5.6)
FPG & FI								
<100 & <13.8	179	−0.24 */−0.24 *	−0.17 */−0.16 *	122	−3.4 (−4.5; −2.3)	57	−5.4 (−7.3; −3.6)	2.0 (0.02;4.0) *
<100 & ≥13.8	75	−0.15/−0.17	−0.14/−0.16	48	−5.6 (−8.2; −2.9)	27	−8.1 (−12.1; −4.1)	2.6 (−2.0;7.2)
≥100 & <13.8	31	−0.47 */−0.47 *	−0.45 */−0.47 *	16	−2.5 (−5.2;0.3)	15	−8.1 (−12.6; −3.5)	5.6 (0.6;10.6) *
≥100 & ≥13.8	32	−0.14/−0.20	−0.01/−0.05	24	−5.8 (−9.6; −2.0)	8	−5.4 (−9.2; −1.6)	−0.4 (−7.2;6.4)
HOMA-IR								
<4.0	251	−0.25 */−0.24 *	−0.19 */−0.19 *	167	−3.8 (−4.9; −2.8)	84	−6.5 (−8.2; −4.7)	2.6 (0.7;4.5) *
>4.0	66	−0.17/−0.16	−0.12/−0.10	43	−5.0 (−7.8; −2.3)	23	−6.5 (−9.7; −3.2)	1.4 (−3.0;5.8)

Abbreviation: FI, Fasting insulin; FPG, Fasting plasma glucose; HOMA-IR, Homeostatic model assessment of insulin resistance. [1] First number is Pearson correlation coefficients (r). Second number is partial correlation coefficients controlled for age, gender and baseline BMI. [2] Based on data from change in dietary fiber intake (g/10 MJ) (intervention − baseline). [3] Based on data from dietary fiber intake (g/10 MJ) during the intervention (not taking baseline dietary fiber intake into consideration). * $p < 0.05$.

4. Discussion

As hypothesized, we found that subjects with normoglycemia lost the most body weight when randomized to the low-fat/high-protein diet, and that subjects with high HOMA-IR lost the most on the high-fat/high-protein diet. Furthermore, we found that participants with the highest intake of dietary fiber lost more body weight during the 24-month dietary intervention period, which was particularly evident among individuals with prediabetes and having below median of FI, where a 5.6 kg difference was observed among those below and above the median of fiber intake. These results are in accordance with previous studies that found that participants with normal FPG lose approximately 1 kg more during a 3–6 month period on a low fat diet [14,17,18]. Participants with impaired fasting glucose lose approximately 4 kg more weight than participants with normal glycaemia over 6 months when exposed to diets higher in dietary fibers [14,17,19]. Furthermore, participants with pretreatment FPG $\geq$ 126 mg/dL have been found to lose approximately 2 kg more body weight after 5 years on a Mediterranean diet compared to subjects with normoglycemia [14,20].

Satiety is a multi-factor construct that is more than just the metabolic effects of nutrients in the gut and intestine. It also includes cognitive and sensory signals generated by the sight, smell, and taste of foods [21]. However, satiety research has typically looked at the physiological effects of food ingredients, where protein exerts satiety through gastrointestinal hormonal signaling by e.g., GLP-1 and PYY, and dietary fiber (dependent of fiber type) provides satiety through increased viscosity, gelling in the stomach, replacing of energy dense foods, and fermentation in the gut are thought to positively affect satiety [13]. Recent evidence confirms the importance of fermentation of dietary fiber by the microbiota to facilitate energy homeostasis possibly through succinate and short chain fatty acids activating intestinal gluconeogenesis signaling to the brain by gastrointestinal nerves [22]. In addition, furthermore, different sources of dietary fiber should be matched with existing microbiota composition of the individual in order to lower body weight [23,24] and improve glucose metabolism [25], as proposed in a recent review stratifying subjects in enterotypes [26]. Furthermore, for non-diabetics, carbohydrates are considered more satiating compared to fats, suggesting that foods should be high in proteins, carbohydrates, and dietary fibers to have the optimal effect on appetite control [21]. However, emerging evidence suggests that carbohydrates will affect satiety primarily among subjects with normoglycemia and, to a lesser extent, among subjects with prediabetes, as less blood glucose will enter the brain (and perhaps other relevant tissues) to generate satiety signals [12]. This concept is supported by the present study, finding that a low-fat/high-protein diet is marginally better among subjects with normoglycemia as long as the glycemic load is keep down and fiber content kept at a minimum (recommending low GI carbohydrates and minimum 20 g/day of dietary fibers), and that a high-fat/high-protein diet is marginally better among the most insulin resistant subjects. These findings support the hypothesis that people with prediabetes/insulin resistance should to a larger extent rely on satiety hormones that are released mainly in response to fats and protein [for example, cholecystokinin (CCK), glucagon-like peptide 1 (GLP-1), and peptide YY (PYY)] reaching the small intestine dietary fat [27] and/or dietary fiber, for glycaemia control [28] and to enable weight loss and combat weight regain [13]. Generally, higher protein intake, as assessed by urea nitrogen/creatinine, has previously been shown to produce larger weight loss after both 6 and 24 months in the present study, and supports our findings that protein contents seem to be important for all phenotypes [29].

Dietary fiber was not a part of the intervention study, and we therefore used self-reported dietary data to investigate the importance of dietary fiber in the subgroups of FPG and FI. Nevertheless, looking at the self-reported fiber intake, it seems as if the randomized diets could have been confounded by dietary fiber intake, as the diets with the highest amount of carbohydrate also had higher fiber intake (among the subgroup that reported their dietary intake). This was perhaps not the case for subjects with normoglycemia as the low fat/high protein diet produced higher weight loss compared to the low-fat/average-protein diet that contained more dietary fiber. However, among subjects with prediabetes, it seems as if dietary fiber is more important than the exact macronutrient composition of the diet at least when recommending low GI carbohydrates, as in the present study. This was seen especially among subjects with prediabetes and FI below the median, which is in good agreement with the three studies in reference [17], but not with all studies [19]. Once the prediabetic state is more advanced, as is likely the case for subjects with prediabetes and high FI, it seems that an adverse effect of carbohydrates overrules the potential beneficial effect of dietary fiber intake, indicating a need to replace carbohydrates in the diet with proteins and fats. This beneficial effect of a diet higher in fats and lower in carbohydrates was observed among subjects with high HOMA-IR in the present study and was observed among subjects with fasting glucose $\geq$126 mg/dL and among type 2 diabetes patient [14,17,20,30,31].

Compliance or adherence is a general problem in long-term dietary intervention studies, as is evident from the overall weight loss and weight regain usually seen after 6 months [32]. The substantial diminished adherence after the first months can also be seen in the present study as weight regain occurred after 6 months, even when being prescribed an energy-restricted diet [15]. In the present study, 750 kcal/day deficit diets were designed based on resting energy expenditure and activity level at baseline. Using the prediction equation developed by Kevin Hall and colleagues [33], subjects in the present study should have lost approximately 33 kg during this 2 year period, had they been adherent to the energy restriction. The actual weight loss was only 4 kg among the 80% completing the study. Overall, these findings suggest that participants in weight-loss programs revert to their customary energy intake, and most likely also macronutrient composition, over time. This lack of adherence makes it difficult to investigate predictors of weight loss from pretreatment personal characteristics. Therefore, a sensitivity analysis was carried out among the half attending the most counseling sessions as those were expected to adhere better to the diets. Although finding those subjects to have lost substantially more weight compared to those attending fewer sessions (as reported previously [15]) FPG, FI, and HOMA-IR were not better predictors of weight loss success on the different diets in this subgroup. Challenges with adherence to the diet were also noted in the 24 month CHO-study that nevertheless found some large differences among a relatively small group of prediabetic obese subjects [34]. Another example highlighting the importance of adherence is from a study that compared an ad libitum low-fat/medium-protein diet with a low-fat/high-protein diet for 24 months among a group of primarily normoglycemic subjects (89% had FPG <100 mg/dL) [35]. In fact, this is the same macronutrient composition found to produce marginally higher weight loss in the present study—especially among normoglycemic subjects. The first 6 months included a strictly controlled dietary intervention with full provision of food from a purpose-built shop where the low-fat/high-protein diet was found to produce a 3.5 kg (p = 0.008) greater weight loss. During the following 6 months, with dietary counseling only, this difference diminished to become an insignificant 1.9 kg. Finally, after an additional 12 months of follow-up, there was no difference between the diets. Therefore, food provision (or other innovative initiatives) that could increase adherence is probably the only way to examine the true effect of different diets on health [5,10,17,19,35]. However, this is very expensive, and cannot be sustained over prolonged periods of time. Therefore, if investigated over a prolonged period of time, it probably needs to be a familiar and common diet in the region. An example of this could be the Mediterranean diet that in Spain was recently found to predict the best weight loss outcome over 5 years among subjects with elevated fasting glucose at baseline [14,20]. In agreement with this, the high-fat diets in the present study have previously been associated with higher levels of dietary adherence compared to low-fat diets [36], likely because the high-fat diets resembled the baseline/habitual diets the most.

Despite the relatively low adherence to the energy-restricted diets, the infrequent dietary reporting, and the expected day-to-day variability in fasting glucose and insulin, we found some evidence for the use of FPG and FI as determinants of weight loss on different diets. However, evidence is still conflicted, and more research is needed. The evidence is incomplete, but it currently suggests that people without diabetes but with normal fasting glucose and insulin sensitivity can achieve marginally greater success on low-fat regimens, preferably higher in protein, provided very high GLs are avoided [14,17,18,35,37]. The results further suggest that people with impaired fasting glucose (especially when FI is low) should have their main dietary focus be the incorporation of more dietary fiber [14,17,19]. Finally, in those with insulin resistance, FPG $\geq$ 126 mg/dL, and type 2 diabetes patients could benefit from increasing protein and fat intake at the expense of carbohydrates [14,17,20,30,31]. These different dietary patterns still need to be compared in randomized trials where the adherence in real-life settings (behavioral support and cultural and social factors) should be removed to investigate the effect of the individual underlying biology. The concepts of personalized nutrition or personalized lifestyle may drive some innovative new research in the area of weight management.

The strengths of our study include the 2-year duration, the consistent findings for both changes and level of dietary fiber consumption during the intervention, and the post-hoc analysis of the study that ensured a completely unbiased observation, whereby neither the investigators nor the participants knew about the background or aim of the current re-analysis. On the other hand, the post-hoc testing involved a relatively large number of statistical comparisons within subgroups of the population, which increases the risk of false positives, as well as leading to an increased risk of failing to detect differences due to power.

5. Conclusions

This study identified modest differences in diet-specific weight loss between glycemic phenotypes, indicating that subjects with normoglycemia could benefit the most from low-fat/high-protein diets, subjects with prediabetes (and low insulin) could benefit the most from diets high in dietary fiber, and subjects with insulin resistance (high HOMA-IR) could benefit the most from high-fat/high-protein diets. However, these findings need to be confirmed in randomized trials with this aim as a primary end-point.

Supplementary Materials: The following are available online at http://www.mdpi.com/2072-6643/11/3/586/s1, Table S1: Two-year weight change according to randomization and stratified on pretreatment FPG and FI among subjects attending at least 44% (median value) of the counseling sessions ($n = 319$).

Author Contributions: G.A.B., D.A.W., D.H.R., J.R., C.M.C., and F.M.S. conceived and carried out the original experiments. C.M.P. and D.C.M. calculated the dietary fiber intake during the intervention. M.F.H. analyzed the data and wrote the first draft of the paper. All authors have contributed to the discussion of analyses, reviewed the manuscript critically and approved the final manuscript.

Funding: The original study was supported by grants from the National Heart, Lung, and Blood Institute (HL073286) and the General Clinical Research Center, National Institutes of Health (RR-02635). The present stratified analysis was supported by a grant from Gelesis, Boston, MA, USA.

Conflicts of Interest: M.F.H., Y.Z., and A.A. are co-inventors on a pending provisional patent application on the use of biomarkers for prediction of weight-loss responses. A.A. is co-inventor of other related patents/patent applications owned by UCPH, in accordance with Danish law. A.A. is consultant for Gelesis Inc. concerning scientific advice unrelated to the current paper. A.A. is furthermore consultant/member of advisory boards for Groupe Éthique et Santé, France, Nestlé Research Center, Switzerland, Weight Watchers, USA, BioCare Copenhagen, Zaluvida, Switzerland, Basic Research, USA, Novo Nordisk, Denmark, and Saniona, Denmark. M.F.H. and A.A. are co-authors of the book "Spis dig slank efter dit blodsukker" (Eat according to your blood sugar and be slim)/Politikens Forlag, Denmark, and of other books about personalized nutrition for weight loss. A.A. is co-owner and member of the Board of the consultancy company Dentacom Aps, Denmark, and co-founder and co-owner of UCPH spin-out Mobile Fitness A/S, Flaxslim ApS. M.F.H. and A.A. are co-founder and co-owner of UCPH spin-out Personalized Weight Management Research Consortium ApS (Gluco-diet.dk). G.B. is on the Nutrition Advisory Board for Herbalife and the Scientific Advisory Board for Medifast. D.C.M. and C.M.C. and F.M.S. have no conflicts of interest.

References

1. Astrup, A.; Grunwald, G.; Melanson, E.; Saris, W.; Hill, J. The role of low-fat diets in body weight control: A meta-analysis of ad libitum dietary intervention studies. *Int. J. Obes.* **2000**, *24*, 1545–1552. [CrossRef]
2. Hall, K.D.; Bemis, T.; Brychta, R.; Chen, K.Y.; Courville, A.; Crayner, E.J.; Goodwin, S.; Guo, J.; Howard, L.; Knuth, N.D.; et al. Calorie for Calorie, Dietary Fat Restriction Results in More Body Fat Loss than Carbohydrate Restriction in People with Obesity. *Cell Metab.* **2015**, *22*, 427–436. [CrossRef] [PubMed]

3. Ebbeling, C.B.; Feldman, H.A.; Klein, G.L.; Wong, J.M.W.; Bielak, L.; Steltz, S.K.; Luoto, P.K.; Wolfe, R.R.; Wong, W.W.; Ludwig, D.S. Effects of a low carbohydrate diet on energy expenditure during weight loss maintenance: Randomized trial. *BMJ* **2018**. [CrossRef] [PubMed]
4. Astrup, A.; Larsen, T.M.; Harper, A. Atkins and other low-carbohydrate diets: Hoax or an effective tool for weight loss? *Lancet* **2004**, *364*, 897–899. [CrossRef]
5. Larsen, T.M.; Dalskov, S.-M.; van Baak, M.; Jebb, S.A.; Papadaki, A.; Pfeiffer, A.F.H.; Martinez, J.A.; Handjieva-Darlenska, T.; Kunešová, M.; Pihlsgård, M. Diets with high or low protein content and glycemic index for weight-loss maintenance. *N. Engl. J. Med.* **2010**, *363*, 2102–2113. [CrossRef] [PubMed]
6. Jensen, M.D.; Ryan, D.H.; Apovian, C.M.; Ard, J.D.; Comuzzie, A.G.; Donato, K.A.; Hu, F.B.; Hubbard, V.S.; Jakicic, J.M.; Kushner, R.F.; et al. 2013 AHA/ACC/TOS Guideline for the Management of Overweight and Obesity in Adults. *J. Am. Coll. Cardiol.* **2014**, *63*, 2985–3023. [CrossRef] [PubMed]
7. Bray, G.A.; Heisel, W.E.; Afshin, A.; Jensen, M.D.; Dietz, W.H.; Long, M.; Kushner, R.F.; Daniels, S.R.; Wadden, T.A.; Tsai, A.G.; et al. The Science of Obesity Management: An Endocrine Society Scientific Statement. *Endocr. Rev.* **2018**, *39*, 79–132. [CrossRef] [PubMed]
8. Brownlee, I.A.; Chater, P.I.; Pearson, J.P.; Wilcox, M.D. Dietary fibre and weight loss: Where are we now? *Food Hydrocoll.* **2017**. [CrossRef]
9. Roager, H.M.; Vogt, J.K.; Kristensen, M.; Hansen, L.B.S.; Ibrügger, S.; Mærkedahl, R.B.; Bahl, M.I.; Lind, M.V.; Nielsen, R.L.; Frøkiær, H.; et al. Whole grain-rich diet reduces body weight and systemic low-grade inflammation without inducing major changes of the gut microbiome: A randomised cross-over trial. *Gut* **2017**. [CrossRef] [PubMed]
10. Poulsen, S.K.; Due, A.; Jordy, A.B.; Kiens, B.; Stark, K.D.; Stender, S.; Holst, C.; Astrup, A.; Larsen, T.M. Health effect of the New Nordic Diet in adults with increased waist circumference: A 6-mo randomized controlled trial. *Am. J. Clin. Nutr.* **2014**, *99*, 35–45. [CrossRef] [PubMed]
11. Woods, S.C. Metabolic signals and food intake. Forty years of progress. *Appetite* **2013**, *71*, 440–444. [CrossRef] [PubMed]
12. Hwang, J.J.; Jiang, L.; Hamza, M.; Sanchez Rangel, E.; Dai, F.; Belfort-DeAguiar, R.; Parikh, L.; Koo, B.B.; Rothman, D.L.; Mason, G.; et al. Blunted rise in brain glucose levels during hyperglycemia in adults with obesity and T2DM. *JCI Insight* **2017**, *2*, 95913. [CrossRef] [PubMed]
13. Slavin, J.L. Dietary fiber and body weight. *Nutrition* **2005**, *21*, 411–418. [CrossRef] [PubMed]
14. Hjorth, M.F.; Zohar, Y.; Hill, J.O.; Astrup, A. Personalized Dietary Management of Overweight and Obesity Based on Measures of Insulin and Glucose. *Annu. Rev. Nutr.* **2018**, *38*, 245–272. [CrossRef] [PubMed]
15. Sacks, F.M.; Bray, G.A.; Carey, V.J.; Smith, S.R.; Ryan, D.H.; Anton, S.D.; McManus, K.; Champagne, C.M.; Bishop, L.M.; Laranjo, N. Comparison of weight-loss diets with different compositions of fat, protein, and carbohydrates. *N. Engl. J. Med.* **2009**, *360*, 859–873. [CrossRef] [PubMed]
16. Association, A.D. 2. Classification and Diagnosis of Diabetes. *Diabetes Care* **2016**, *39* (Suppl. 1), S13–S22.
17. Hjorth, M.F.; Ritz, C.; Blaak, E.E.; Saris, W.H.; Langin, D.; Poulsen, S.K.; Larsen, T.M.; Sørensen, T.I.; Zohar, Y.; Astrup, A. Pretreatment fasting plasma glucose and insulin modify dietary weight loss success: Results from 3 randomized clinical trials. *Am. J. Clin. Nutr.* **2017**, *106*, 499–505. [CrossRef] [PubMed]
18. Wan, Y.; Wang, F.; Yuan, J.; Li, J.; Jiang, D.; Zhang, J.; Huang, T.; Zheng, J.; Mann, J.; Li, D. Effects of Macronutrient Distribution on Weight and Related Cardiometabolic Profile in Healthy Non-Obese Chinese: A 6-month, Randomized Controlled-Feeding Trial. *EBioMedicine* **2017**, *22*, 200–207. [CrossRef] [PubMed]
19. Hjorth, M.F.; Due, A.; Larsen, T.M.; Astrup, A. Pretreatment Fasting Plasma Glucose Modifies Dietary Weight Loss Maintenance Success: Results from a Stratified, R.C.T. *Obesity* **2017**, *25*, 2045–2048. [CrossRef] [PubMed]
20. Estruch, R.; Corella, D.; Salas-Salvado, J.; Hjorth, M.F.; Astrup, A.; Zohar, Y.; Urban, L.; Serra-Majem, L.; Lapetra, J.; Aros, F.; et al. Pretreatment fasting plasma glucose determines weight loss on high-fat diets: The PREDIMED Study. *Obesity* **2017**, *25*, 2045–2048.
21. Chambers, L.; McCrickerd, K.; Yeomans, M.R. Optimising foods for satiety. *Trends Food Sci. Technol.* **2015**, *41*, 149–160. [CrossRef]
22. de Vadder, F.; Mithieux, G. Gut-brain signaling in energy homeostasis: The unexpected role of microbiota-derived succinate. *J. Endocrinol.* **2018**, *236*, R105–R108. [CrossRef] [PubMed]

23. Hjorth, M.F.; Blædel, T.; Bendtsen, L.Q.; Lorenzen, J.K.; Holm, J.B.; Kiilerich, P.; Roager, H.M.; Kristiansen, K.; Larsen, L.H.; Astrup, A. Prevotella-to-Bacteroides ratio predicts body weight and fat loss success on 24-week diets varying in macronutrient composition and dietary fiber: Results from a post-hoc analysis. *Int. J. Obes.* **2018**, *43*, 149–157. [CrossRef] [PubMed]
24. Hjorth, M.F.; Roager, H.M.; Larsen, T.M.; Poulsen, S.K.; Licht, T.R.; Bahl, M.I.; Zohar, Y.; Astrup, A. Pre-treatment microbial Prevotella-to-Bacteroides ratio, determines body fat loss success during a 6-month randomized controlled diet intervention. *Int. J. Obes.* **2018**, *42*, 580–583. [CrossRef] [PubMed]
25. Gu, Y.; Wang, X.; Li, J.; Zhang, Y.; Zhong, H.; Liu, R.; Zhang, D.; Feng, Q.; Xie, X.; Hong, J.; et al. Analyses of gut microbiota and plasma bile acids enable stratification of patients for antidiabetic treatment. *Nat. Commun.* **2017**, *8*, 1785. [CrossRef] [PubMed]
26. Christensen, L.; Roager, H.M.; Astrup, A.; Hjorth, M.F. Microbial enterotypes in personalized nutrition and obesity management. *Am. J. Clin. Nutr.* **2018**, *108*, 645–651. [CrossRef] [PubMed]
27. Belza, A.; Ritz, C.; Sørensen, M.Q.; Holst, J.J.; Rehfeld, J.F.; Astrup, A. Contribution of gastroenteropancreatic appetite hormones to protein-induced satiety. *Am. J. Clin. Nutr.* **2013**, *97*, 980–989. [CrossRef] [PubMed]
28. Goff, H.D.; Repin, N.; Fabek, H.; El Khoury, D.; Gidley, M.J. Dietary fibre for glycaemia control: Towards a mechanistic understanding. *Bioact. Carbohydr. Diet Fibre* **2018**, *14*, 39–53. [CrossRef]
29. Bray, G.A.; Ryan, D.H.; Johnson, W.; Champagne, C.M.; Johnson, C.M.; Rood, J.; Williamson, D.A.; Sacks, F.M. Markers of dietary protein intake are associated with successful weight loss in the POUNDS LOST trial. *Clin. Obes.* **2017**, *7*, 166–175. [CrossRef] [PubMed]
30. Ajala, O.; English, P.; Pinkney, J. Systematic review and meta-analysis of different dietary approaches to the management of type 2 diabetes. *Am. J. Clin. Nutr.* **2013**, *97*, 505–516. [CrossRef] [PubMed]
31. Snorgaard, O.; Poulsen, G.M.; Andersen, H.K.; Astrup, A. Systematic review and meta-analysis of dietary carbohydrate restriction in patients with type 2 diabetes. *BMJ Open Diabetes Res. Care* **2017**, *5*, e000354. [CrossRef] [PubMed]
32. Lean, M.E.J.; Astrup, A.; Roberts, S.B. Making progress on the global crisis of obesity and weight management. *Br. Med. J.* **2018**, *361*, k2538. [CrossRef] [PubMed]
33. Hall, K.D.; Sacks, G.; Chandramohan, D.; Chow, C.C.; Wang, Y.C.; Gortmaker, S.L.; Swinburn, B.A. Quantification of the effect of energy imbalance on bodyweight. *Lancet* **2011**, *378*, 826–837. [CrossRef]
34. Hjorth, M.F.; Astrup, A.; Zohar, Y.; Urban, L.E.; Sayer, R.D.; Patterson, B.W.; Herring, S.J.; Klein, S.; Zemel, B.S.; Foster, G.D.; et al. Personalized nutrition: Pretreatment glucose metabolism determines individual long-term weight loss responsiveness in individuals with obesity on low-carbohydrate versus low-fat diet. *Int. J. Obes.* **2018**. [CrossRef] [PubMed]
35. Due, A.; Toubro, S.; Skov, A.R.; Astrup, A. Effect of normal-fat diets, either medium or high in protein, on body weight in overweight subjects: A randomised 1-year trial. *Int. J. Obes.* **2004**, *28*, 1283–1290. [CrossRef] [PubMed]
36. Williamson, D.A.; Anton, S.D.; Han, H.; Champagne, C.M.; Allen, R.; Leblanc, E.; Ryan, D.H.; McManus, K.; Laranjo, N.; Carey, V.J.; et al. Adherence is a multi-dimensional construct in the POUNDS LOST trial. *J. Behav. Med.* **2010**, *33*, 35–46. [CrossRef] [PubMed]
37. Astrup, A.; Hjorth, M.F. Low-Fat or Low Carb for Weight Loss? It Depends on Your Glucose Metabolism. *EBioMedicine* **2017**, *22*, 20–21. [CrossRef] [PubMed]

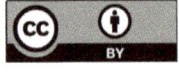 © 2019 by the authors. Licensee MDPI, Basel, Switzerland. This article is an open access article distributed under the terms and conditions of the Creative Commons Attribution (CC BY) license (http://creativecommons.org/licenses/by/4.0/).

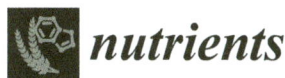

Review

A Scientific Perspective of Personalised Gene-Based Dietary Recommendations for Weight Management

Theresa Drabsch and Christina Holzapfel *

Institute for Nutritional Medicine, University Hospital Klinikum rechts der Isar, Technical University of Munich, Georg-Brauchle-Ring 62, 80992 Munich, Germany; theresa.drabsch@tum.de
* Correspondence: christina.holzapfel@tum.de; Tel.: +49-89-289-249-23

Received: 31 January 2019; Accepted: 9 March 2019; Published: 14 March 2019

Abstract: Various studies showed that a "one size fits all" dietary recommendation for weight management is questionable. For this reason, the focus increasingly falls on personalised nutrition. Although there is no precise and uniform definition of personalised nutrition, the inclusion of genetic variants for personalised dietary recommendations is more and more favoured, whereas scientific evidence for gene-based dietary recommendations is rather limited. The purpose of this article is to provide a science-based viewpoint on gene-based personalised nutrition and weight management. Most of the studies showed no clinical evidence for gene-based personalised nutrition. The Food4Me study, e.g., investigated four different groups of personalised dietary recommendations based on dietary guidelines, and physiological, clinical, or genetic parameters, and resulted in no difference in weight loss between the levels of personalisation. Furthermore, genetic direct-to-consumer (DTC) tests are widely spread by companies. Scientific organisations clearly point out that, to date, genetic DTC tests are without scientific evidence. To date, gene-based personalised nutrition is not yet applicable for the treatment of obesity. Nevertheless, personalised dietary recommendations on the genetic landscape of a person are an innovative and promising approach for the prevention and treatment of obesity. In the future, human intervention studies are necessary to prove the clinical evidence of gene-based dietary recommendations.

Keywords: gene-based; personalised nutrition; dietary recommendation; nutrigenetics; direct-to-consumer test; genotype; gene–diet interaction; weight loss; obesity

---

1. Body Weight Regulation

The regulation of body weight is of a complex nature. In addition to energy intake and expenditure, physiological parameters, feedback, and interaction systems of hormones, as well as the central nervous system, play a major role in body weight regulation. Signals of hunger and satiety are transmitted from fat tissue, muscles, and the gastrointestinal tract to brain areas. One of the satiety hormones is leptin, which is released by the adipose tissue and regulates the neuropeptide expression in the hypothalamus [1,2]. Leptin deficiency leads to extreme obesity and presents the most popular form of monogenic obesity [3]. Another hormone of hunger and satiety is ghrelin, which is secreted in the gastrointestinal tract after energy intake, and which is involved in glucose, lipid, and energy metabolism [4]. There are many other hormones which are involved in the regulation of hunger and satiety such as insulin, cholecystokinin, or glucagon-like peptide 1 [1,5,6]. For body weight maintenance, a balanced energy homeostasis is necessary. Therefore, lifestyle factors leading to a positive or negative energy balance result in weight gain or loss, respectively.

2. Dietary Intervention and Weight Loss

Lifestyle changes based on increasing physical activity and reducing energy intake are the basic therapeutic approaches for weight loss and weight maintenance. It is well known that not the macronutrient composition of a diet, but the energy content resulting in a negative energy balance plays the major role for weight loss. This guarantees a higher flexibility for experts and patients in the choice of a dietary concept in order to reach a hypocaloric diet for weight loss. Additionally, food preferences and wishes of patients, as well as the suitability of the dietary strategy for the daily routine can be taken into account. An evaluation of 48 studies showed that, regardless of the macronutrient composition of a diet, the extent of weight loss was similar within six and 12 months [7]. In another study, four diets consisting of different macronutrient compositions were investigated. After two years, there was no significant difference in weight loss between the four intervention groups [8]. Another study by Shai et al. showed that weight reduction after two years was independent of the macronutrient composition of the diet [9]. This effect was confirmed in a study on 609 adults with a body mass index (BMI) between 28 and 40 kg/m^2 [10]. Gardner et al. found out that, after one year of dietary intervention, mean weight loss was not significantly different as individuals lost 6.0 kg of weight in the low-carbohydrate diet group and 5.3 kg of weight in the low-fat diet group [10]. A meta-analysis of 16 randomised controlled trials including 3436 individuals suggests that a Mediterranean diet leads to a significantly higher weight loss compared to a control diet (mean difference between diet groups: -1.75 kg), especially if diet was energy-reduced and was associated with an increased physical activity [11]. Based on this finding and further studies, it might be concluded that alternative diets such as the plant-based form of the Atkins diet or the Mediterranean diet may lead to a moderate weight loss [9,12,13]. However, due to the saturation effect of protein-rich diets, an increased protein intake is also often aimed at in nutritional weight loss concepts. Another aspect is the quality of fats. Studies showed that an increased consumption of omega-3 or omega-6 polyunsaturated fatty acids improves plasma lipid levels as well as the risk for cardiovascular events [14,15]. In addition, new information and communication technologies such as mobile applications are popular for making self-help recommendations for weight loss [16]. Due to eating preferences, as well as individual metabolic responses on dietary intake and large variations in weight loss success, the need of an individual nutritional recommendation instead of a "one size fits all" is increasing. Personalised dietary recommendations are of high potential for an improved and more successful weight management. However, the nature and the extent of personalised dietary recommendations are still unknown.

3. Individual Metabolic Response to Dietary Intervention

In the last few years, studies showed that persons individually respond to predefined meal challenges. In the Human Metabolome (HuMet) study, 15 males were investigated for metabolic responses to specific challenges [17]. After a fasting period of 36 h, participants underwent an oral glucose and lipid test, liquid test meals, and exercises, and they were exposed to cold. Due to deep phenotyping and the healthy nature of the participants, Krug et al. could show large variability in metabolic responses between phenotypically similar individuals after challenges by test meals or exercise programmes [17]. Another study investigated the metabolic response to identical meals in 800 participants. In this Israeli study, blood glucose levels of the participants, aged 18–70 years, were analysed during a standardised meal resulting likewise in a large inter-individual variability [18]. The average postprandial glycaemic response (PPGR) differed largely between individuals (e.g., bread: 44 ± 31 mg/dL·h (mean $\pm$ standard deviation). This inter-individual difference of glycaemic response validated the fact that the same meal may lead to another or even the opposite metabolic response when comparing different individuals. In a sub-study, participants were assigned to a predicted "good" or "bad" diet based on the glucose levels. The results showed that personalised dietary interventions can lead to improved PPGR [18]. Another study by the same research group analysed the individual PPGR to different types of bread [19]. In that randomised cross-over trial, participants received a white or sourdough-leavened bread. A large inter-individual variability in PPGR to the two kinds of bread was confirmed. Some subjects had a higher glycaemic response to one bread and some to the other [19]. In a cross-over study, the metabolic response of 20 healthy male volunteers and 20 male patients with type 2 diabetes to a PhenFlex test drink or glucose drink (OGTT) was investigated [20]. The PhenFlex test used a drink consisting of 60 g of fat, 75 g of glucose, and 20 g of protein. OGTT corresponds to the commonly used drink with 75 g of glucose. A total of 132 metabolic parameters were quantified as markers for 26 different metabolic processes. The results showed a significant difference between the two groups, indicating different phenotypic flexibility, especially in metabolically impaired individuals [20]. The explanations for the differences in metabolic response are complex and widely discussed. Genetic parameters, as well as the microbiome, might play a role and are of high potential to explain a certain amount of the inter-individual metabolic differences upon meal challenges.

4. Purpose of This Work

The purpose of this article was to provide a science-based viewpoint on gene-based personalised nutrition and weight management. This means that the scientific background of the commercially available direct-to-consumer (DTC) genetic tests was questioned. Furthermore, human intervention studies investigating the effect of gene-based dietary recommendations on weight change are described in order to present the ongoing research. This viewpoint combines different perspectives (science, clinical evidence, practical issues) and various aspects (scientific results, commercially available offers) and discusses recent issues aiming to highlight the current evidence of gene-based personalised nutrition.

5. Definition of a Gene-Based Personalised Diet

To date, there is no single definition of a personalised diet. Personalised nutrition is also called precision or tailored nutrition [21]. Nizel et al. defined personalised nutrition with a personal consultation of patients in order to achieve an improvement in dietary habits [22]. Subsequently, further tools were included, such as online available platforms or applications based on dietary and behavioural habits of each patient as a kind of computer-generated personalised nutrition [23]. Another concept defined as "personalised, gene-based nutrition" combines genetic information with specific dietary recommendations. In 2013, Stewart-Knox et al. described a personalised nutrition as a healthy dietary recommendation tailored to the health status, lifestyle, and/or the genetic information of an individual [24]. Lifestyle data included age, gender, height, weight, and clinical facts such as disease history, food allergies, or intolerances, as well as dietary habits and exercise behaviour. Wang and Hu included at least the microbial composition to improve dietary recommendations [25]. Furthermore, personalised nutrition is directly related to nutrigenetics [26]. However, direct translation from a genetic profile to the phenotypic characterisation of a person is of a complex nature. Therefore, the concept of personalised dietary recommendations has to follow a multi-dimensional approach considering, e.g., social, lifestyle, genetic, and metabolic parameters. Different aspects of a personalised nutrition are described in Figure 1.

The major aim of a personalised nutrition, according to Daniel and Klein, should be a dietary recommendation adjusted to an individual's requirements by including, if necessary, dietary recommendations based on phenotype and genotype to maintain the health status and to counteract risks for diseases or their comorbidities [27]. In a double-blinded randomised controlled trial, short- and long-term effects on dietary intake of a gene-based personalised nutrition were investigated [28]. In this study, Nielsen and El-Sohemy showed that there was no significant difference in dietary intake after three months of intervention between the intervention group receiving information on their genetic background and, additionally, a corresponding gene-based dietary recommendation and the control group. After 12 months, some significant improvements in dietary intake such as a reduced intake of sodium in the personalised nutrition group were observed, suggesting a long-term change in dietary habits [28]. Nevertheless, the exact mechanisms and factors influencing the long-term effect of a personalised nutrition are still unclear.

Another aspect is the psychological effect of a personalised dietary recommendation. In a survey, 9381 participants from nine European countries were interviewed [29]. The questionnaire was based on results of an explorative analysis and data from the literature. The study showed that the greater the participant's benefit of a personalised dietary recommendation is, the more positive the respective attitudes are and the greater the probability that such a recommendation will be accepted [29]. The results of this study also indicate that the provider's presentation of the potential benefits, the efficacy of regulatory control, and the protection of consumers' personal data are major concerns for the adoption of personalised dietary recommendations. These aspects are also in line with the Health Belief Model [30]. This model describes that changes in health behaviour are more likely if the associated benefits are experienced as high, while individual burdens ("costs") are perceived as low. Another point, suggested by Anderson, is the consideration of the social environment for personalised dietary recommendations to maximise the individual success and the change to healthy eating behaviour [31]. The social network, e.g., contact with a partner or a group, could prevent unhealthy eating behaviour through regular contact, monitoring of each other's weight change, and solving problems together.

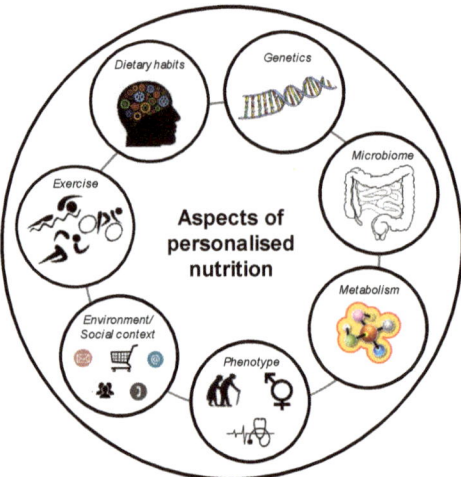

Figure 1. Aspects of personalised nutrition.

6. Genetics and Obesity

The first studies investigating the association between a genetic background and body weight were focused on the heritability of body weight by analysing twins or adopted children. Bouchard et al. could show that, after overfeeding, the differences in increasing body weight were higher between twin pairs than within one twin pair [32]. In adoption studies, the BMI of adopted children was more associated with the BMI of their biological parents than with the BMI of their non-biological parents [33]. However, in hypothesis-driven candidate gene studies, a significant association between genetic loci and body weight was identified. The investigated genes were mainly chosen due to biological plausibility and had a function in regulating food intake, played a role in lipid metabolism, or were involved in the excretion of intestinal hormones. For instance, the fatty-acid-binding protein 2 (*FABP2*) is expressed by epithelial cells of the small intestine where it is mainly related to fat absorption. Variants in the *FABP2* genetic locus lead to increased fat absorption and are associated with obesity [34,35]. Another example is the peroxisome proliferator-activated receptor-gamma (*PPARG*) gene, which is expressed in fat cells and, thus, plays a key role in the differentiation of adipocytes [36,37]. Deeb et al. could show that the *PPARG* gene is associated with BMI and insulin sensitivity [38]. In hypothesis-free, genome-wide association studies (GWAS), many genetic loci were identified for an association with body weight [39–42]. However, only 2.7% of the variation in BMI might be explained by these genetic loci [40]. Up to now, around 500 genetic loci are described for associations with adiposity traits such as BMI or waist-to-hip ratio [43]. To date, the fat mass and obesity associated (*FTO*) locus is the gene with the strongest effect on body weight. Frayling et al. could show that carriers of two risk alleles of the single nucleotide polymorphism (SNP) rs9939609 at the *FTO* locus weighed up to three kilograms more than the non-risk allele carriers [44]. This finding was confirmed by Dina et al. in French individuals [45] but not in African Americans [46]. Scuteri et al. explained this non-significant finding in African Americans by the ethnic-based differences of the genetic architecture of obesity. The *FTO* SNP rs9939609 might be quite common in Europeans but rare in African Americans [46]. Claussnitzer et al. showed that the *FTO* SNP rs1421085 influences the expression of two proxies of the iroquois homeobox family, resulting in the promotion of the expression of energy-storing white adipocytes and in the inhibition of energy-burning beige adipocytes [47]. Therefore, weight gain may not necessarily be the result of higher energy intake, but may be related to a reduced proportion of energy-burning adipocytes [47]. In addition to the *FTO* locus, further genetic variants at different loci were shown to be associated with body weight. One of these is the transmembrane protein 18 (*TMEM18*) gene. *TMEM18* is expressed throughout the body and plays a role in the regulation of body weight, appetite, and even in the development of obesity [48,49]. Another gene on chromosome 18 is the melanocortin-4 receptor (*MC4R*), whose risk allele is associated with 0.23 kg/m^2 higher BMI [42]. This effect might be explained by the role of *MC4R* in the regulation of dietary intake [50]. Moreover, a deficiency of this gene leads to the most common monogenic form of obesity [51]. However, the biological function of most of the obesity-associated genetic loci remains unclear [43]. In the future, the identification of rare and causal genetic variants might serve for drug development for weight loss.

7. Genetics and Weight Loss

It seems plausible that obesity-associated genetic variants are also associated with weight loss. Therefore, studies investigated the association between SNPs and weight change. In a systematic review and meta-analysis, Xiang et al. meta-analysed 10 weight loss intervention studies [52]. In this meta-analysis, the *FTO* risk allele A carriers had significantly greater weight loss than non-risk allele carriers. However, in another systematic review and meta-analysis on the association between the *FTO* gene and weight loss, Livingstone et al. summarised the findings of eight randomised controlled trials including 9563 adults [53]. Results of that meta-analysis showed that people carrying the *FTO* risk allele of SNP rs9939609 achieved a similar weight loss compared to non-risk allele carriers after dietary intervention. Livingstone et al. justified the different outcomes of the two meta-analyses with the fact that, despite a small overlap of the included studies, the population size in the work of Livingstone et al. was considerably larger and only randomised trials were considered for inclusion [53]. This non-significant difference between risk and non-risk allele carriers is in line with an intervention study which investigated 26 obesity-related loci and their association with weight loss [54]. In this randomised controlled trial conducted in eight clinical centres in Europe, 771 adults with obesity underwent a 10-week dietary hypocaloric intervention. There were no significant differences in weight loss when risk allele carriers were compared to non-risk allele carriers [54]. Results of the recently published randomised controlled Diet Intervention Examining the Factors Interacting with Treatment Success (DIETFITS) study showed again that weight reduction of 609 adults with overweight was independent of genotypes [10]. In addition to the non-significant findings, a pooled analysis of studies showed a significant positive association between the risk G allele of the mitochondrial translational initiation factor 3 SNP rs1885988 and weight loss [55].

8. Genetics and Dietary Intake

The regulation of food intake, selection of macronutrients, and total energy intake is very complex. Some epidemiological and intervention studies investigated associations between genetic variants and dietary intake.

A systematic review and meta-analysis analysed data from epidemiological studies which investigated the association between the *FTO* genotype and macronutrient intake [56]. In this review,

Livingstone et al. provided evidence for a significant association between carriers of *FTO* risk alleles and a reduced energy intake of around six kilocalories per day [56]. Another published systematic review provided an overview of a wide range of genetic loci and confirmed an inconsistency of findings concerning the relationship between genetic variants and energy intake [57]. A recently published GWAS investigated the relationship between genetic loci and energy intake in 18,773 individuals of European ancestry [58]. No significant association between genetic variants of the *FTO* gene and energy intake was found.

Livingstone et al. could further show a significant association between *FTO* risk allele carriers and an increased fat and protein intake [56]. In contrast to Livingstone et al. [56], the systematic review by Drabsch et al. [57] did not provide clear evidence of an association between *FTO* and carbohydrate or fat intake. This result was confirmed by Merino et al. who provided data of a large GWAS based on 91,114 individuals from 24 epidemiological studies [59]. No genome-wide significance for an association between the *FTO* SNP rs1421085 and carbohydrate or fat intake was shown. Only the association between the *FTO* SNP rs421085 and a higher protein intake was confirmed. In addition to the *FTO* genotype, further genetic loci were investigated for associations with macronutrient intake. Merino et al. identified two genetic loci, the retinoic acid receptor beta (*RARB*) locus and the deoxyribonucleic acid (DNA) damage regulated autophagy modulator 1 (*DRAM1*) locus, which showed genome-wide significance concerning a relation to macronutrient intake. The *RARB* SNP rs7619139 was positively associated with carbohydrate intake. Similarly, a significant association between rs77694286 at the *DRAM1* locus and a higher protein intake was shown. In addition to these findings, Merino et al. confirmed that the fibroblast growth factor 21 SNP rs838133 was associated with all macronutrient intakes [59].

In addition to epidemiological findings, results from intervention studies are of interest (Table 1). In the Nutrient–Gene Interactions in Human Obesity (NUGENOB) randomised trial, 771 adults with obesity were assigned to a 10-week dietary intervention based on two different hypocaloric diets [54]. A total of 42 SNPs at 26 genetic loci were examined. The results showed no significant interaction between genetic variants and dietary intervention on weight change [54]. This result was confirmed by the Diet, Obesity, and Genes (DiOGenes) study [60], in which 742 participants were randomly assigned to one of five diets based on different levels of glycaemic indices. However, findings could not provide significant evidence for 651 different SNPs and an interaction with diet on weight change [60]. In 2012, results of the randomised controlled trial Preventing Overweight Using Novel Dietary Strategies (POUNDS LOST) were published [61]. In this study, *FTO* risk allele carriers showed a significantly increased improvement in body weight change, body composition, and fat distribution compared to carriers of the non-risk allele. However, this effect was only observed if risk allele carriers of the *FTO* SNP rs1558902 followed a high-protein diet [61]. In a prospective analysis of this trial, Qi et al. described that homozygous risk allele C carriers of the insulin receptor substrate 1 SNP rs2943641 had higher weight loss than those with the non-risk genotype in the high-carbohydrate and low-fat diet group [62]. Furthermore, results of the Food4Me [63] and the DIETFITS [10] study were not significant (Table 1). In conclusion, none of the selected studies presented in Table 1 could show either a significant SNP-diet interaction on weight loss or a genotype-dependent effect on weight loss.

Table 1. Examples of studies investigating associations between genetic variants, dietary intake, and weight change.

Study	Investigated SNPs	Intervention	Result	Reference
NUGENOB	42 SNPs at 26 genetic loci	Ten-week dietary intervention based on two hypocaloric diets of 600 kcal/d each and percentage of energy derived from fat of 20–25% (low fat) or 40–45% (high fat)	No SNP–diet interaction on weight change	Sorensen et al. (2006) [54]
DiOGenes	651 SNPs at 69 genetic loci	Five different ad libitum diets consisting of different glycaemic indices (GI) and contents of dietary protein (P): low P/low GI vs. low P/high GI vs. high P/.ow GI vs. high P/high GI vs. control diet	No SNP–diet interaction on weight change	Larsen et al. (2012) [60]
Food4Me	5 SNPs at 5 genetic loci (FTO, FADS1, TCF7L2, ApoE(e4), MTHFR)	Four different diet groups: (1) Non-personalised dietary recommendation (2) Personalised dietary advice based on dietary habit (3) Personalised dietary advice based on dietary habit and phenotypic data (4) Personalised dietary advice based on dietary habit, phenotypic and genotypic data	No significant difference of weight change between risk and non-risk allele carriers; level of personal dietary advice had no effect on weight change	Celis-Morales et al. (2015) [63]
DIETFITS	3 SNPs at 3 genetic loci (PPARG, ADRB2, FABP2)	Low-fat diet or a low-carbohydrate diet	Similar weight change between groups independent of genetic pattern	Gardner et al. (2018) [10]

Examples for studies investigating associations between genetic variants, dietary intake and weight change. ADRB2, adrenoreceptor beta 2; ApoE(e4), apolipoprotein E (e4); DIETFITS, the Diet Intervention Examining the Factors Interacting with Treatment Success randomised clinical trial; DiOGenes, the Diet, Obesity, and Genes study; FABP2, fatty-acid-binding protein 2; FADS1, fatty-acid desaturase 1; FTO, fat mass and obesity associated; MTHFR, methylenetetrahydrofolate reductase; NUGENOB, Nutrient–Gene Interactions in Human Obesity: Implications for Dietary Guidelines; PPARG, peroxisome proliferator-activated receptor-gamma; SNP, single nucleotide polymorphism; TCF7L2, transcription factor 7 like 2.

9. Direct-to-Consumer Tests

Gene-based dietary recommendations represent potential for commercial purposes. A number of companies already offer so-called DTC genetic tests (Table 2). The given dietary recommendation is based on the customer's DNA sample. The genetic profile, which is determined by the commercial providers, is mainly based on gene variants, which were investigated in candidate gene studies and for which associations with metabolic functions or certain disease risks are known (Table 2). One example might be the *PPARG* locus, which is associated with insulin sensitivity and body weight [38].

In general, a DTC test is defined as genetic test which is purchased directly by the consumer mostly via the internet [64]. In this case, genetic tests typically use saliva samples. Some companies only investigate one single genetic variant, while other DTC genetic test companies analyse several hundred SNPs [64]. The general pattern according to which these companies proceed is shown in Figure 2. After registration (online profile), the customer receives a box with tools, with which the genotype of each individual can be analysed using saliva samples. Based on the customer's profile and the genetic background, the company provides a personalised dietary recommendation. Subsequently, customers receive their specific results of the genetic test, as well as the dietary recommendation by email or by downloading the material in the online account on the company's website. In some cases, customers also receive a proposal for supplements that they can purchase directly from the company and that support the compliance of the gene-based dietary recommendations. The costs of a genetic DTC test vary largely between companies. In Table 2 some companies and their concepts are listed.

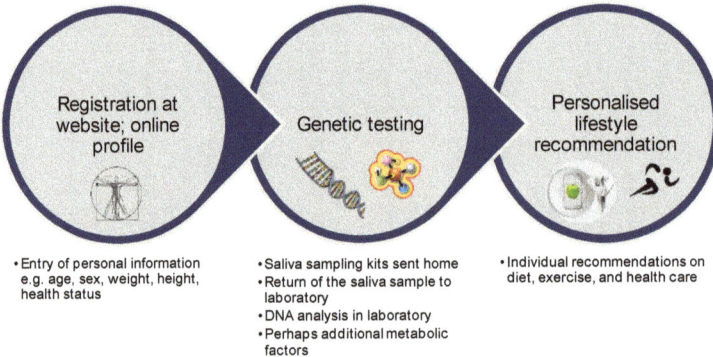

Figure 2. Schematic workflow of a commercially available gene-based dietary recommendation. DNA, deoxyribonucleic acid.

Studies investigated the effect of commercially available gene-based dietary recommendations on weight loss. In a prospective study sponsored by a company providing genetic DTC tests, 51 individuals with overweight or obesity were randomly assigned to a nutrigenetic guided diet or a standard control diet [65]. Focusing on the number of participants who lost 5% of body weight at eight or 24 weeks, there was no significant difference between the two diet groups [65]. This study was limited by a small sample size and a short duration. Another study using a commercially available genetic test also had several methodological limitations [66].

Table 2. Examples of companies offering gene-based dietary recommendations for weight loss.

Company	Genetic Approach	Dietary Recommendation Based on	Homepage
Pathway Genomics	SNPs at genetic loci such as *ADIPOQ* (rs17300539, rs17366568), *APOA2* (rs5082), *FADS1* (rs174547), *FTO* (rs9939609, rs1121980), *MC4R* (rs17782313), *PPARG* (rs1801282)	Genetic profile matched to a low-fat, low-carbohydrate, Mediterranean or balanced diet, including genetic risks for metabolic health factors (e.g., blood sugar, lipids)	https://www.pathway.com
Thinner Gene	SNPs at genetic loci such as *FTO*, *PPARG*, *PLIN*, *ADRB2*, *ADIPOQ*, *FABP2*, *PPARG*, *IRS1*, *APOA2/5*, *TCF7L2*	Genetic profile and sensitivity for carbohydrates, fats, and proteins matched with healthy food and fat control	http://www.thinnergene.com
Genetic Balance	SNPs at genetic loci associated with fat and carbohydrate metabolism	Genetic make-up matched to good or bad burning of carbohydrates or fats	https://www.genetic-balance.com
Bodykey by NUTRILITE	SNPs at genetic loci such as *FABP2* (rs1799883), *PPARG* (rs1801282), *ADRB2* (rs1042713), *ADRB2* (rs1042714), *ADRB3* (rs4994)	Genetic profile matched to diets with different macronutrient compositions	https://www.bodykey.at
Nutrigenes	100 SNPs at genetic loci such as *FADS1*	Genetic predisposition to food and nutrient needs, intolerances and sensitivities	http://www.nutrigenes.ch
My Kirée	Eight genetic loci associated with body weight	Genetic profile for fat or carbohydrate sensitivity, including supplementation with fat and carbohydrate blockers	https://my-kiree.com

All homepages were visited on 25th January 2019. *ADIPOQ*, adiponectin, C1Q, and collagen domain containing; *ADRB2/3*, adrenoceptor beta 2/3; *APOA2/5*, apolipoprotein A2/5; *FABP2*, fatty-acid-binding protein 2; *FADS1*, fatty-acid desaturase 1; *FTO*, fat mass and obesity associated; *IRS1*, insulin receptor substrate 1; *LIPC*, lipase C, hepatic type; *MC4R*, melanocortin 4 receptor; *PLIN*, perilipin 1; *PPARG*, peroxisome proliferator-activated receptor-gamma; *TCF7L2*, transcription factor 7 like 2.

In addition to the genetic profile, some companies also include other aspects of human metabolism into their dietary recommendations. The company Habit (https://habit.com) investigates the metabolic response on carbohydrates, fats, and proteins (shakes) and includes this information into the personalised dietary recommendation. Another commercially available personalised dietary programme is provided by the Million Friends company (https://www.millionfriends.de), which includes continuous glucose monitoring and the analysis of the microbiome into the personalised dietary recommendations.

In a systematic review by Covolo et al., different aspects of DTC tests were summarised [67]. The clinical validity of the genetic tests and the benefits are still limited. Furthermore, a lack of scientific evidence is clearly pointed out. In addition, contradictions in the results of genetic tests on the same individuals were identified. Due to missing counselling, a high risk of misinterpretation of the genetic result is given. Covolo et al. concluded that the practical experiences are limited, and that this market is still in a premature state [67].

10. Current Opinions for Gene-Based Diets

As described above, there is little scientific evidence for genetic DTC tests. This is also reflected by the opinions of nutritional and genetic societies. The German Society for Human Genetics rejects the use of genetic tests in their positioning paper [68], and the American Society of Dietetics and Nutrition declined the use of gene-based dietary recommendations in clinical settings [69]. In their position paper they stated, *"The practical application of nutritional genomics for complex chronic disease is an emerging science and the use of nutrigenetic testing to provide dietary advice is not ready for routine dietetics practice. Registered dietitian nutritionists need basic competency in genetics as a foundation for understanding nutritional genomics; proficiency requires advanced knowledge and skills"*. A systematic review of 17 European position statements, policies, guidelines, and recommendations described the concerns of societies about the DTC tests referring to the quality, genetic understanding, and protection of privacy [70]. Despite the concerns of societies, the mentioned review points out that the concept should be strictly regulated and that a common European regulation on the use of genetic data is crucial [70]. In addition, medical staff should be given the best possible training in the field of genetic DTC tests. In addition to the opinions of public societies, even the personal opinions, wishes, and concerns of individuals should be taken into account [71]. Furthermore, ethnic-based genetic differences should be considered.

11. Outlook

Bray and colleagues clearly pointed out in their article that personalised dietary recommendations are a hot topic for future obesity therapy and that clinical studies are necessary [72]. The whole area of personalised nutrition is very complex, and it is of urgent need to focus on several aspects (Figure 1), and not only on the person´s genetic background. Therefore, it is indispensable to conduct multidisciplinary studies in order to bring all potential factors together for a valid personalised dietary recommendation. The topic of personalised nutrition was picked up in the framework of the *enable* cluster (http://www.enable-cluster.de), which is funded by the Federal Ministry of Education and Research in Germany. The aim of the lifestyle intervention (LION) study is to identify, e.g., genetic, epigenetic, metabolic, and psychological predictors and barriers for weight loss and weight loss maintenance.

Author Contributions: T.D. and C.H. wrote the manuscript and approved the final version of the manuscript.

Funding: This article was supported by a grant of the German Federal Ministry of Education and Research (Bundesministerium für Bildung und Forschung, BMBF) (funding code: 01EA1709, *enable* publication number: 039). This article was written by the Junior Research Group "Personalised Nutrition & eHealth" within the Nutrition Cluster *enable*.

Acknowledgments: The authors thank the German Federal Ministry of Education and Research (BMBF) for funding.

Conflicts of Interest: The authors declare no conflicts of interests.

References

1. Lam, Y.Y.; Ravussin, E. Analysis of energy metabolism in humans: A review of methodologies. *Mol. Metab.* **2016**, *5*, 1057–1071. [CrossRef] [PubMed]
2. Crowley, V.E. Overview of human obesity and central mechanisms regulating energy homeostasis. *Ann Clin. Biochem.* **2008**, *45*, 245–255. [CrossRef] [PubMed]
3. Montague, C.T.; Farooqi, I.S.; Whitehead, J.P.; Soos, M.A.; Rau, H.; Wareham, N.J.; Sewter, C.P.; Digby, J.E.; Mohammed, S.N.; Hurst, J.A.; et al. Congenital leptin deficiency is associated with severe early-onset obesity in humans. *Nature* **1997**, *387*, 903–908. [CrossRef] [PubMed]
4. Wiedmer, P.; Nogueiras, R.; Broglio, F.; D'Alessio, D.; Tschop, M.H. Ghrelin, obesity and diabetes. *Nat. Clin. Pract. Endocrinol. Metab.* **2007**, *3*, 705–712. [CrossRef] [PubMed]
5. Woods, S.C.; D'Alessio, D.A. Central control of body weight and appetite. *J. Clin. Endocrinol. Metab.* **2008**, *93*, S37–S50. [CrossRef] [PubMed]
6. Raybould, H.E. Mechanisms of CCK signaling from gut to brain. *Curr. Opin. Pharmacol.* **2007**, *7*, 570–574. [CrossRef] [PubMed]
7. Johnston, B.C.; Kanters, S.; Bandayrel, K.; Wu, P.; Naji, F.; Siemieniuk, R.A.; Ball, G.D.; Busse, J.W.; Thorlund, K.; Guyatt, G.; et al. Comparison of weight loss among named diet programs in overweight and obese adults: A meta-analysis. *JAMA* **2014**, *312*, 923–933. [CrossRef] [PubMed]
8. Sacks, F.M.; Bray, G.A.; Carey, V.J.; Smith, S.R.; Ryan, D.H.; Anton, S.D.; McManus, K.; Champagne, C.M.; Bishop, L.M.; Laranjo, N.; et al. Comparison of weight-loss diets with different compositions of fat, protein, and carbohydrates. *N. Engl. J. Med.* **2009**, *360*, 859–873. [CrossRef] [PubMed]
9. Shai, I.; Schwarzfuchs, D.; Henkin, Y.; Shahar, D.R.; Witkow, S.; Greenberg, I.; Golan, R.; Fraser, D.; Bolotin, A.; Vardi, H.; et al. Weight Loss with a Low-Carbohydrate, Mediterranean, or Low-Fat Diet. *N. Engl. J. Med.* **2008**, *359*, 229–241. [CrossRef] [PubMed]
10. Gardner, C.D.; Trepanowski, J.F.; Del Gobbo, L.C.; Hauser, M.E.; Rigdon, J.; Ioannidis, J.P.A.; Desai, M.; King, A.C. Effect of Low-Fat vs Low-Carbohydrate Diet on 12-Month Weight Loss in Overweight Adults and the Association with Genotype Pattern or Insulin Secretion: The DIETFITS Randomized Clinical Trial. *JAMA* **2018**, *319*, 667–679. [CrossRef] [PubMed]
11. Esposito, K.; Kastorini, C.M.; Panagiotakos, D.B.; Giugliano, D. Mediterranean diet and weight loss: Meta-analysis of randomized controlled trials. *Metab. Syndr. Relat. Disord.* **2011**, *9*, 1–12. [CrossRef]
12. Jenkins, D.J.; Wong, J.M.; Kendall, C.W.; Esfahani, A.; Ng, V.W.; Leong, T.C.; Faulkner, D.A.; Vidgen, E.; Greaves, K.A.; Paul, G.; et al. The effect of a plant-based low-carbohydrate ("Eco-Atkins") diet on body weight and blood lipid concentrations in hyperlipidemic subjects. *Arch. Intern. Med.* **2009**, *169*, 1046–1054. [CrossRef]
13. Jenkins, D.J.; Wong, J.M.; Kendall, C.W.; Esfahani, A.; Ng, V.W.; Leong, T.C.; Faulkner, D.A.; Vidgen, E.; Paul, G.; Mukherjea, R.; et al. Effect of a 6-month vegan low-carbohydrate ('Eco-Atkins') diet on cardiovascular risk factors and body weight in hyperlipidaemic adults: A randomised controlled trial. *BMJ Open* **2014**, *4*, e003505. [CrossRef]
14. Harris, W.S.; Mozaffarian, D.; Rimm, E.; Kris-Etherton, P.; Rudel, L.L.; Appel, L.J.; Engler, M.B.; Sacks, F. Omega-6 fatty acids and risk for cardiovascular disease: A science advisory from the American Heart Association Nutrition Subcommittee of the Council on Nutrition, Physical Activity, and Metabolism; Council on Cardiovascular Nursing; and Council on Epidemiology and Prevention. *Circulation* **2009**, *119*, 902–907. [CrossRef]
15. Bamberger, C.; Rossmeier, A.; Lechner, K.; Wu, L.; Waldmann, E.; Stark, R.G.; Altenhofer, J.; Henze, K.; Parhofer, K.G. A Walnut-Enriched Diet Reduces Lipids in Healthy Caucasian Subjects, Independent of Recommended Macronutrient Replacement and Time Point of Consumption: A Prospective, Randomized, Controlled Trial. *Nutrients* **2017**, *9*, 097. [CrossRef]
16. Holzmann, S.L.; Pröll, K.; Hauner, H.; Holzapfel, C. Nutrition apps: Quality and limitations. An explorative investigation on the basis of selected apps. *Ernaehrungs Umsch.* **2017**, *64*, 80–89. [CrossRef]
17. Krug, S.; Kastenmuller, G.; Stuckler, F.; Rist, M.J.; Skurk, T.; Sailer, M.; Raffler, J.; Romisch-Margl, W.; Adamski, J.; Prehn, C.; et al. The dynamic range of the human metabolome revealed by challenges. *FASEB J. Off. Publ. Fed. Am. Soc. Exp. Biol.* **2012**, *26*, 2607–2619. [CrossRef]

18. Zeevi, D.; Korem, T.; Zmora, N.; Israeli, D.; Rothschild, D.; Weinberger, A.; Ben-Yacov, O.; Lador, D.; Avnit-Sagi, T.; Lotan-Pompan, M.; et al. Personalized Nutrition by Prediction of Glycemic Responses. *Cell* **2015**, *163*, 1079–1094. [CrossRef]
19. Korem, T.; Zeevi, D.; Zmora, N.; Weissbrod, O.; Bar, N.; Lotan-Pompan, M.; Avnit-Sagi, T.; Kosower, N.; Malka, G.; Rein, M.; et al. Bread Affects Clinical Parameters and Induces Gut Microbiome-Associated Personal Glycemic Responses. *Cell Metab.* **2017**, *25*, 1243.e1245–1253.e1245. [CrossRef]
20. Wopereis, S.; Stroeve, J.H.M.; Stafleu, A.; Bakker, G.C.M.; Burggraaf, J.; van Erk, M.J.; Pellis, L.; Boessen, R.; Kardinaal, A.A.F.; van Ommen, B. Multi-parameter comparison of a standardized mixed meal tolerance test in healthy and type 2 diabetic subjects: The PhenFlex challenge. *Genes Nutr.* **2017**, *12*, 21. [CrossRef]
21. De Toro-Martin, J.; Arsenault, B.J.; Despres, J.P.; Vohl, M.C. Precision Nutrition: A Review of Personalized Nutritional Approaches for the Prevention and Management of Metabolic Syndrome. *Nutrients* **2017**, *9*, 913. [CrossRef] [PubMed]
22. Nizel, A.E. Personalized nutrition counseling. *ASDC J. Dent. Child.* **1972**, *39*, 353–360. [PubMed]
23. Brug, J.; Campbell, M.; van Assema, P. The application and impact of computer-generated personalized nutrition education: A review of the literature. *Patient Educ. Couns.* **1999**, *36*, 145–156. [CrossRef]
24. Stewart-Knox, B.; Kuznesof, S.; Robinson, J.; Rankin, A.; Orr, K.; Duffy, M.; Poinhos, R.; de Almeida, M.D.; Macready, A.; Gallagher, C.; et al. Factors influencing European consumer uptake of personalised nutrition. Results of a qualitative analysis. *Appetite* **2013**, *66*, 67–74. [CrossRef] [PubMed]
25. Wang, D.D.; Hu, F.B. Precision nutrition for prevention and management of type 2 diabetes. *Lancet. Diabetes Endocrinol.* **2018**, *6*, 416–426. [CrossRef]
26. Van Ommen, B.; van den Broek, T.; de Hoogh, I.; van Erk, M.; van Someren, E.; Rouhani-Rankouhi, T.; Anthony, J.C.; Hogenelst, K.; Pasman, W.; Boorsma, A.; et al. Systems biology of personalized nutrition. *Nutr. Rev.* **2017**, *75*, 579–599. [CrossRef] [PubMed]
27. Daniel, H.; Klein, U. Personalisierte Ernährung. *J. Für Ernährungsmedizin* **2016**, *13*, 6–9.
28. Nielsen, D.E.; El-Sohemy, A. Disclosure of genetic information and change in dietary intake: A randomized controlled trial. *PLoS ONE* **2014**, *9*, e112665. [CrossRef]
29. Poinhos, R.; van der Lans, I.A.; Rankin, A.; Fischer, A.R.; Bunting, B.; Kuznesof, S.; Stewart-Knox, B.; Frewer, L.J. Psychological determinants of consumer acceptance of personalised nutrition in 9 European countries. *PLoS ONE* **2014**, *9*, e110614. [CrossRef]
30. Janz, N.K.; Becker, M.H. The Health Belief Model: A decade later. *Health Educ. Q.* **1984**, *11*, 1–47. [CrossRef]
31. Anderson, A.S. How to implement dietary changes to prevent the development of metabolic syndrome. *Br. J. Nutr.* **2000**, *83* (Suppl. 1), S165–S168. [CrossRef]
32. Bouchard, C.; Tremblay, A. Genetic influences on the response of body fat and fat distribution to positive and negative energy balances in human identical twins. *J. Nutr.* **1997**, *127*, 943s–947s. [CrossRef]
33. Stunkard, A.J.; Sorensen, T.I.; Hanis, C.; Teasdale, T.W.; Chakraborty, R.; Schull, W.J.; Schulsinger, F. An adoption study of human obesity. *N. Engl. J. Med.* **1986**, *314*, 193–198. [CrossRef]
34. Levy, E.; Menard, D.; Delvin, E.; Stan, S.; Mitchell, G.; Lambert, M.; Ziv, E.; Feoli-Fonseca, J.C.; Seidman, E. The polymorphism at codon 54 of the FABP2 gene increases fat absorption in human intestinal explants. *J. Biol. Chem.* **2001**, *276*, 39679–39684. [CrossRef]
35. Hegele, R.A.; Harris, S.B.; Hanley, A.J.; Sadikian, S.; Connelly, P.W.; Zinman, B. Genetic variation of intestinal fatty acid-binding protein associated with variation in body mass in aboriginal Canadians. *J. Clin. Endocrinol. Metab.* **1996**, *81*, 4334–4337. [CrossRef]
36. Tontonoz, P.; Hu, E.; Graves, R.A.; Budavari, A.I.; Spiegelman, B.M. mPPAR gamma 2: Tissue-specific regulator of an adipocyte enhancer. *Genes Dev.* **1994**, *8*, 1224–1234. [CrossRef]
37. Tontonoz, P.; Hu, E.; Spiegelman, B.M. Stimulation of adipogenesis in fibroblasts by PPAR gamma 2, a lipid-activated transcription factor. *Cell* **1994**, *79*, 1147–1156. [CrossRef]
38. Deeb, S.S.; Fajas, L.; Nemoto, M.; Pihlajamaki, J.; Mykkanen, L.; Kuusisto, J.; Laakso, M.; Fujimoto, W.; Auwerx, J. A Pro12Ala substitution in PPARgamma2 associated with decreased receptor activity, lower body mass index and improved insulin sensitivity. *Nat. Genet.* **1998**, *20*, 284–287. [CrossRef]
39. Hagg, S.; Ganna, A.; Van Der Laan, S.W.; Esko, T.; Pers, T.H.; Locke, A.E.; Berndt, S.I.; Justice, A.E.; Kahali, B.; Siemelink, M.A.; et al. Gene-based meta-analysis of genome-wide association studies implicates new loci involved in obesity. *Hum. Mol. Genet.* **2015**, *24*, 6849–6860. [CrossRef]

40. Locke, A.E.; Kahali, B.; Berndt, S.I.; Justice, A.E.; Pers, T.H.; Day, F.R.; Powell, C.; Vedantam, S.; Buchkovich, M.L.; Yang, J.; et al. Genetic studies of body mass index yield new insights for obesity biology. *Nature* **2015**, *518*, 197–206. [CrossRef]
41. Thorleifsson, G.; Walters, G.B.; Gudbjartsson, D.F.; Steinthorsdottir, V.; Sulem, P.; Helgadottir, A.; Styrkarsdottir, U.; Gretarsdottir, S.; Thorlacius, S.; Jonsdottir, I.; et al. Genome-wide association yields new sequence variants at seven loci that associate with measures of obesity. *Nat. Genet.* **2009**, *41*, 18–24. [CrossRef]
42. Speliotes, E.K.; Willer, C.J.; Berndt, S.I.; Monda, K.L.; Thorleifsson, G.; Jackson, A.U.; Lango Allen, H.; Lindgren, C.M.; Luan, J.; Magi, R.; et al. Association analyses of 249,796 individuals reveal 18 new loci associated with body mass index. *Nat. Genet.* **2010**, *42*, 937–948. [CrossRef]
43. Loos, R.J. The genetics of adiposity. *Curr. Opin. Genet. Dev.* **2018**, *50*, 86–95. [CrossRef]
44. Frayling, T.M.; Timpson, N.J.; Weedon, M.N.; Zeggini, E.; Freathy, R.M.; Lindgren, C.M.; Perry, J.R.; Elliott, K.S.; Lango, H.; Rayner, N.W.; et al. A common variant in the FTO gene is associated with body mass index and predisposes to childhood and adult obesity. *Science* **2007**, *316*, 889–894. [CrossRef]
45. Dina, C.; Meyre, D.; Gallina, S.; Durand, E.; Korner, A.; Jacobson, P.; Carlsson, L.M.; Kiess, W.; Vatin, V.; Lecoeur, C.; et al. Variation in FTO contributes to childhood obesity and severe adult obesity. *Nat. Genet.* **2007**, *39*, 724–726. [CrossRef]
46. Scuteri, A.; Sanna, S.; Chen, W.M.; Uda, M.; Albai, G.; Strait, J.; Najjar, S.; Nagaraja, R.; Orru, M.; Usala, G.; et al. Genome-wide association scan shows genetic variants in the FTO gene are associated with obesity-related traits. *PLoS Genet.* **2007**, *3*, e115. [CrossRef] [PubMed]
47. Claussnitzer, M.; Dankel, S.N.; Kim, K.H.; Quon, G.; Meuleman, W.; Haugen, C.; Glunk, V.; Sousa, I.S.; Beaudry, J.L.; Puviindran, V.; et al. FTO Obesity Variant Circuitry and Adipocyte Browning in Humans. *N. Engl. J. Med.* **2015**, *373*, 895–907. [CrossRef]
48. Larder, R.; Sim, M.F.M.; Gulati, P.; Antrobus, R.; Tung, Y.C.L.; Rimmington, D.; Ayuso, E.; Polex-Wolf, J.; Lam, B.Y.H.; Dias, C.; et al. Obesity-associated gene TMEM18 has a role in the central control of appetite and body weight regulation. *Proc. Natl. Acad. Sci. USA* **2017**, *114*, 9421–9426. [CrossRef]
49. Wiemerslage, L.; Gohel, P.A.; Maestri, G.; Hilmarsson, T.G.; Mickael, M.; Fredriksson, R.; Williams, M.J.; Schioth, H.B. The Drosophila ortholog of TMEM18 regulates insulin and glucagon-like signaling. *J. Endocrinol.* **2016**, *229*, 233–243. [CrossRef]
50. Cone, R.D. Anatomy and regulation of the central melanocortin system. *Nat. Neurosci.* **2005**, *8*, 571–578. [CrossRef]
51. Farooqi, I.S.; Keogh, J.M.; Yeo, G.S.; Lank, E.J.; Cheetham, T.; O'Rahilly, S. Clinical spectrum of obesity and mutations in the melanocortin 4 receptor gene. *N. Engl. J. Med.* **2003**, *348*, 1085–1095. [CrossRef] [PubMed]
52. Xiang, L.; Wu, H.; Pan, A.; Patel, B.; Xiang, G.; Qi, L.; Kaplan, R.C.; Hu, F.; Wylie-Rosett, J.; Qi, Q. FTO genotype and weight loss in diet and lifestyle interventions: A systematic review and meta-analysis. *Am. J. Clin. Nutr.* **2016**, *103*, 1162–1170. [CrossRef]
53. Livingstone, K.M.; Celis-Morales, C.; Papandonatos, G.D.; Erar, B.; Florez, J.C.; Jablonski, K.A.; Razquin, C.; Marti, A.; Heianza, Y.; Huang, T.; et al. FTO genotype and weight loss: Systematic review and meta-analysis of 9563 individual participant data from eight randomised controlled trials. *BMJ* **2016**, *354*, i4707. [CrossRef] [PubMed]
54. Sorensen, T.I.; Boutin, P.; Taylor, M.A.; Larsen, L.H.; Verdich, C.; Petersen, L.; Holst, C.; Echwald, S.M.; Dina, C.; Toubro, S.; et al. Genetic polymorphisms and weight loss in obesity: A randomised trial of hypo-energetic high- versus low-fat diets. *PLoS Clin. Trials* **2006**, *1*, e12. [CrossRef]
55. Papandonatos, G.D.; Pan, Q.; Pajewski, N.M.; Delahanty, L.M.; Peter, I.; Erar, B.; Ahmad, S.; Harden, M.; Chen, L.; Fontanillas, P.; et al. Genetic Predisposition to Weight Loss and Regain with Lifestyle Intervention: Analyses From the Diabetes Prevention Program and the Look AHEAD Randomized Controlled Trials. *Diabetes* **2015**, *64*, 4312–4321. [CrossRef]
56. Livingstone, K.M.; Celis-Morales, C.; Lara, J.; Ashor, A.W.; Lovegrove, J.A.; Martinez, J.A.; Saris, W.H.; Gibney, M.; Manios, Y.; Traczyk, I.; et al. Associations between FTO genotype and total energy and macronutrient intake in adults: A systematic review and meta-analysis. *Obes. Rev.* **2015**, *16*, 666–678. [CrossRef] [PubMed]

57. Drabsch, T.; Gatzemeier, J.; Pfadenhauer, L.; Hauner, H.; Holzapfel, C. Associations between Single Nucleotide Polymorphisms and Total Energy, Carbohydrate, and Fat Intakes: A Systematic Review. *Adv. Nutr.* **2018**, *9*, 425–453. [CrossRef] [PubMed]
58. Jiang, L.; Penney, K.L.; Giovannucci, E.; Kraft, P.; Wilson, K.M. A genome-wide association study of energy intake and expenditure. *PLoS ONE* **2018**, *13*, e0201555. [CrossRef]
59. Merino, J.; Dashti, H.S.; Li, S.X.; Sarnowski, C.; Justice, A.E.; Graff, M.; Papoutsakis, C.; Smith, C.E.; Dedoussis, G.V.; Lemaitre, R.N.; et al. Genome-wide meta-analysis of macronutrient intake of 91,114 European ancestry participants from the cohorts for heart and aging research in genomic epidemiology consortium. *Mol. Psychiatry* **2018**. [CrossRef]
60. Larsen, L.H.; Angquist, L.; Vimaleswaran, K.S.; Hager, J.; Viguerie, N.; Loos, R.J.; Handjieva-Darlenska, T.; Jebb, S.A.; Kunesova, M.; Larsen, T.M.; et al. Analyses of single nucleotide polymorphisms in selected nutrient-sensitive genes in weight-regain prevention: The DIOGENES study. *Am. J. Clin. Nutr.* **2012**, *95*, 1254–1260. [CrossRef]
61. Zhang, X.; Qi, Q.; Zhang, C.; Smith, S.R.; Hu, F.B.; Sacks, F.M.; Bray, G.A.; Qi, L. FTO genotype and 2-year change in body composition and fat distribution in response to weight-loss diets: The POUNDS LOST Trial. *Diabetes* **2012**, *61*, 3005–3011. [CrossRef] [PubMed]
62. Qi, Q.; Bray, G.A.; Smith, S.R.; Hu, F.B.; Sacks, F.M.; Qi, L. Insulin receptor substrate 1 gene variation modifies insulin resistance response to weight-loss diets in a 2-year randomized trial: The Preventing Overweight Using Novel Dietary Strategies (POUNDS LOST) trial. *Circulation* **2011**, *124*, 563–571. [CrossRef] [PubMed]
63. Celis-Morales, C.; Livingstone, K.M.; Marsaux, C.F.; Forster, H.; O'Donovan, C.B.; Woolhead, C.; Macready, A.L.; Fallaize, R.; Navas-Carretero, S.; San-Cristobal, R.; et al. Design and baseline characteristics of the Food4Me study: A web-based randomised controlled trial of personalised nutrition in seven European countries. *Genes Nutr.* **2015**, *10*, 450. [CrossRef]
64. Saukko, P. State of play in direct-to-consumer genetic testing for lifestyle-related diseases: Market, marketing content, user experiences and regulation. *Proc. Nutr. Soc.* **2013**, *72*, 53–60. [CrossRef]
65. Frankwich, K.A.; Egnatios, J.; Kenyon, M.L.; Rutledge, T.R.; Liao, P.S.; Gupta, S.; Herbst, K.L.; Zarrinpar, A. Differences in Weight Loss Between Persons on Standard Balanced vs Nutrigenetic Diets in a Randomized Controlled Trial. *Clin. Gastroenterol. Hepatol. Off. Clin. Pract. J. Am. Gastroenterol. Assoc.* **2015**, *13*, 1625–1632.e1621. [CrossRef] [PubMed]
66. Steinberg, G.; Scott, A.; Honcz, J.; Spettell, C.; Pradhan, S. Reducing Metabolic Syndrome Risk Using a Personalized Wellness Program. *J. Occup. Environ. Med.* **2015**, *57*, 1269–1274. [CrossRef] [PubMed]
67. Covolo, L.; Rubinelli, S.; Ceretti, E.; Gelatti, U. Internet-Based Direct-to-Consumer Genetic Testing: A Systematic Review. *J. Med. Internet Res.* **2015**, *17*, e279. [CrossRef]
68. Reis, A. Stellungnahme der Deutschen Gesellschaft fuer Humangenetik (GfH) zu "Direct-to-Consumer" (DTC)-Gentests. Dtsch. Ges. Fuer Humangenet. E.V., 2011. Available online: https://www.gfhev.de/de/leitlinien/LL_und_Stellungnahmen/2011_12_02_GfH-Stellungnahme_DTC-Gentests.pdf (accessed on 25 January 2019).
69. Camp, K.M.; Trujillo, E. Position of the Academy of Nutrition and Dietetics: Nutritional genomics. *J. Acad. Nutr. Diet.* **2014**, *114*, 299–312. [CrossRef]
70. Rafiq, M.; Ianuale, C.; Ricciardi, W.; Boccia, S. Direct-to-consumer genetic testing: A systematic review of european guidelines, recommendations, and position statements. *Genet. Test. Mol. Biomark.* **2015**, *19*, 535–547. [CrossRef]
71. Bloss, C.S.; Ornowski, L.; Silver, E.; Cargill, M.; Vanier, V.; Schork, N.J.; Topol, E.J. Consumer perceptions of direct-to-consumer personalized genomic risk assessments. *Genet. Med. Off. J. Am. Coll. Med. Genet.* **2010**, *12*, 556–566. [CrossRef]
72. Bray, M.S.; Loos, R.J.; McCaffery, J.M.; Ling, C.; Franks, P.W.; Weinstock, G.M.; Snyder, M.P.; Vassy, J.L.; Agurs-Collins, T. NIH working group report-using genomic information to guide weight management: From universal to precision treatment. *Obesity* **2016**, *24*, 14–22. [CrossRef] [PubMed]

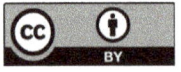

© 2019 by the authors. Licensee MDPI, Basel, Switzerland. This article is an open access article distributed under the terms and conditions of the Creative Commons Attribution (CC BY) license (http://creativecommons.org/licenses/by/4.0/).

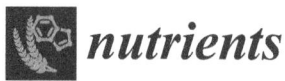

Article

Assessment of the Effectiveness of a Computerised Decision-Support Tool for Health Professionals for the Prevention and Treatment of Childhood Obesity. Results from a Randomised Controlled Trial

George Moschonis [1,2,*], Maria Michalopoulou [2], Konstantina Tsoutsoulopoulou [2], Elpis Vlachopapadopoulou [3], Stefanos Michalacos [3], Evangelia Charmandari [4,5], George P. Chrousos [4] and Yannis Manios [2]

[1] Department of Dietetics, Nutrition and Sport, School of Allied Health, Human Services and Sport, La Trobe University, Melbourne, VIC 3086, Australia
[2] Department of Nutrition and Dietetics, Harokopio University of Athens, 70 El Venizelou Avenue, Kallithea, 17671 Athens, Greece; mariamichal95@gmail.com (M.M.); kontsou@gmail.com (K.T.); manios@hua.gr (Y.M.)
[3] Department of Endocrinology-Growth and Development, Children's Hospital P. A. Kyriakou, 11527 Athens, Greece; elpis.vl@gmail.com (E.V.); stmichalakos@gmail.com (S.M.)
[4] Division of Endocrinology, Metabolism, and Diabetes, First Department of Pediatrics, University of Athens Medical School, Aghia Sophia Children's Hospital, 11527 Athens, Greece; echarmand@med.uoa.gr (E.C.); chrousge@med.uoa.gr (G.P.C.)
[5] Division of Endocrinology and Metabolism, Center of Clinical, Experimental Surgery and Translational Research, Biomedical Research Foundation of the Academy of Athens, 11527 Athens, Greece
* Correspondence: g.moschonis@latrobe.edu.au; Tel.: +61-03-9479-3482

Received: 16 February 2019; Accepted: 22 March 2019; Published: 26 March 2019

Abstract: We examined the effectiveness of a computerised decision-support tool (DST), designed for paediatric healthcare professionals, as a means to tackle childhood obesity. A randomised controlled trial was conducted with 65 families of 6–12-year old overweight or obese children. Paediatricians, paediatric endocrinologists and a dietitian in two children's hospitals implemented the intervention. The intervention group (IG) received personalised meal plans and lifestyle optimisation recommendations via the DST, while families in the control group (CG) received general recommendations. After three months of intervention, the IG had a significant change in dietary fibre and sucrose intake by 4.1 and −4.6 g/day, respectively. In addition, the IG significantly reduced consumption of sweets (i.e., chocolates and cakes) and salty snacks (i.e., potato chips) by −0.1 and −0.3 portions/day, respectively. Furthermore, the CG had a significant increase of body weight and waist circumference by 1.4 kg and 2.1 cm, respectively, while Body Mass Index (BMI) decreased only in the IG by −0.4 kg/m^2. However, the aforementioned findings did not differ significantly between study groups. In conclusion, these findings indicate the dynamics of the DST in supporting paediatric healthcare professionals to improve the effectiveness of care in modifying obesity-related behaviours. Further research is needed to confirm these findings.

Keywords: personalised; nutrition; intervention; children; obesity; healthcare professionals

1. Introduction

A plethora of epidemiological data reports the high prevalence of obesity, an "epidemic" that represents a huge public health burden for many countries. Besides the increased risk for chronic diseases, obesity is also related to nutrient insufficiencies, a paradox that has been characterised as the "double burden of malnutrition" [1]. This "double burden" paradox can be interpreted by the existence of a chronic, low-grade inflammation state that is produced and sustained in obese children [2], leading to low blood concentration of essential micronutrients, such as iron [3] and vitamin D [4]. Considering the important roles of these micronutrients in several cellular, metabolic and physiological processes, their long-term insufficiency in obese individuals may become detrimental for children's optimal growth and development.

Due to the huge dimensions and detrimental effects of obesity and related complications, these conditions have been the major focus of public health research over the past decade. However, existing tools, programmes and strategies to counteract the "obesity epidemic" have only experienced limited success [5]. This is mainly due to the inadequate understanding of the complex mosaic of mechanistic pathways leading to obesity. In this regard, excess body weight is not only the product of a positive energy balance, but also an interaction of a plethora of other etiological factors, such as environmental ones that exert their effects even from very early life stages, such as the prenatal period and the first 5 years of life. By acting "in utero" (e.g., maternal obesity, smoking during pregnancy, etc.) or during infancy (infant formula feeding, growth velocity, etc.), perinatal factors can cause permanent endocrine adaptations, usually expressed as increased hunger, adipogenesis and consequently obesity at later life stages [6,7]. Another important reason for the limited or only short-term effectiveness of weight management programs is usually their delayed implementation in already obese children or in adulthood, when the energy-balance-related behaviours (EBRBs) and consequently the obesity phenotype are already established [8]. As such, the implementation of intervention initiatives as early in life as possible, when EBRBs and their determinants are still flexible, is promising for the prevention of obesity and related cardiometabolic complications [9].

Health professionals (i.e., general practitioners, family doctors, paediatricians, dietitians, nutritionists) have a key role among health experts, in prospectively and frequently monitoring children [10,11]. Furthermore, this key role places them into a central position, with regards to childhood obesity prevention and treatment, since they are also the ones guiding parents in providing the appropriate healthcare to their children. However, these professionals on many occasions they require additional and appropriate support to conduct a thorough assessment and provide tailor-made diet and lifestyle optimisation advice to families with children in need of weight management [12,13].

As such, the objective of this study was to examine the effectiveness of a computerised decision-support tool (DST), developed to assist paediatricians and paediatric endocrinologists in delivering personalised nutrition and lifestyle optimisation advice to children and their families, as a means of childhood obesity management.

2. Materials and Methods

2.1. Development of the Decision Support Tool

The development of the computerised DST is based on decision-tree algorithms (Supplementary Figure S1 provides an example of these algorithms), which include five different levels, namely the "assessment of children's current weight status" (level 1), the "assessment of the likelihood for the future manifestation of obesity in normal-weight children" (level 2), the "evaluation of the most appropriate body weight management goal" (level 3), the "estimation of children's dietary energy and macronutrients intake needs" (level 4) and the delivery of "personalised diet and lifestyle optimisation advice" (level 5).

The first level of the decision tree algorithms ("assessment of children's current weight status") is based on the measurement of body weight in all age groups from infancy to adolescence and of the recumbent length in infants and children until the age of 2 years or standing height in all children and adolescents after the age of 2 years. The international Body Mass Index (BMI)-for-age growth curves and the relevant reference values proposed by the WHO are further used to finalise the assessment of children's weight status [14] and categorise them into "underweight" (BMI-for-age < 5th percentile), "normal weight" (5th percentile ≤ BMI-for-age < 85th percentile), "overweight" (85th percentile ≤ BMI-for-age < 95th percentile) and "obese" (BMI-for-age ≥ 95th percentile).

The second level of the decision tree algorithms ("assessment of the likelihood for the future manifestation of obesity in normal-weight children") is important because even if a child's current body weight is normal, this does not exclude the likelihood of the future manifestation of obesity, especially in children that are subjected to the combined effect of obesity risk factors. In an attempt to examine the likelihood for the future occurrence of obesity in normal weight children, due to the combined effect of individual obesity risk factors, including socio-demographic and perinatal ones, the CORE (Childhood Obesity Risk Evaluation) index [15], was included as another component of the DST. More specifically, the CORE index represents a simple, easy-to-use and valid score [16], which provides an estimation of the future likelihood of obesity manifestation as early as the age of 6 months. This estimation achieved through the combined use and scoring of easily collected data on specific perinatal risk factors, such as maternal pre-pregnancy weight status, maternal smoking during pregnancy, infant's weight gain during the first 6 months of life, as well as simple socio-demographic indices, namely the child's gender and mother's educational level.

In the third level ("evaluation of the most appropriate body weight management goal") the decision tree algorithms use the recommendations of the American Pediatric Association as a basis for the prevention and treatment of child and adolescent overweight and obesity [17]. More specifically, data collected on children's age and current weight status, as well as on the presence of obesity-related comorbidities (i.e., hyperglycaemia, insulin resistance, dyslipidaemia, hypertension) in children and of obesity in one or both parents, are combined to inform each one of the following weight management pathways: (i) body weight maintenance, which aims to the progressive reduction of BMI due to the increase in height stemming from children's growth, or (ii) body weight loss, whenever this is deemed appropriate, such as in cases where comorbidities and/or parental obesity co-exist with childhood obesity.

Following the evaluation of the most appropriate weight management goal, the fourth level of the decision tree algorithms ("estimation of children's dietary energy and macronutrients intake needs") is necessary to facilitate weight maintenance or weight loss as well as children's growth. The mathematical formulas provided by the Institute of Medicine (IOM) for infants, children and adolescents [18] were used to assess estimated energy requirements (EER). After the estimation of dietary energy intake requirements, the DST calculates the percent distribution of energy into macronutrients, within the Acceptable Macronutrient Distribution Ranges (AMDRs) proposed by the IOM for carbohydrates, fat and protein for infants, children and adolescents [18].

In the fifth level ("personalised diet and lifestyle optimisation advice"), the decision tree algorithms analyse all aforementioned data and deliver a report providing the assessment of the examined child, as well as body weight, diet and lifestyle recommendations that will support the decision of health professionals. The report includes (a) the assessment of children's current weight status and the need for body weight maintenance or loss, (b) the assessment of the likelihood for the future manifestation of obesity in normal-weight children, (c) children's total dietary energy requirements based on the anticipated body weight management (i.e., weight maintenance or loss) target, (d) children's dietary needs in carbohydrates, total fat and protein, (e) personalised meal plans, as well as (f) diet and lifestyle optimisation recommendations, tailored to the specific needs and weight management goals set for each child. The recommendations include practical advice to the family on how (i) to achieve an energy and nutrients' balanced diet, via an increase in the consumption of foods that are rich sources of dietary fibre and complex carbohydrates and a reduction in the consumption of foods that have a high content of simple sugars, total and saturated dietary fat, cholesterol and sodium, (ii) to become more physically active, (iii) to reduce sedentary activities and (iv) to improve children's sleep patterns [19].

2.2. Operational Components of the DST

The DST comprises of two operational components, namely the data entry and the data processing component. Regarding data entry, paediatric healthcare professionals collect information on the child's gender and birth date and conduct anthropometric measurements of body weight, recumbent length or standing height (depending on the child's age). Healthcare professionals also collect perinatal, socio-demographic and parental data, as well as some additional information on characteristics related to the child. In terms of perinatal factors, data is collected on maternal pre-pregnancy body weight (in kg), maternal smoking habits during pregnancy, while the child's health record is used to copy information with regards to the child's weight (in kg) at birth and at six months of age. Regarding socio-demographic and parental data, information is collected on self-reported mother's educational level (in years of education), and on measured mother's and father's body weight (in kg) and height (in cm). Furthermore, healthcare professionals use a set of validated questions [20] to collect appropriate data that will allow them to categorise the child's physical activity level, into light (<4 METs), moderate (4–7 METs) or vigorous (>7 METs). Lastly, information on the presence of obesity-related comorbidity indices, such as insulin resistance, dyslipidaemias and hypertension is also collected, either based on the child's physical examination or based on biochemical or clinical indices from the child's medical record that is available to the paediatric healthcare professionals.

As far as data processing is concerned, all data are uploaded to the DST, which processes them and extracts a report with the child's assessment and the personalised diet and lifestyle optimisation recommendations. More specifically, the DST uses the birth and examination dates to calculate child's age (in months and years), it then calculates child's BMI (in kg/m^2) and consequently estimates the child's weight status, through its categorisation into underweight, normal-weight, overweight or obese. In normal-weight children, the DST also calculates the CORE index score, based on which children with a higher (i.e., CORE index score $\geq$ 4) likelihood for obesity manifestation in childhood or adolescence are identified [16]. In addition, the DST calculates the estimated dietary energy requirement (in kcals per day) for the child, so as to achieve the desired body weight management (i.e., weight maintenance or loss) goal, while relevant calculations are also made with regards to dietary protein, carbohydrates and fat needs (in grams per day). Furthermore, the DST processes the data uploaded for parents, thus calculating parental BMI (in kg/m^2) and categorising parents as non-obese or obese (i.e., BMI > 30 kg/m^2). Finally, the DST proposes diet and lifestyle optimisation advice recommendations for the child and/or the entire family (Supplementary Table S1 provides examples of the recommendations), as well as personalised weekly meal plans adjusted to the estimated energy requirements calculated for each child (Supplementary Table S2 provides examples of the meal plans).

2.3. Personalised Lifestyle Optimisations Recommendations and Weekly Meal Plans

The DST follows five steps dictated by the decision tree algorithms (Supplementary Figure S1 provides the relevant steps) to propose personalised lifestyle optimisation recommendations and weekly meal plans.

In step 1, children are categorised based on their BMI into normal-weight, overweight or obese, while in step 2 the CORE index score is calculated for normal-weight children. In normal-weight children with a lower likelihood for the future manifestation of obesity, the DST proposes diet and physical activity recommendations, which support the maintenance of normal body weight and growth (recommendation 1).

In step 3, the DST focuses on normal-weight children with a higher likelihood for the future obesity manifestation and evaluates the co-existence of clinical disorders (i.e., hyperglycaemia, insulin resistance, dyslipidaemia and/or hypertension). In normal-weight children with no clinical disorders and with non-obese parents, the DST advises health professionals to provide recommendation 1 (i.e., similar to step 2 above). In normal-weight children with no clinical disorders but with at least one obese parent, the DST advises health professionals to provide specialised recommendations, aiming to improve diet and physical activity habits for the entire family (recommendation 2).

In normal-weight children with at least one clinical disorder but with non-obese parents, the DST provides recommendations, aiming at maintaining the child's normal body weight, but also delivering practical advice that supports the consumption of foods rich in dietary fibre and complex carbohydrates, but simultaneously the reduction in the consumption of foods high in simple sugars, total and saturated fat, dietary cholesterol and sodium (recommendation 3). Finally, in normal-weight children with at least one clinical disorder and with at least one obese parent, the DST provides recommendations targeting the entire family and aiming to improve physical activity and dietary habits for all family members (recommendation 4). The DST also proposes a periodic re-evaluation every 6 months for high-risk normal-weight children with at least one clinical disorder and/or at least one obese parent and every 12 months for children with no clinical disorders and/or non-obese parents.

In step 4 the DST focuses on overweight children. In overweight children with no clinical disorders and with non-obese parents, the DST advises health professionals to provide recommendation 1, but also an isocaloric weekly meal plan, aiming to maintain the child's body weight (meal plan 1) and consequently to progressively decrease its BMI (as the child grows and height increases), ideally below the 85th percentile. In overweight children with no clinical disorders and at least one obese parent, the DST provides recommendation 2, that targets the entire family, as well as the isocaloric meal plan 1, which aims for the maintenance of the child's body weight. In overweight children with at least one clinical disorder and with non-obese parents, the DST proposes recommendation 3, as well as an isocaloric meal plan (meal plan 2), aiming for the maintenance of the child's body weight via the consumption of foods rich in dietary fibre and complex carbohydrates, but also with a lower content of simple sugars, total and saturated fat, dietary cholesterol and sodium, compared to meal plan 1. Finally, in overweight children with at least one clinical disorder and with at least one obese parent, the DST advises health professionals to provide recommendation 4 to the entire family, as well as meal plan 2. The DST also suggests a periodic re-evaluation every 3 months for overweight children with at least one clinical disorder and/or at least one obese parent and every 6 months for children with no clinical disorders and/or non-obese parents. If the re-evaluation shows no reduction of BMI below the 85th percentile, the DST follows the same process described under Step 4. If the re-evaluation shows a reduction of BMI below the 85th percentile, the DST follows the process described under Step 3.

In step 5, the DST focuses on obese children. In the case of 2–5-year-old obese children, the DST follows exactly the same approach dictated by Step 4 for overweight children. The main differentiation occurs in 6–15-year-old obese children to whom mild weight loss is also prescribed. In this regard, in 6–15-year-old obese children with no clinical disorders and at least one obese parent, the DST targets the family and proposes recommendation 2 and a hypocaloric meal plan (meal plan 3). In 6–15-year-old obese children with at least one clinical disorder and non-obese parents, the DST proposes recommendation 3, as well as a hypocaloric meal plan (meal plan 4), via the consumption of foods rich in dietary fibre and complex carbohydrates, but also the decrease in the consumption of foods rich in simple sugars, total and saturated fat, dietary cholesterol and sodium. Finally, in 6–15-year-old obese children with at least one clinical disorder and with at least one obese parent, the DST targets the family and proposes recommendation 4 and a hypocaloric meal plan 4. The DST also proposes a periodic re-evaluation every 3 months for obese children with at least one clinical disorder and/or at least one obese parent and every 6 months for children with no clinical disorders and/or non-obese parents. If the re-evaluation shows no reduction of BMI below the 95th percentile, the DST follows the same approach described under Step 4 or Step 5, depending on the child's age (i.e., 2–5 or 6–15 years old). If the re-evaluation shows a reduction of BMI below the 95th percentile, but BMI remains higher than the 85th percentile, the DST follows the pathway dictated by Step 4. If the re-evaluation shows a reduction of BMI below the 85th percentile, the DST proposes the process described under Step 3.

Table 1 summarises the target population and the behavioural change goals and lifestyle optimisation advice provided by each level of recommendations through the DST.

Table 1. Population and behavioural change goals of diet and lifestyle optimisation advice provided through the decision support tool.

	Recommendation 1	Recommendation 2	Recommendation 3	Recommendation 4
Target population *:				
Children	☑		☑	
Children and Family		☑		☑
Behavioural change goals				
Keep a balanced diet, increase physical activity and Improve sleep habits	☑	☑	☑	☑
Increase consumption of foods rich in dietary fibre and complex carbohydrates			☑	☑
Reduce consumption of foods rich in simple sugars, total and saturated dietary fat, cholesterol and sodium			☑	☑

* Both the content and style of recommendations were adjusted to promote behavioural change to children only or to the entire family.

2.4. Randomised Controlled Trial to Assess the Effectiveness of the Computerised DST

The effectiveness of the DST was assessed through a pilot randomised controlled intervention trial (RCT). The RCT was initiated on May 2018 and was conducted in the Endocrinology Department of the "P. and A. Kyriakou" Children's Hospital and in the Division of Endocrinology, Metabolism, and Diabetes of the "Aghia Sophia" Children's Hospital in Athens, Greece. Before the study initiation, a statistical power calculation indicated that a total sample size of 64 children (50% females) would be adequate to observe a mean BMI difference of 1.5 kg/m^2 between the two study groups (statistical power of 80% and level of statistical significance at 5%). Taking into account an attrition rate of 20%, a screening conducted in the premises of the aforementioned settings managed to recruit a total sample of 80 children, who were identified as eligible to be included in the RCT. The main eligibility criteria for inclusion in the RCT were children aged 6–12 years old, as well as overweight or obese status (i.e., BMI-for-age $\geq$ 85th percentile). Signed informed consent forms were obtained from all parents of eligible children, before their participation to the study. The study was conducted in accordance with the rules of the Declaration of Helsinki of 1975, revised in 2013 and the protocol was approved by the Bioethics Committee of Harokopio University, Athens (approval no.: 61/30-3-2018). Finally, the RCT was registered to clinicaltrials.gov (NCT03819673).

2.5. Study Groups

The 80 overweight or obese children that were eligible to participate in the RCT, were randomly and equally allocated to two study groups. Those children that were randomly allocated to the intervention group (IG), were examined by paediatricians (i.e., general paediatricians and paediatric endocrinologists) and a dietitian, who were all trained in the use of the DST. A manual of operation with detailed instructions on the use of the DST was prepared and distributed to medical practitioners prior to the commencement of the study. The dietitian also assisted the paediatricians to assess children's weight status, to set appropriate weight management goals and to provide personalised meal plans and/or recommendations to children and their families. In contrast, those families whose children were randomly allocated to the control group (CG), were provided with general recommendations of diet and physical activity and follow-up appointments were made for weight checks. The effectiveness of the intervention was evaluated through the collection of data at baseline and at a follow-up examination after 3 months.

2.6. Data Collection: Parental Socio-Demographic and Anthropometric Characteristics

Data on specific socio-demographic characteristics were collected from parents (most preferably from the mother) during the scheduled face-to-face interviews. All interviews were conducted by the paediatricians or the dietitian with the use of a standardized questionnaire. The socio-demographic data collected by parents included father's and mother's age, educational level (years of education) and occupation. In addition, parents also reported or had their body weight and height measured, from which BMI was calculated and used to categorise each parent based on their weight status.

2.7. Dietary Intake

Dietary intake data were obtained by the dietitian with the use of a 24-h recall of one typical day in terms of children's dietary intake and with a short food frequency questionnaire (FFQ), via interviews conducted with parents of children younger than 10 years of age or directly with children older than 10 years old.

According to the data recorded from the 24h-recall, all study participants were asked to describe the type and amount of foods and beverages consumed, during the previous day, provided that it was a typical day according to the participant's perception. To improve the accuracy of food description, standard household measures (cups, tablespoons, etc.) and food models were used to define amounts. At the end of each interview, the dietitian reviewed the collected data with the respondent in order to clarify entries, servings and possible forgotten foods. Dietary intake data were analysed using the Nutritionist V diet analysis software (version 2.1, 1999, First Databank, San Bruno, CA, USA), which was modified to include traditional Greek dishes and recipes [18]. Furthermore, the database was updated with nutritional information of processed foods provided by independent research institutes, food companies and fast-food chains.

In addition, a short semi-quantitative valid FFQ [21] was used to collect data on children's dietary intake of foods representing all main food groups (i.e., fruits, vegetables, grains, dairy and protein foods). The FFQ included questions that evaluate the consumption frequency of foods during the previous 3 months in frequencies ranging from less than 1 portion/month to more than 4 portions per day.

2.8. Perinatal Data

Regarding perinatal data, mothers were asked to recall information on their pre-pregnancy body weight and smoking practices during pregnancy. Additionally, mothers were asked to report their child's body weight and recumbent length at birth and 6 months of age, as this was recorded at their child's health record.

2.9. Physical Activity Levels

Organised and leisure time physical activities were assessed using a standardized questionnaire, that was also used and validated in the multicentre Feel4Diabetes study that was conducted in six European countries, including Greece [20]. Respondents reported the type, time (in minutes) and frequency (in times per week) spent by children on organised and/or leisure time physical activities.

2.10. Anthropometric Data

Body weight was measured to the nearest 0.1 kg using a digital weight scale (Seca Alpha, Model 770, Hamburg, Germany). Subjects were weighed without shoes in minimal clothing. Height was measured to the nearest 0.1 cm using a commercial stadiometer with subjects not wearing shoes, their shoulders in a relaxed position, their arms hanging freely and their head aligned according to the Frankfort plane. Weight and height were converted to BMI using Quetelet's equation (weight $(kg)/height^2$ (m^2)), while the international BMI-for-age growth curves and the relevant reference values proposed by the WHO [14] were issued to calculate BMI z-score. Waist circumference (WC) was also measured to the nearest 0.1 cm with the use of a non-elastic tape and with the child standing, at the end of a gentle expiration. The measuring tape was placed around the trunk, at the level of the umbilicus, midway between the lower rib margin and the iliac crest.

2.11. Statistical Analysis

Normality of the distribution of continuous variables was analysed using the Kolmogorov-Smirnov test. Normally distributed continuous variables were expressed as Mean values (+/−Standard Error of the Mean: SEM) and categorical variables were reported as frequencies (%). Associations between continuous and categorical variables were examined using Student's *t*-test for normally distributed variables or the non-parametric Mann-Whitney test for skewed variables even though logarithmic transformations were made. The associations between categorical variables were assessed using the chi square (χ^2) test. Repeated-measures ANOVA was used to evaluate the significance of the differences among study groups at baseline and at the 3-month follow-up (treatment effect), the significance of the change from baseline to follow-up observed within each group (time effect) and the treatment × time interaction effect. The between-group factor was the study groups (i.e., IG compared to CG) and the within-group factor was the time point of measurement. Adjustments were also made for potential possible confounding factors. All reported *p*-values were based on two-sided tests. The level of statistical significance in all analyses was set at $p < 0.05$. The SPSS vs. 24.0 (SPSS Inc., Chicago, IL, USA) software was used for all statistical analyses.

3. Results

From the initial total sample of 80 children randomly allocated to the two study groups, 15 children (5 from the IG and 10 from the CG) could not be re-examined at follow-up. Figure 1 provides the flow diagram of the study according to the CONSORT guidelines.

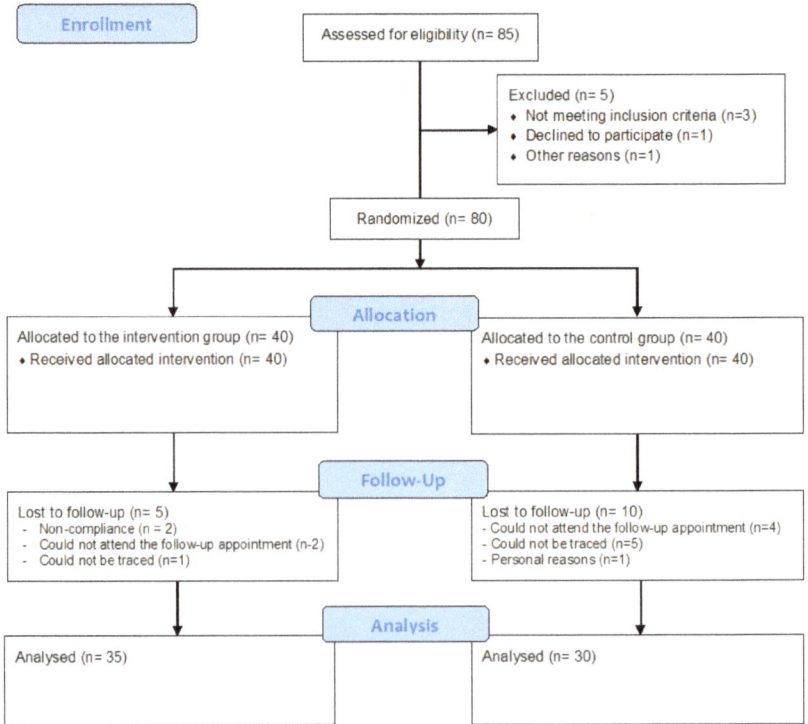

Figure 1. Flow diagram of study participants.

The attrition resulted in a total sample of 65 children (35 in the IG and 30 in the CG) with full data at baseline and follow-up. The descriptive characteristics of these children and their parents at baseline are summarised as mean (+/−SEM) or as percentages in Table 2. Regarding demographic indices, the mean age of children participating in the study was 9.7 (0.2) years, while the mean age of fathers and mothers was 46.1 (0.3) and 41.2 (0.3) years, respectively. Furthermore, 24.6% of mothers had <9 years of education, which is the compulsory education level in Greece, while 42.6% had a higher education of >12 years. Regarding behavioural indices, the mean dietary energy intake recorded for children was 1535.6 (81.3) kcal per day with the percentage of energy coming in a descending order from carbohydrates (47.4%), fat (35.4%) and protein (18.5%), while the mean daily time spent by children on physical activity was 21.6 (2.3) min. As far as perinatal indices were concerned, the mean birth weight and recumbent length of children was 3.2 (0.1) kg and 50.7 (0.4) cm, respectively, while mean maternal pre-pregnancy BMI was 24.9 (0.4) kg/m^2, with 15.5% of mothers being obese before conception. Regarding anthropometric indices, children's mean body weight, height, BMI and WC was 51.9 (1.9) kg, 142.4 (1.4) cm, 25.1 (0.5) kg/m^2 and 79.9 (1.5) cm, respectively, with 60.7% of children being obese. In addition, the mean BMI of fathers was 28.6 (0.4) kg/m^2, with 27.6% of them being obese, while the mean BMI of mothers was 27.3 (0.4) kg/m^2, with 31.6% of them being obese. Regarding differences between study groups, the mean BMI of mothers of children in the CG was higher than that of mothers of children in the IG (28.9 (1.2) vs. 26.0 (0.8) kg/m^2; $p = 0.045$). No other statistically significant differences were observed between study groups.

Table 2. Descriptive characteristics of children and their parents at baseline.

	Total Sample (n = 65)	Intervention Group (n = 35)	Control Group (n = 30)	p-Value [2]
Data [1] on children				
Age (years)	9.7 (0.2)	9.8 (0.3)	9.6 (0.2)	0.447
Dietary energy intake (kcal/day)	1535.6 (81.3)	1552.2 (65.6)	1548.3 (74.1)	0.969
Dietary protein intake (% of kcal)	18.5 (0.6)	18.3 (0.9)	19.2 (1.0)	0.511
Dietary carbohydrates intake (% of kcal)	47.4 (1.5)	47.1 (1.9)	46.3 (2.3)	0.790
Dietary fat intake (% of kcal)	35.4 (1.4)	36.2 (1.8)	35.6 (2.1)	0.840
Physical activity (min/day)	21.6 (2.3)	22.6 (3.0)	20.4 (3.5)	0.631
Birth weight (kg)	3.2 (0.1)	3.2 (0.1)	3.2 (0.1)	0.986
Recumbent length at birth (cm)	50.7 (0.4)	50.7 (0.5)	50.6 (0.6)	0.905
Body weight (kg)	51.9 (1.9)	54.3 (2.4)	48.6 (2.7)	0.127
BMI (kg/m^2)	25.1 (0.5)	25.6 (0.7)	25.2 (0.7)	0.172
Overweight children (%)	39.3	42.4	35.7	0.593
Obese children (%)	60.7	57.6	64.3	0.593
Height (cm)	142.4 (1.4)	143.5 (1.9)	141.3 (2.0)	0.415
Waist circumference (cm)	79.9 (1.5)	81.0 (2.3)	78.3 (2.1)	0.388
Data [1] on parents				
Mother's pre-pregnancy BMI (kg/m^2)	24.9 (0.4)	23.8 (0.7)	26.2 (1.0)	0.055
Obese mothers before pregnancy (%)	15.5	9.1	24.0	0.163
Father's age (years)	46.1 (0.3)	45.5 (0.8)	46.7 (1.0)	0.341
Mother's age (years)	41.2 (0.3)	40.9 (0.9)	41.6 (1.0)	0.656
Mother's education < 9 years (%)	24.6	24.2	25.0	0.535
Mother's education > 12 years (%)	42.6	48.5	35.7	0.535
Father's BMI (kg/m^2)	28.6 (0.4)	29.1 (1.0)	28.1 (0.9)	0.452
Obese father (%)	27.6	37.5	15.4	0.084
Mother's BMI (kg/m^2)	27.3 (0.4)	26.0 (0.8)	28.9 (1.2)	**0.045**
Obese mother (%)	31.6	24.2	41.7	0.303

[1] Data are presented as Mean (SEM) in the case of continuous variables and as percentages (%) in the case of categorical variables, [2] p-values derived from Student's t-test or the non-parametric Mann-Whitney test in the case of continues variables and the Pearson chi-square test in the case of categorical variables. Figures in bold highlight statistically significant p-values.

The mean (SEM) values at baseline and follow-up examination, as well as the mean (95% CI) changes from baseline to follow-up, for both study groups with regards to children's dietary intake of energy, macro- and micro-nutrients are presented in Table 3. Regarding dietary energy intake, no significant differences were observed between groups regarding the changes from baseline to follow-up, despite the decrease observed in the IG and the increase in the CG. As far as macronutrient intake was concerned, the increase observed in the IG for dietary fibre intake (4.1, 95% CI: 1.4 to 6.8) was higher than the non-significant change recorded in the CG (p = 0.005). In addition, sucrose intake decreased significantly only in the IG (−4.6, 95% CI: −8.8 to −0.3), although no significant differences were observed between study groups. Regarding micronutrient intake, significant increases were observed in the IG for iron (2.6, 95% CI: 0.2 to 5.0), zinc (1.7, 95% CI: 0.1 to 3.3) and magnesium intake (36.6, 95% CI: 9.4 to 63.8). In the case of magnesium, the significant increase observed in the IG was also higher than the change observed in the CG (p = 0.011). Lastly, a significant decrease was observed for vitamin C intake in the CG (−28.4, 95% CI: −53.6 to −3.1), although no group difference was found with regards to the changes from baseline to follow-up. No other significant changes within groups or differences between study groups were observed in the dietary intake of the rest of macro- and micro-nutrients, despite the fact that some of the changes were more favourable in the IG than the CG (e.g., for calcium, potassium, sodium, vitamin A and vitamin D).

Table 3. Changes in dietary intake indices from baseline to follow-up.

	Baseline Mean (SEM)	Follow-Up Mean (SEM)	Mean Change (95% CI) (Time Effect)	p-Value [†]
Dietary energy intake (kcal/day)				0.207
Intervention Group (n = 35)	1552.2 (65.6)	1467.6 (73.5)	−84.7 (−229.7 to 60.3)	
Control Group (n = 30)	1548.3 (74.1)	1605.9 (83.0)	57.6 (−106.3 to 221.5)	
p-value (Treatment effect)	0.969	0.225		
Dietary protein intake (% of kcal)				0.712
Intervention Group (n = 35)	18.3 (0.9)	17.5 (1.0)	−0.8 (−3.1 to 1.5)	
Control Group (n = 30)	19.2 (1.0)	19.1 (1.1)	−0.1 (−2.8 to 2.1)	
p-value	0.511	0.308		
Dietary carbohydrates intake (% of kcal)				0.777
Intervention Group (n = 35)	47.1 (1.9)	46.4 (1.6)	−0.7 (−4.5 to 3.1)	
Control Group (n = 30)	46.3 (2.3)	44.7 (1.9)	−1.6 (−6.1 to 2.9)	
p-value (Treatment effect)	0.790	0.514		
Dietary fat intake (% of kcal)				0.796
Intervention Group (n = 35)	37.5 (1.7)	36.2 (1.8)	−1.3 (−4.8 to 2.2)	
Control Group (n = 30)	35.6 (2.1)	37.7 (2.0)	2.1 (−2.1 to 6.2)	
p-value (Treatment effect)	0.840	0.953		
Saturated fat intake (% of kcal)				0.123
Intervention Group (n = 35)	13.0 (0.8)	12.6 (0.7)	−0.4 (−2.0 to 1.2)	
Control Group (n = 30)	12.9 (0.9)	14.4 (0.8)	1.5 (−0.3 to 3.3)	
p-value (Treatment effect)	0.887	0.099		
Dietary cholesterol intake (mg/day)				0.733
Intervention Group (n = 35)	288.9 (25.2)	245.1 (27.5)	−43.6 (−112.7 to 25.5)	
Control Group (n = 30)	239.0 (22.3)	211.5 (24.4)	−27.5 (−88.6 to 33.6)	
p-value (Treatment effect)	0.152	0.373		
Dietary fibre intake (g/day)				**0.047**
Intervention Group (n = 35)	13.0 (1.2)	17.1 (1.5)	**4.1 (1.4 to 6.8)**	
Control Group (n = 30)	11.9 (1.3)	12.0 (1.7)	0.2 (−2.9 to 3.3)	
p-value (Treatment effect)	0.534	**0.033**		
Sucrose intake (g/day)				0.680
Intervention Group (n = 35)	16.0 (2.4)	11.4 (1.6)	**−4.6 (−8.8 to −0.3)**	
Control Group (n = 30)	11.9 (2.7)	8.7 (1.8)	−3.2 (−8.0 to 1.7)	
p-value (Treatment effect)	0.279	0.267		

Table 3. Cont.

	Baseline Mean (SEM)	Follow-Up Mean (SEM)	Mean Change (95% CI) (Time Effect)	p-Value [†]
Calcium intake (mg/day)				0.067
Intervention Group (n = 35)	769.0 (143.6)	913.8 (60.1)	144.9 (−165.0 to 454.6)	
Control Group (n = 30)	1203.3 (162.4)	903.9 (67.9)	−299.3 (−649.5 to 50.9)	
p-value (Treatment effect)	0.053	0.915		
Iron intake (mg/day)				0.099
Intervention Group (n = 35)	10.7 (0.9)	13.3 (1.0)	**2.6 (0.2 to 5.0)**	
Control Group (n = 30)	11.9 (1.3)	11.4 (1.1)	−0.5 (−3.2 to 2.2)	
p-value (Treatment effect)	0.370	0.211		
Potassium intake (mg/day)				0.116
Intervention Group (n = 35)	1888.1 (141.6)	2052.6 (147.3)	169.5 (−110.4 to 449.4)	
Control Group (n = 30)	2119.2 (160.1)	1945.6 (166.5)	−173.6 (−490.0 to 142.7)	
p-value (Treatment effect)	0.292	0.622		
Magnesium intake (mg/day)				**0.011**
Intervention Group (n = 35)	192.1 (13.2)	228.7 (13.4)	**36.6 (9.4 to 63.8)**	
Control Group (n = 30)	228.0 (14.9)	209.8 (15.1)	−18.2 (−49.0 to 12.5)	
p-value (Treatment effect)	0.081	0.359		
Zinc intake (mg/day)				0.066
Intervention Group (n = 35)	7.6 (0.6)	9.3 (0.7)	**1.7 (0.1 to 3.3)**	
Control Group (n = 30)	9.6 (0.7)	9.0 (0.8)	−0.6 (−2.3 to 1.2)	
p-value (Treatment effect)	0.031	0.768		
Sodium intake (mg/day)				0.135
Intervention Group (n = 35)	1717.1 (210.4)	1426.2 (129.2)	−290.9 (−745.4 to 163.7)	
Control Group (n = 30)	1550.4 (237.8)	1788.3 (146.1)	238.0 (−275.9 to 751.8)	
p-value (Treatment effect)	0.608	0.073		
Vitamin A intake (RE/day)				0.137
Intervention Group (n = 35)	616.7 (122.9)	888.2 (243.5)	271.5 (−256.1 to 799.1)	
Control Group (n = 30)	670.4 (139.0)	330.5 (275.3)	−339.9 (−936.2 to 256.5)	
p-value (Treatment effect)	0.777	0.141		
Vitamin C intake (µg/day)				0.655
Intervention Group (n = 35)	81.5 (11.3)	60.9 (8.9)	−20.6 (−42.9 to 1.7)	
Control Group (n = 30)	70.2 (12.9)	41.9 (10.0)	**−28.4 (−53.6 to −3.1)**	
p-value (Treatment effect)	0.522	0.168		
Vitamin D intake (IU/day)				0.120
Intervention Group (n = 35)	93.2 (21.3)	107.9 (16.6)	14.6 (−29.2 to 58.4)	
Control Group (n = 30)	145.2 (24.1)	106.8 (18.7)	−38.4 (−87.9 to 11.1)	
p-value (Treatment effect)	0.117	0.965		

[†] p-values indicate the significance of the treatment × time interaction effects; adjustments were made for maternal BMI. Figures in bold highlight statistically significant p-values or statistically significant mean changes from baseline to follow-up.

Table 4 depicts the changes in the consumption of specific food items and the relevant differences between the two study groups. More specifically, children in the IG had a higher mean consumption of cereals at follow-up than children in the CG (0.78 (0.11) vs. 0.43 (0.12), p = 0.041). In addition, the consumption of yogurt decreased significantly only in the CG (−0.23, 95% CI: −0.42 to −0.50), while the consumption of chocolates (−0.32, 95% CI: −0.52 to −0.11), cakes (−0.13, 95% CI: −0.23 to −0.02) and chips (−0.08, 95% CI: −0.13 to −0.03) decreased significantly only in the IG. The changes observed for the consumption of yogurt (p = 0.005) and chocolates (p = 0.025) were significantly different between the two study groups.

Table 4. Food intake from baseline to follow-up.

	Baseline Mean (SEM)	Follow-Up Mean (SEM)	Mean Change (95% CI) (Time Effect)	p-Value [†]
Fruits intake (portions/day)				0.236
Intervention Group (n = 35)	1.14 (0.15)	1.26 (0.14)	0.12 (−0.18 to 0.41)	
Control Group (n = 30)	1.25 (0.18)	1.09 (0.17)	−0.16 (−0.52 to 0.19)	
p-value (Treatment effect)	0.643	0.455		
Vegetables intake (portions/day)				0.941
Intervention Group (n = 35)	0.94 (0.11)	0.93 (0.07)	−0.01 (−0.25 to 0.23)	
Control Group (n = 30)	0.87 (0.13)	0.88 (0.09)	0.03 (−0.27 to 0.29)	
p-value (Treatment effect)	0.701	0.665		
Cereals intake (portions/day)				0.446
Intervention Group (n = 35)	0.62 (0.10)	0.78 (0.11)	0.16 (−0.09 to 0.41)	
Control Group (n = 30)	0.42 (0.12)	0.43 (0.12)	−0.01 (−0.29 to 0.30)	
p-value (Treatment effect)	0.208	**0.041**		
Fish intake (portions/day)				0.502
Intervention Group (n = 35)	0.16 (0.02)	0.35 (0.11)	0.19 (−0.04 to 0.41)	
Control Group (n = 30)	0.15 (0.02)	0.22 (0.13)	0.07 (−0.20 to 0.33)	
p-value (Treatment effect)	0.565	0.440		
Milk intake (portions/day)				0.272
Intervention Group (n = 35)	1.05 (0.11)	1.17 (0.15)	0.11 (−0.21 to 0.43)	
Control Group (n = 30)	1.02 (0.17)	1.18 (0.13)	0.17 (−0.21 to 0.54)	
p-value (Treatment effect)	0.819	0.955		
Yogurt intake (portions/day)				**0.005**
Intervention Group (n = 35)	0.22 (0.07)	0.34 (0.04)	0.12 (−0.04 to 0.27)	
Control Group (n = 30)	0.50 (0.08)	0.26 (0.04)	**−0.23 (−0.42 to −0.50)**	
p-value (Treatment effect)	**0.017**	0.177		
Chocolates intake (portions/day)				**0.025**
Intervention Group (n = 35)	0.70 (0.09)	0.39 (0.06)	**−0.32 (−0.52 to −0.11)**	
Control Group (n = 30)	0.55 (0.10)	0.59 (0.08)	0.05 (−0.19 to 0.28)	
p-value (Treatment effect)	0.268	**0.044**		
Fizzy drinks intake (portions/day)				0.707
Intervention Group (n = 35)	0.08 (0.03)	0.08 (0.03)	0.004 (−0.05 to 0.06)	
Control Group (n = 30)	0.11 (0.03)	0.10 (0.03)	−0.01 (−0.08 to 0.06)	
p-value (Treatment effect)	0.366	0.676		
Cakes intake (portions/day)				0.317
Intervention Group (n = 35)	0.18 (0.05)	0.05 (0.01)	**−0.13 (−0.23 to −0.02)**	
Control Group (n = 30)	0.10 (0.07)	0.06 (0.01)	−0.04 (−0.17 to 0.08)	
p-value (Treatment effect)	0.268	**0.044**		
Chips intake (portions/day)				0.397
Intervention Group (n = 35)	0.14 (0.03)	0.06 (0.01)	**−0.08 (−0.13 to −0.03)**	
Control Group (n = 30)	0.09 (0.03)	0.04 (0.01)	−0.05 (−0.11 to 0.02)	
p-value (Treatment effect)	0.249	0.221		

[†] p-values indicate the significance of the treatment × time interaction effects; adjustments were made for maternal BMI. Figures in bold highlight statistically significant p-values or statistically significant mean changes from baseline to follow-up.

The changes from baseline to follow-up, as well as the differences between study groups with regards to anthropometric indices are presented in Table 5. Body weight and WC increased significantly only in the CG by 1.4 kg (95% CI 0.3 to 2.6) and 2.1 cm (95% CI 0.7 to 3.5), respectively, height increased significantly in both study groups by 2.0 cm (95% CI 1.5 to 2.5) in the IG and by 1.6 cm (95% CI 1.0 to 2.1) in the CG, while BMI and BMI z-score decreased significantly only in the IG by 0.4 kg (95% CI −0.9 to −0.1) and 0.2 standard deviations (−0.3 to 0.05). Nevertheless, these changes were not found to differentiate significantly between the two study groups.

Table 5. Anthropometric indices from baseline to follow-up.

	Baseline Mean (SEM)	Follow-Up Mean (SEM)	Mean Change (95% CI) (Time Effect)	p-Value [†]
Body weight (kg)				0.360
Intervention Group (n = 35)	54.3 (2.4)	55.0 (2.4)	0.7 (−0.3 to 1.7)	
Control Group (n = 30)	48.6 (2.7)	50.0 (2.7)	**1.4 (0.3 to 2.6)**	
p-value (Treatment effect)	0.127	0.174		
Height (cm)				0.120
Intervention Group (n = 35)	143.5 (1.9)	145.5 (1.8)	**2.0 (1.5 to 2.5)**	
Control Group (n = 30)	141.3 (2.0)	142.7 (2.0)	**1.6 (1.0 to 2.1)**	
p-value (Treatment effect)	0.415	0.304		
BMI (kg/m^2)				0.112
Intervention Group (n = 35)	25.6 (0.7)	25.2 (0.7)	**−0.4 (−0.9 to −0.1)**	
Control Group (n = 30)	24.1 (0.9)	24.3 (0.8)	0.2 (−0.4 to 0.8)	
p-value (Treatment effect)	0.172	0.389		
BMI z-score				0.318
Intervention Group (n = 35)	2.6 (0.2)	2.5 (0.1)	−0.2 (−0.3 to 0.05)	
Control Group (n = 30)	2.8 (0.2)	2.8 (0.2)	0.1 (−0.02 to 0.2)	
p-value (Treatment effect)				
Waist circumference (cm)				0.144
Intervention Group (n = 35)	81.0 (2.3)	81.6 (2.3)	0.6 (−0.9 to 2.1)	
Control Group (n = 30)	78.3 (2.1)	80.4 (2.1)	**2.1 (0.7 to 3.5)**	
p-value (Treatment effect)	0.388	0.705		

[†] p-values indicate the significance of the treatment × time interaction effects; adjustments were made for maternal BMI. Figures in bold highlight statistically significant p-values or statistically significant mean changes from baseline to follow-up.

4. Discussion

The current randomised controlled trial showed that a computerised DST designed to assist paediatric healthcare professionals in providing personalised nutrition and lifestyle optimisation recommendations to overweight or obese children and their parents, can result in favourable changes to certain dietary intake and anthropometric indices in the children that received the intervention. The findings of this study support the growing, although still limited, body of evidence regarding the effectiveness of computerised or eHealth DSTs used in primary care settings for improving clinicians' performance on childhood obesity management outcomes [22,23].

Health professionals have the potential to influence large numbers of patients. Up to date there has been little evidence on how clinical practice can be enhanced in order to assist children (and their parents) in achieving appropriate to their weight status and sustainable weight management. The role of new technology, through the development of appropriate computerised or e-Health tools, seems to be the way forward. Although there are currently several computerised or e-Health tools designed to promote personalised advice on weight management in children, the vast majority of those do not involve health professionals in the implementation process [24]. Even in the case of e-Health tools that are targeting health professionals, in most of the occasions their usability has been described as difficult [22,24]. As such, in the HopSCOTCH Shared-Care Obesity Trial in Australia, the general practitioners (GPs) that used the relevant e-Health tool to deliver the personalised intervention to children and their parents, characterised implementation as challenging and usability of the tool as poor, mainly due to technical reasons, such as out-dated hardware, software installation difficulties and poor internet connections [22].

Despite the scarcity of tools supporting paediatric healthcare professionals on children's weight management, Taveras et al. [23,25] developed a computerised tool very similar to the DST developed in the current study. The effectiveness of this tool was examined in the "Study of Technology to Accelerate Research" (STAR), which was a three-arm, cluster-randomised controlled trial that was implemented in 14 paediatric offices in Massachusetts and on 800, 6 to 12-year-old, obese children [25]. After 12 months of intervention, the STAR trial reported a lower increase in BMI in children randomised in the study group that received the personalised advice via the use of the DST by paediatric healthcare professionals compared to the control group that received the usual care offered in the participating paediatric offices (mean adjusted BMI change difference: -0.51 kg/m^2; 95% CI -0.91 to -0.11) [23]. The aforementioned results of the STAR study agree with the findings of our study, which -although they included a smaller sample size of 65 children and had a shorter duration of 3 months- reported a mean adjusted BMI change difference of -0.6 kg/m^2 in the IG, compared to the CG. Similarly to the STAR trial, the effect of the intervention implemented in the current study on BMI also exceeded the mean adjusted change difference observed in other primary-care intervention trials, such as the "Live, Eat and Play" (LEAP) study (mean adjusted BMI change difference: -0.20 after 9 months) [26], the LEAP-2 study (mean adjusted BMI change difference: -0.11 after 12 months) [27] and the "Shared-Care Obesity Trial in Children" (HopSCOTCH) study (mean adjusted BMI change difference: (-0.10 after 12 months) [28]. In addition to BMI, the significant increase in waist circumference observed only in the CG is another indication of the effectiveness of the current RCT in controlling children's central body fat deposition more effectively than in the CG. The mean adjusted difference of -1.5 cm observed in this study, in the changes of WC between the IG and the CG, is similar to the relevant difference of -1.7 cm, observed in the HopSCOTCH study. However, considering that the HopSCOTCH study was also conducted with a greater sample size (i.e., 107 children) and had a longer duration (i.e., 12 months), this probably highlights the promising potential of the tools that were developed and tested in this study, with regards to the effective management of childhood obesity.

The changes observed in the IG on BMI and WC, could be partly a reflection of the relevant favourable dietary changes recorded for the IG, compared to the CG. In this regard, the higher increase in dietary fibre intake in the IG than the CG and the significant decrease of dietary sucrose intake only in the IG are probably indicative of the effectiveness of the intervention in increasing the consumption of high-fibre foods that promote satiety and at the same time in decreasing the consumption of foods with a high sugar and, thus, high energy content. The aforementioned changes were also evidenced by the higher consumption of cereals at follow-up in the IG than the CG, as well as the significant decrease in the consumption of chocolates and cakes only in the IG. The above, in conjunction with the decrease in the consumption of chips in the IG, could possibly provide a basis that supports a lower dietary energy intake and consequently the favourable anthropometric changes observed for children in the IG. In line with the findings of the present study, the HopSCOTCH study also reported a higher diet quality score (reflected by the higher consumption of fruit, vegetables and water and by the lower consumption of fatty/sugary foods and non-diet sweet drinks) among 3–10-year-old obese children that received dietary and lifestyle optimisation advice for their weight management through a web-based software [28]. The fact that the HopSCOTCH study reported no significant differences between groups in the change of children's physical activity levels from baseline to follow-up, indicates that any favourable changes observed in this study on the examined anthropometric indices are mainly attributed to the improvement of dietary habits in the intervention compared to the control treatment arm. To some extent, the same also applies in our study, as physical activity levels did not differentiate between the IG and the CG (data not shown).

Obesity in children has been strongly linked to important micronutrient insufficiencies, which is usually the outcome of a chronic, low-grade inflammation induced by the elevated levels of visceral adipose tissue [2]. As such, the DST was designed to assist children that received the personalised advice to achieve, not only a better management of their body weight, but also a higher intake of several essential micronutrients. This was evidenced by the significant increases in the dietary intakes of iron, magnesium and zinc observed only in the IG, which can correct potential obesity-related insufficiencies [3] and can subsequently support children's growth, motor and cognitive function [29–31]. In addition, since hypertension is another common comorbidity of obesity in children [32], the dietary recommendations provided to children (particularly to those diagnosed with elevated blood pressure) and their parents via the DST, were also aiming to reduce the use of table salt, as well as the consumption of foods that are rich sources of salt in the diet. The significant decrease in dietary sodium intake observed in the present study only in the IG provides evidence that this additional aim of the intervention was partially achieved.

Our study has both strengths and limitations. The main strength was its randomised controlled design resulting in a homogeneity of children's characteristics at baseline in both treatment arms. Another strength was the use of the DST to guide clinicians on effectively managing children's elevated body weight, by accurately assessing their nutritional status and needs and by providing appropriate dietary and lifestyle optimisation advice to children and their families, encouraging family self-management of behavioural changes. As evidenced by the current and the STAR study [23], intervention approaches that involve self-guided behavioural changes by families may be better suited to sustain the intensity required for effective behavioural change than those that primarily rely on healthcare professionals to deliver the main bulk of the intervention [27]. In this context, the meal plans delivered by the health professionals to the families in the present study were only a guide for healthier eating and not a prescriptive pathway that was compulsory for the children and their families to follow. The emphasis was given mainly to the recommendations and how families can adopt and embed as many of these suggestions as possible to their daily life. Regarding additional strengths, according to qualitative feedback collected from the clinicians that used the DST, the paediatricians reported that the tool was quite easy to use (it runs with Microsoft Excel and/or Access) and represented a well-structured and quick procedure that helped them provide tailored advice to children and families. As far as limitations are concerned, although the study initially recruited 80 children, only 65 were examined at follow-up, resulting in a drop-out rate of approximately 19%. Nevertheless, the fact that only 5 out of 15 study participants that dropped out were originally allocated to the IG is an indication that the intervention was better accepted, increasing retention rates in the IG children and their families, compared to the CG that received only generic advice.

5. Conclusions

The current study showed that a computerised DST, designed to support paediatric healthcare professionals in the delivery of personalised diet and lifestyle optimisation advice to overweight or obese children and their families, resulted in improvement of the children's dietary intake and BMI. These changes are indicative of the dynamics of the tool in supporting clinicians to improve the effectiveness of care. Interventions of longer duration and larger sample sizes are needed to confirm the findings of our study and to demonstrate their long-term sustainability.

Supplementary Materials: The following are available online at http://www.mdpi.com/2072-6643/11/3/706/s1, Figure S1: Decision-tree algorithms, Table S1: Dietary and Lifestyle Optimisation Recommendations, Table S2: Weekly Meal Plans.

Author Contributions: Conceptualization and project administration, G.M. and Y.M.; Methodology preparation, software preparation, statistical analyses and funding acquisition, G.M.; Investigation, G.M., M.M., E.V., S.M., E.C., G.P.C. and Y.M.; Resources, G.M., E.V., S.M., E.C., G.P.C., K.T. and Y.M.; writing—original draft preparation, All authors; supervision, G.M., M.M., E.V., S.M., E.C., G.P.C. and Y.M.

Funding: This research is implemented through IKY scholarships programme and co-financed by the European Union (European Social Fund—ESF) and Greek national funds through the action entitled "Reinforcement of Postdoctoral Researchers", in the framework of the Operational Programme "Human Resources Development Program, Education and Lifelong Learning" of the National Strategic Reference Framework (NSRF) 2014–2020.

Acknowledgments: The authors would like to thank all research members involved in the data collection as well as all study participants for their collaboration. The authors would also like to thank Konstantina Tsoutsoulopoulou, dietitian, and Sofia Tanagra, nutrition expert, for their contribution in the development of the personalised recommendations and meal plans at the different caloric levels.

Conflicts of Interest: The authors declare no conflict of interest.

References

1. Waxman, A. WHO global strategy on diet, physical activity and health. *Food Nutr. Bull.* **2004**, *25*, 292–302. [CrossRef]

2. Subramanian, V.; Ferrante, A.W., Jr. Obesity, inflammation, and macrophages. *Nestle Nutr. Workshop Ser. Pediatr. Program* **2009**, *63*, 151–159.
3. Manios, Y.; Moschonis, G.; Chrousos, G.P.; Lionis, C.; Mougios, V.; Kantilafti, M.; Tzotzola, V.; Skenderi, K.P.; Petridou, A.; Tsalis, G.; et al. The double burden of obesity and iron deficiency on children and adolescents in Greece: The Healthy Growth Study. *J. Hum. Nutr. Diet.* **2013**, *26*, 470–478. [CrossRef] [PubMed]
4. Moschonis, G.; Androutsos, O.; Hulshof, T.; Dracopoulou, M.; Chrousos, G.P.; Manios, Y. Vitamin D insufficiency is associated with insulin resistance independently of obesity in primary schoolchildren. The healthy growth study. *Pediatr. Diabetes* **2018**, *19*, 866–873. [CrossRef] [PubMed]
5. Dombrowski, S.U.; Knittle, K.; Avenell, A.; Araujo-Soares, V.; Sniehotta, F.F. Long term maintenance of weight loss with non-surgical interventions in obese adults: Systematic review and meta-analyses of randomised controlled trials. *BMJ* **2014**, *348*, g2646. [CrossRef] [PubMed]
6. Birbilis, M.; Moschonis, G.; Mougios, V.; Manios, Y. Obesity in adolescence is associated with perinatal risk factors, parental BMI and sociodemographic characteristics. *Eur. J. Clin. Nutr.* **2013**, *67*, 115–121. [CrossRef] [PubMed]
7. Desai, M.; Beall, M.; Ross, M.G. Developmental origins of obesity: Programmed adipogenesis. *Curr. Diab. Rep.* **2013**, *13*, 27–33. [CrossRef]
8. Booth, H.P.; Prevost, T.A.; Wright, A.J.; Gulliford, M.C. Effectiveness of behavioural weight loss interventions delivered in a primary care setting: A systematic review and meta-analysis. *Fam. Pract.* **2014**, *31*, 643–653. [CrossRef]
9. Dattilo, A.M.; Birch, L.; Krebs, N.F.; Lake, A.; Taveras, E.M.; Saavedra, J.M. Need for early interventions in the prevention of pediatric overweight: A review and upcoming directions. *J. Obes.* **2012**, *2012*, 123023. [CrossRef] [PubMed]
10. Vignolo, M.; Rossi, F.; Bardazza, G.; Pistorio, A.; Parodi, A.; Spigno, S.; Torrisi, C.; Gremmo, M.; Veneselli, E.; Aicardi, G. Five-year follow-up of a cognitive-behavioural lifestyle multidisciplinary programme for childhood obesity outpatient treatment. *Eur. J. Clin. Nutr.* **2008**, *62*, 1047–1057. [CrossRef]
11. Visram, S.; Hall, T.D.; Geddes, L. Getting the balance right: Qualitative evaluation of a holistic weight management intervention to address childhood obesity. *J. Public Health* **2013**, *35*, 246–254. [CrossRef] [PubMed]
12. Barratt, J. Diet-related knowledge, beliefs and actions of health professionals compared with the general population: An investigation in a community Trust. *J. Hum. Nutr. Diet.* **2001**, *14*, 25–32. [CrossRef] [PubMed]
13. Hankey, C.R.; Eley, S.; Leslie, W.S.; Hunter, C.M.; Lean, M.E.J. Eating habits, beliefs, attitudes and knowledge among health professionals regarding the links between obesity, nutrition and health. *Public Health Nutr.* **2007**, *7*, 337–343. [CrossRef] [PubMed]
14. World Health Organization. Nutrition for Health and Development. In *WHO Child Growth Standards: Length/Height-for-Age, Weight-for-Age, Weight-for-Length, Weight-for-Height and Body Mass Index-for-Age: Methods and Development*; World Health Organization: Geneva, Switzerland, 2006.
15. Manios, Y.; Birbilis, M.; Moschonis, G.; Birbilis, G.; Mougios, V.; Lionis, C.; Chrousos, G.P.; Healthy Growth Study Group. Childhood Obesity Risk Evaluation based on perinatal factors and family sociodemographic characteristics: CORE index. *Eur. J. Pediatr.* **2013**, *172*, 551–555. [CrossRef] [PubMed]
16. Manios, Y.; Vlachopapadopoulou, E.; Moschonis, G.; Karachaliou, F.; Psaltopoulou, T.; Koutsouki, D.; Bogdanis, G.; Carayanni, V.; Hatzakis, A.; Michalacos, S. Utility and applicability of the "Childhood Obesity Risk Evaluation" (CORE)-index in predicting obesity in childhood and adolescence in Greece from early life: The "National Action Plan for Public Health". *Eur. J. Pediatr.* **2016**, *175*, 1989–1996. [CrossRef] [PubMed]
17. Barlow, S.E.; Expert, C. Expert committee recommendations regarding the prevention, assessment, and treatment of child and adolescent overweight and obesity: Summary report. *Pediatrics* **2007**, *120*, S164–S192. [CrossRef]
18. Institute of Medicine. *Dietary Reference Intakes for Energy, Carbohydrate, Fiber, Fat, Fatty Acids, Cholesterol, Protein and Amino Acids*; National Academies Press: Washington, DC, USA, 2005.
19. National Dietary Guidelines for Infants, Children and Adolescents. Available online: http://www.diatrofikoiodigoi.gr/?page=summary-children (accessed on 18 January 2018).

20. Manios, Y.; Androutsos, O.; Lambrinou, C.P.; Cardon, G.; Lindstrom, J.; Annemans, L.; Mateo-Gallego, R.; de Sabata, M.S.; Iotova, V.; Kivela, J.; et al. A school- and community-based intervention to promote healthy lifestyle and prevent type 2 diabetes in vulnerable families across Europe: Design and implementation of the Feel4Diabetes-study. *Public Health Nutr.* **2018**, *21*, 3281–3290. [CrossRef]
21. Roumelioti, M.; Leotsinidis, M. Relative validity of a semiquantitative food frequency questionnaire designed for schoolchildren in western Greece. *Nutr. J.* **2009**, *8*, 8. [CrossRef] [PubMed]
22. Lycett, K.; Wittert, G.; Gunn, J.; Hutton, C.; Clifford, S.A.; Wake, M. The challenges of real-world implementation of web-based shared care software: The HopSCOTCH Shared-Care Obesity Trial in Children. *BMC Med. Inform. Decis. Mak.* **2014**, *14*, 61. [CrossRef]
23. Taveras, E.M.; Marshall, R.; Kleinman, K.P.; Gillman, M.W.; Hacker, K.; Horan, C.M.; Smith, R.L.; Price, S.; Sharifi, M.; Rifas-Shiman, S.L.; et al. Comparative effectiveness of childhood obesity interventions in pediatric primary care: A cluster-randomized clinical trial. *JAMA Pediatr.* **2015**, *169*, 535–542. [CrossRef]
24. Flodgren, G.; Goncalves-Bradley, D.C.; Summerbell, C.D. Interventions to change the behaviour of health professionals and the organisation of care to promote weight reduction in children and adults with overweight or obesity. *Cochrane Database Syst. Rev.* **2017**, *11*, CD000984. [CrossRef] [PubMed]
25. Taveras, E.M.; Marshall, R.; Horan, C.M.; Gillman, M.W.; Hacker, K.; Kleinman, K.P.; Koziol, R.; Price, S.; Simon, S.R. Rationale and design of the STAR randomized controlled trial to accelerate adoption of childhood obesity comparative effectiveness research. *Contemp. Clin. Trials* **2013**, *34*, 101–108. [CrossRef] [PubMed]
26. McCallum, Z.; Wake, M.; Gerner, B.; Baur, L.A.; Gibbons, K.; Gold, L.; Gunn, J.; Harris, C.; Naughton, G.; Riess, C.; et al. Outcome data from the LEAP (Live, Eat and Play) trial: A randomized controlled trial of a primary care intervention for childhood overweight/mild obesity. *Int. J. Obes.* **2007**, *31*, 630–636. [CrossRef] [PubMed]
27. Wake, M.; Baur, L.A.; Gerner, B.; Gibbons, K.; Gold, L.; Gunn, J.; Levickis, P.; McCallum, Z.; Naughton, G.; Sanci, L.; et al. Outcomes and costs of primary care surveillance and intervention for overweight or obese children: The LEAP 2 randomised controlled trial. *BMJ* **2009**, *339*, b3308. [CrossRef] [PubMed]
28. Wake, M.; Lycett, K.; Clifford, S.A.; Sabin, M.A.; Gunn, J.; Gibbons, K.; Hutton, C.; McCallum, Z.; Arnup, S.J.; Wittert, G. Shared care obesity management in 3–10 year old children: 12 month outcomes of HopSCOTCH randomised trial. *BMJ* **2013**, *346*, f3092. [CrossRef]
29. Huma, N.; Salim Ur, R.; Anjum, F.M.; Murtaza, M.A.; Sheikh, M.A. Food fortification strategy—Preventing iron deficiency anemia: A review. *Crit. Rev. Food Sci. Nutr.* **2007**, *47*, 259–265. [CrossRef]
30. Kawade, R. Zinc status and its association with the health of adolescents: A review of studies in India. *Glob. Health Action* **2012**, *5*, 7353. [CrossRef] [PubMed]
31. Kurpad, A.V.; Edward, B.S.; Aeberli, I. Micronutrient supply and health outcomes in children. *Curr. Opin. Clin. Nutr. Metab. Care* **2013**, *16*, 328–338. [CrossRef] [PubMed]
32. Manios, Y.; Karatzi, K.; Moschonis, G.; Ioannou, G.; Androutsos, O.; Lionis, C.; Chrousos, G. Lifestyle, anthropometric, socio-demographic and perinatal correlates of early adolescence hypertension: The Healthy Growth Study. *Nutr. Metab. Cardiovasc. Dis.* **2018**. [CrossRef]

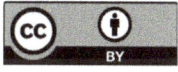

© 2019 by the authors. Licensee MDPI, Basel, Switzerland. This article is an open access article distributed under the terms and conditions of the Creative Commons Attribution (CC BY) license (http://creativecommons.org/licenses/by/4.0/).

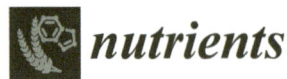

Article

The Type 2 Diabetes Susceptibility PROX1 Gene Variants Are Associated with Postprandial Plasma Metabolites Profile in Non-Diabetic Men

Edyta Adamska-Patruno [1],*, Joanna Godzien [1], Michal Ciborowski [1], Paulina Samczuk [1], Witold Bauer [1], Katarzyna Siewko [2], Maria Gorska [2], Coral Barbas [3] and Adam Kretowski [1,2]

1. Clinical Research Centre, Medical University of Bialystok, 15-089 Bialystok, Poland; joannagodzien@gmail.com (J.G.); michal.ciborowski@umb.edu.pl (M.C.); paulina.samczuk@gmail.com (P.S.); witold.bauer@umb.edu.pl (W.B.); adamkretowski@wp.pl (A.K.)
2. Department of Endocrinology, Diabetology and Internal Medicine, Medical University of Bialystok, 15-089 Bialystok, Poland; katarzynasiewko@o2.pl (K.S.); mgorska25@wp.pl (M.G.)
3. Center for Metabolomics and Bioanalysis (CEMBIO), Universidad CEU San Pablo, 28003 Madrid, Spain; cbarbas@ceu.es
* Correspondence: edyta.adamska@umb.edu.pl; Tel.: +48-85-746-8153

Received: 11 March 2019; Accepted: 17 April 2019; Published: 19 April 2019

Abstract: The prospero homeobox 1 (PROX1) gene may show pleiotropic effects on metabolism. We evaluated postprandial metabolic alterations dependently on the rs340874 genotypes, and 28 non-diabetic men were divided into two groups: high-risk (HR)-genotype (CC-genotype carriers, $n = 12$, 35.3 ± 9.5 years old) and low-risk (LR)-genotype (allele T carriers, $n = 16$, 36.3 ± 7.0 years old). Subjects participated in two meal-challenge-tests with high-carbohydrate (HC, carbohydrates 89%) and normo-carbohydrate (NC, carbohydrates 45%) meal intake. Fasting and 30, 60, 120, and 180 min after meal intake plasma samples were fingerprinted by liquid chromatography quadrupole time-of-flight mass spectrometry (LC-QTOF-MS). In HR-genotype men, the area under the curve (AUC) of acetylcarnitine levels was higher after the HC-meal [+92%, variable importance in the projection (VIP) = 2.88] and the NC-meal (+55%, VIP = 2.00) intake. After the NC-meal, the HR-risk genotype carriers presented lower AUCs of oxidized fatty acids (−81−66%, VIP = 1.43–3.16) and higher linoleic acid (+80%, VIP = 2.29), while after the HC-meal, they presented lower AUCs of ornithine (−45%, VIP = 1.83), sphingosine (−48%, VIP = 2.78), linoleamide (−45%, VIP = 1.51), and several lysophospholipids (−40−56%, VIP = 1.72–2.16). Moreover, lower AUC (−59%, VIP = 2.43) of taurocholate after the HC-meal and higher (+70%, VIP = 1.42) glycodeoxycholate levels after the NC-meal were observed. Our results revealed differences in postprandial metabolites from inflammatory and oxidative stress pathways, bile acids signaling, and lipid metabolism in PROX1 HR-genotype men. Further investigations of diet–genes interactions by which PROX1 may promote T2DM development are needed.

Keywords: nutrigenetics; nutrimetabolomics; high-carbohydrate meal; normo-carbohydrate meal; postprandial metabolic fingerprinting; ultra-high performance liquid chromatography; PROX1 gene; type 2 diabetes mellitus risk

---

1. Introduction

Type 2 diabetes mellitus (T2DM) is a major public health issue affecting 415 million people worldwide in 2015 [1], and it is expected that it will affect over 439 million people by 2030 [2] and 642 million by 2040 [1]. The T2DM is characterized by impaired β-cell function and insulin resistance, which leads to chronic hyperglycemia [3].

The Genome-Wide Association Studies (GWAS) and other, different scale meta-analyses and studies have indicated that the rs340874 single nucleotide polymorphism (SNP) in the prospero homeobox 1 (PROX1) gene is a strong genetic susceptibility factor for T2DM [4–6]. It has been shown that allele C of rs340874 is associated with reduced insulin sensitivity, β-cell function, insulin secretion, and fasting glucose levels [7–9]. PROX1 encodes a key transcription factor (TF), which is involved in the development of tissues such as pancreas [10]. It has been also suggested that reduced expression of PROX1 results in altered β-cell insulin secretion and thereby confers the T2DM susceptibility [5]. In one of our previous studies [11], we noted that carriers of the rs340874 PROX1 CC genotype presented higher free fatty acids levels after a high-fat meal intake and lower glucose utilization after a high-carbohydrate meal intake. Moreover, in subjects carrying the CC genotype, we found higher visceral fat accumulation despite lower daily food consumption, which indicates that another potential pathway may be involved in T2DM development in people at high genetic risk. Taken together, the studies show that PROX1 variants may have a pleiotropic effect on metabolism; however, the link between PROX1 and T2DM has not been established to date. Detailed characterization of PROX1 genetic variability can help to elucidate the role of PROX1 gene variations in T2DM development and to explore its potential pathways.

We hypothesize that one of the pathways involved in the T2DM development in subjects with the PROX1 rs340874 CC genotype may be a lipid metabolism path, and its further oxidative stress consequences can be modulated by different diets with varying macronutrients content. In our previous studies, we found that some subtle metabolism alterations are detectable only postprandially, and since most of the daytime people spend in the post absorptive state, the postprandial metabolism may play a crucial role in metabolic disorders development and/or progression [12]. We observed in our studied group that the differences in the postprandial metabolic response depend on many factors such as actual nutritional status [13–15] but also depend on genotype [11,16,17].

Studies carried out so far—as well as our own observations—indicate that the mechanisms by which the PROX1 gene affects the susceptibility to T2DM seem to be more complex. Therefore, for further investigation, we used the metabolomics approach. We used a liquid chromatography quadrupole time-of-flight mass spectrometry (LC-QTOF-MS) to evaluate postprandial changes in serum metabolites during the high-carbohydrate (HC) and normo-carbohydrate (NC) meal-challenge-tests in non-diabetic men dependent on the PROX1 rs340874 genotypes.

2. Materials and Methods

2.1. Subjects

The volunteers for our meal test study [14–17] were recruited from the 1000PLUS cohort study of Polish origin Caucasian population [11,18,19]. This trial was registered at www.clinicaltrials.gov as NCT03792685. Only males were enrolled into the meal-challenge-tests because of the possible sexual dimorphism of investigated factors [20]. The study participants ($n = 28$) were divided into 2 groups dependent on the PROX1 rs340874 genotypes: the homozygous carriers of high-risk (HR) allele C (CC genotype, $n = 12$) and carriers of low-risk (LR) allele T (both CT and TT genotypes, $n = 16$). None of the participants suffered from T2DM, prediabetes, or other disorders, nor did they report any treatments that might affect the tests results. Subjects who followed any special diet or dietary patterns (vegetarian, high-fat, etc.) were excluded from the experiment.

2.2. Ethics

The study procedures were conducted in accordance with all of the ethical standards of human experimentation and with the Declaration of Helsinki. The study protocol was approved by the local Ethics Committee (Medical University of Bialystok, Poland, R-I-002/35/2009), and before any study procedures, all of the participants signed informed consent.

2.3. Study Procedures

At the screening visit, the demographic data and anthropometric measurements, body weight, body composition analysis, oral glucose tolerance test (OGGT), and blood collections for biochemical and genotype analyses were performed as described previously [11,18]. Only men were enrolled into the meal-challenge-tests. Participants were instructed to maintain their regular lifestyle throughout the study and to avoid alcohol, coffee, and excessive physical exercise at least on the day before each test. The meal-challenge-test visits were conducted as described previously [14–17,21]. Briefly, the volunteers participated in two meal-challenge-tests visits in crossover design at an interval of 2–3 weeks. After an overnight fast, the participants arrived at the laboratory, and after fasting blood collection, they received (in random order) a standardized HC-meal (300 mL, Nutridrink Juice Style, Fat Free, Nutricia, Poland), which provided 450 kcal (89% of energy from carbohydrate, 11% from protein, and 0% from fat), or NC-meal (360mL, Cubitan, Nutricia, Poland), providing 450 kcal (45% of energy from carbohydrate, 30% from protein, and 25% from fat). During the whole experiment, men stayed in bed in a quiet room with thermoneutral conditions (22–25 °C). The metabolomics analyses were performed on plasma samples from the blood collected at fasting and at 30, 60, 120, and 180 min after meal intake.

2.4. Metabolomics Analysis

The metabolomics analysis is described in detail in the Supplementary Materials. Briefly, metabolic fingerprinting was performed on an HPLC system (1290 Infinity, Agilent Technologies, Santa Clara, CA, USA) coupled to an iFunnel Q-TOF (6550, Agilent Technologies, Santa Clara, CA, USA) mass spectrometer. Plasma samples were prepared and analyzed (in positive and negative ion modes) following previously described protocols and methods [22].

Data treatment included cleaning of background noise and unrelated ions through molecular feature extraction (MFE) tool in Mass Hunter Qualitative Analysis Software (B.06.00, Agilent, Santa Clara, CA, USA). Mass Profiler Professional (B.12.61, Agilent Technologies, Santa Clara, CA, USA) software was used to perform quality assurance (QA) procedure and data filtration. QA procedure covered a selection of metabolic features with good repeatability. To achieve the features detected in >80% in quality control (QC) samples and with RSD <30% (as calculated for the QC samples) in NC- and/or HC-meals, the dataset was kept for further data treatment. Additional data filtering was performed considering biological samples. Data were divided into ten sets with five time-points: 0, 30, 60, 120, and 180 min in two meal challenge groups. Metabolic features present in ≥80% of samples in at least one of these datasets were accepted. Moreover, a dedicated filtering for each comparison was performed—metabolic features present in a minimum of 80% of samples from one group were forwarded for statistical analysis. Detailed information about analytical conditions is available in the Supplementary Materials.

2.5. Calculations

Based on the relation between time points and the signal intensity of each metabolite, the areas under the curve (AUCs) were calculated using a trapezoid rule in R software environment (version 3.4.3, https://www.R-project.org/). The Homeostatic Model Assessment of Insulin Resistance (HOMA-IR) was calculated using the standard formula [23]:

$$\text{HOMA-IR} = \text{fasting plasma glucose concentration (mmol/L)} \times \text{fasting insulin concentration (µU/mL)}/22.5$$

The Homeostatic Model Assessment of β-cell function (HOMA-B) was calculated using the following formula [23]:

$$\text{HOMA-B} = 20 \times \text{fasting insulin (µU/mL)}/\text{fasting glucose (mmol/L)} - 3.5$$

2.6. Statistical Analysis

Statistical analysis was performed on each metabolite's mean AUCs within different strata. Patients with the HR-genotype (CC genotype) were compared to patients with the LR-genotype carrying the protective allele T (CT/TT genotypes) in rs340874 of the PROX1 gene. NC- and HC-meal groups were analyzed independently. Selection of statistically significant metabolites was performed implementing both, uni-, and multivariate analyses. For each significant metabolite, p-value was calculated in Matlab (MathWorks Inc.). The Shapiro-Wilk test was used for normality testing and then, dependent on the data distribution, the t-test or the Mann-Whitney test were performed. Partial least square discriminant analysis (PLS-DA) models were computed using the SIMCA software (Umetrics). Based on PLS-DA models, volcano plots were created plotting variable importance in the projection (VIP) against corrected p-values [p(corr), loading values scaled as correlation coefficients values]. Variables with VIP >1.0 and absolute p(corr) >0.4 were considered significant.

2.7. Identification

Statistically significant metabolites were annotated by matching the spectral data from public databases (HMDB, METLIN, and LIPIDMAPS) with spectral data obtained through MSMS (tandem MS—mass spectrometry) analysis for metabolites present in plasma samples. Detailed information about identified metabolites is included in the Supplementary Materials (Table S1).

3. Results

3.1. Baseline Characteristics

The baseline characteristic of the studied population is presented in Table 1. The studied genotypes groups were well matched without any between-group differences in age, anthropometric measurements, body mass index (BMI), body fat and fat free mass content, fasting glucose and insulin concentrations, HOMA-IR, HOMA-B, and glycated hemoglobin (HbA1c).

Table 1. The baseline characteristic of studied population by the rs340874 PROX1 genotypes.

	CC Genotype	CT/TT	p-Value *
Age (years)	35.3 ± 9.5	36.3 ± 7.0	0.75
Weight (kg)	93.6 ± 24.5	89.1 ± 16.1	0.95
Body mass index (BMI) (kg/m^2)	29.1 ± 8.1	27.3 ± 4.2	0.74
Body fat content (%)	23.8 ± 10.1	23.2 ± 7.8	0.87
Fat free mass (%)	69.6 ± 11.0	67.6 ± 8.3	0.60
Waist (cm)	99.6 ± 21.1	95.7 ± 13.6	0.77
Hip (cm)	104.3 ± 14.8	99.6 ± 8.7	0.76
WHR	0.9 ± 0.1	1.0 ± 0.1	0.81
Fasting glucose concentration (mg/dl)	86.2 ± 8.0	86.7 ± 6.4	0.85
Fasting insulin concentration (IU/mL)	10.4 ± 9.1	8.9 ± 5.4	0.84
HOMA-IR	2.2 ± 2.0	1.9 ± 1.3	0.81
HOMA-B	188.2 ± 163.3	143.7 ± 88.9	0.78
HbA1c	5.2 ± 0.5	5.2 ± 0.2	0.90

* For quantitative variables with normal distribution, the parametric t-test was used; for the other variables, the non-parametric Mann–Whitney test was applied. The data are represented as the mean ± STD, and p-values < 0.05 were considered significant. * HOMA-IR = Homeostatic Model Assessment of Insulin Resistance; HOMA-B = Homeostatic Model Assessment of β-cell function; HbA1c = glycated hemoglobin; CC = high risk genotype; CT/TT = low risk genotype; WHR = waist-hip ratio.

3.2. Genotype Effects on Metabolites Profiles

Samples were divided into two groups according to the type of meal taken, NC- and HC-meals, and then analyzed in independent analytical batches in both polarity modes. This resulted in four datasets, which were aligned according to their polarity: ESI+ for both meals and ESI- for both meals. After application of the QA procedure, there were 1717 metabolic features in ESI+ and 848 in ESI- past QA procedure from both data sets (NC- and HC-meals). Principal component analysis (PCA) was implemented to visualize the results of the QA procedure. For each analytical sequence, the QC samples clustered tightly (Figure S1), which indicated the system's stability and therefore the good quality of the data.

Final datasets contained only features presented in ≥80% of the samples in at least one of the two studied groups (CC versus CT/TT). It resulted in 1494 and 843 features for the NC- and HC-meals in ESI+ mode and the NC- and HC-meal in ESI- mode, respectively.

To select discriminating metabolites, volcano plots (Figure 1) were built based on PLS-DA models (Figure 2). Studied genotypes did not differ significantly in fasting metabolite profiles, however, metabolic profiles changed and differed between genotypes after the meal intake.

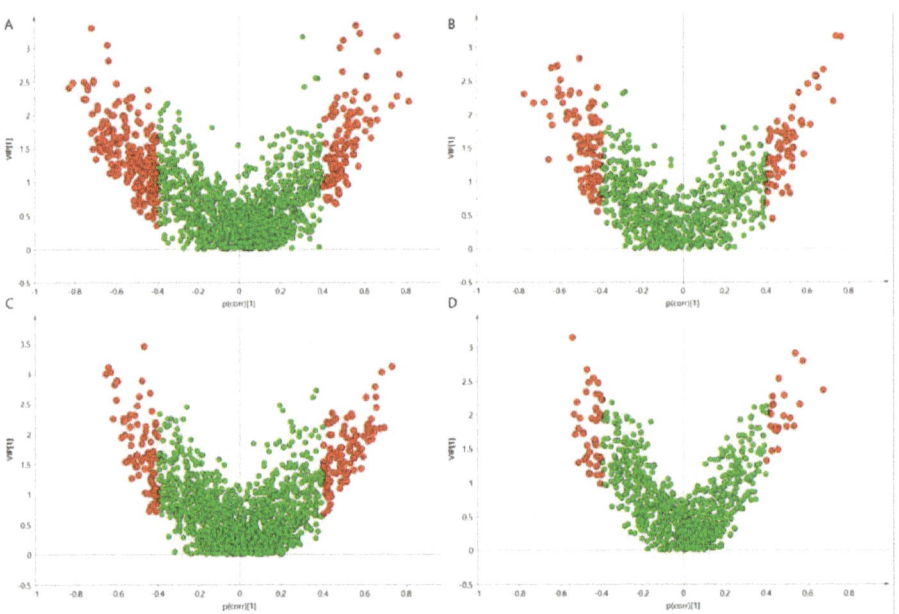

Figure 1. Volcano plots build on the Partial least square discriminant analysis (PLS-DA) models computed based on the area under the curves (AUCs) of plasma metabolites after norma-carbohydrate (NC)-meal for ESI+ (**A**) and ESI- (**B**) and high carbohydrate (HC)-meal for ESI+ (**C**) and ESI- (**D**). Red color marks metabolic features significantly differing HR-genotype (CC) and LR-genotype (CT/TT) carriers.

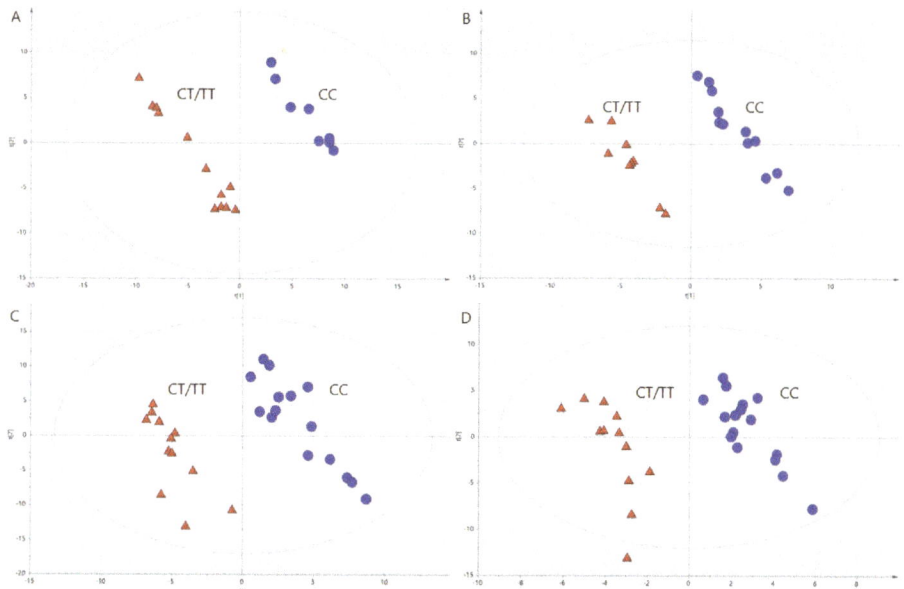

Figure 2. PLS-DA models computed based on AUCs of plasma metabolites illustrating clear separation between men carrying CC (blue dots) and CT/TT (red triangles) genotypes after NC-meal for ESI+ (**A**) and ESI- (**B**), and HC-meal for ESI+ (**C**) and ESI- (**D**). The parameters of the models: $R2 = 0.989$, $Q2 = 0.279$ for NC-meal for ESI+; $R2 = 0.989$, $Q2 = 0.433$ for NC-meal for ESI-; $R2 = 0.947$, $Q2 = 0.490$ for HC-meal for ESI+; $R2 = 0.943$, $Q2 = 0.109$ for HC-meal for ESI-. R2 = explained variance, Q = predictive capability of the model.

Metabolites discriminating studied genotypes after both meals are presented in Table 2. For all of the identified metabolites, the calculated error of the measured mass in comparison to the theoretical monoisotopic mass was ≤4 ppm.

Global overview of all the samples revealed that there was a difference in the metabolic response to the meal between men carrying CC and CT/TT genotypes (Figure 3). Interestingly, the direction of these changes was different between the two polarity modes applied and therefore was related to the type of molecules measured. In ESI+ lipids, different lipid classes were changing (in majority of the cases) opposite to the way they were changing between men with different genotypes. In ESI-, most of the molecules exhibited the same direction of change but with differences in the magnitude of the change.

We did not observe any crucial differences between studied genotypes in the fasting plasma metabolites profile, as mentioned above. Postprandially, we noted that the AUCs of the postprandial very long chain unsaturated PC36:5 levels were lower after NC-meals, while the AUCs of PE38:6 levels were significantly higher after both meal intakes in the HR-group. The HR-genotype carriers presented lower AUCs after the HC-meal and higher AUCs after the NC-meal for postprandial levels of polyunsaturated LysoPC and LysoPE with 18-22-carbon chain length. Conversely, the AUCs of the monounsaturated and the saturated LysoPCs postprandial levels (18 and 16 carbons in length) after the NC-meal intake in the HR-genotype men were lower compared to the LR-genotype carriers. We also noted higher AUCs of postprandial linoleic acid (LA) levels, lower AUCs of hydroxyeicosatetraenoic acids (HETE), and hydroxyoctadecenoic acid (HODE) levels after NC-meal intake, and after both meals, we noted lower AUCs of postprandial hydroxydocosahexaenoic acid (HDoHe) levels. After the HC-meal intake in HR-genotype men, we observed higher AUCs of postprandial tetradecanedioic acid. The HR-genotype men presented lower AUCs of postprandial leukotriene A4 (LTA4) and sphingosines levels and higher AUCs of postprandial acylcarnitines levels after both meal intakes. Lower AUCs of postprandial linoleamide levels after the HC-meal, and for dodecanamide levels, after both meal intakes, were observed. The AUCs of postprandial taurocholic acid levels were lower after the HC-meal intake, while the AUCs of deoxycholic acid glycine conjugated were higher after the NC-meal intake. Moreover, we noticed lower AUCs of postprandial ornithine levels after the HC-meal intake in the HR-genotype men.

Table 2. The percentage differences in AUCs of postprandial plasma metabolite levels after NC-meal and HC-meal intake in the PROX1 high-risk-genotype (CC) men compared to the low-risk genotype carriers (CT/TT).

Name	Molecular Weight, Da	RT, Min	NC-Meal				HC-Meal			
			Change, %	p-Value	p (corr)	VIP	Change, %	p-Value	p (corr)	VIP
PE 38:6	763.5152	9.40	50	0.25	0.43	1.38	62	0.18	−0.56	1.98
PC 36:5	779.5465	7.95	−4	0.93	−0.51	1.35	−48	0.19	0.30	1.43
PC O-18:0/20:4	795.6141	10.20			−0.45	1.52			−0.16	1.34
LysoPC O-18:1	507.3689	5.95	−42	0.17	−0.59	2.21	59	0.45	0.27	0.46
LysoPC O-16:0	481.3532	5.80	−34	0.50	−0.64	2.81	−22	0.61	0.34	1.30
LysoPC 18:2 sn-2	519.3325	5.40	69	0.30	0.30	1.07	−56	0.049	0.55	1.90
LysoPC 18:3	517.3168	5.05	79	0.28	0.16	0.71	−53	0.26	0.53	1.72
LysoPC 22:4	571.3638	5.85	28	0.47	0.55	1.51	−40	0.018	0.56	1.96
LysoPC 20:4	543.3325	5.40	42	0.46	0.21	1.01	−42	0.01	0.62	2.16
LysoPC 20:4 sn-2	543.3325	5.35	49	0.07	−0.50	1.43	−27	0.11	0.45	1.76
LysoPC 20:4 sn-1	543.3325	5.35	20	0.74	−0.01	0.07	−72	0.02	0.54	2.91
LysoPC 22:6	567.3325	5.40	101	0.04	0.81	2.21	−18	0.40	0.26	1.11
LysoPE 22:6 sn-2	525.2855	5.35	80	0.23	−0.54	2.35	−45	0.29	−0.34	1.26
LysoPE 22:6 sn-1	525.2855	5.35	118	0.09	−0.56	2.03	−4	0.86	−0.27	1.10
Tetradecanedioic acid	258.1831	4.35	21	0.44	−0.20	0.78	51	0.005	−0.53	2.01
Linoleic acid	280.2402	7.05	80	0.01	−0.59	2.29	−65	0.13	−0.12	0.67
HETE	320.2351	5.70	−66	0.10	0.64	2.56	−4	0.93	0.38	1.69
HETE	320.2351	5.70	−62	0.10	0.57	1.89	−65	0.13	0.43	2.15
HODE	298.2508	5.85	−33	0.09	0.51	1.43	20	0.43	−0.26	1.06
HDoHE	344.2351	5.70	−61	0.11	0.57	1.90	−28	0.53	0.43	2.15
C18:2 Sphingosine	297.2668	5.85	−37	0.25	−0.41	1.60	−48	0.01	0.65	2.78
Leukotriene A4	318.2195	5.45	−81	0.02	0.74	3.16	−43	0.21	0.16	0.79
Leukotriene A4	318.2195	5.45	−71	0.01	0.64	2.58	−15	0.71	0.24	1.14
Leukotriene A4	318.2195	5.45	−52	0.10	0.58	1.40	−41	0.14	0.41	2.03
Acetylcarnitine	203.1158	0.25	55	0.06	0.54	2.00	92	0.002	−0.60	2.88
Linoleamide	279.2562	5.30	6	0.93	−0.01	0.05	−45	0.09	0.53	1.51
Dodecanamide	199.1936	5.20	−28	0.49	−0.81	2.48	−38	0.16	0.48	1.10
Taurocholic acid	515.2917	2.30	−27	0.35	−0.39	0.39	−59	0.07	0.66	2.43
Deoxycholic acid glycine conjugate	449.3141	4.30	70	0.14	0.55	1.42	6	0.75	−0.29	0.91
Ornithine	132.0899	0.25	4	0.83	0.12	0.05	−45	0.047	0.53	1.83

VIP = variable importance in the projection, RT = retention time.

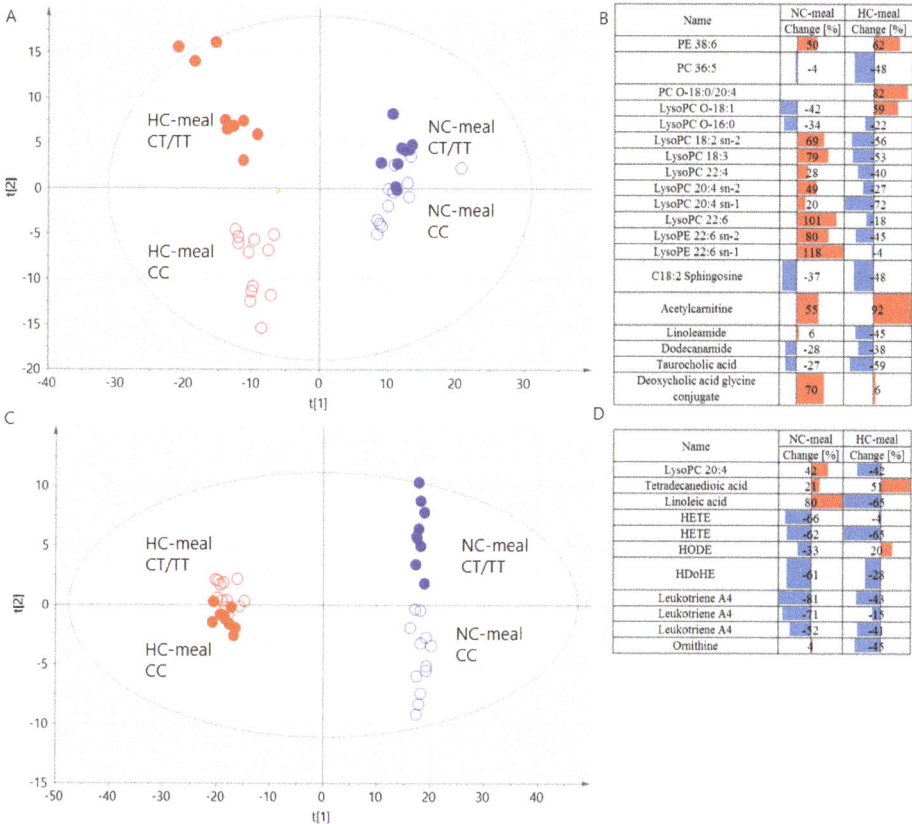

Figure 3. PLS-DA models computed based on AUCs of plasma metabolites illustrating clear separation between men carrying CC (empty dots) and CT/TT (full dots) genotypes after NC- (blue color) and HC-meal (red color) for ESI+ (panel **A**) and ESI- (panel **C**) with the summary of the differentiating signals and their change in ESI+ (panel **B**) and ESI- (panel **D**). The parameters of the models: R2 = 0.581, Q2 = 0.318 for ESI+; R2 = 0.594, Q2 = 0.0.264 for ESI-. R2 = explained variance, Q = predictive capability of the model.

4. Discussion

We evaluated the metabolomics analyses at fasting and postprandial states to explore the impacts of the rs340874 SNP in the PROX1 gene on the human metabolism. At the fasting state, we did not observe any crucial differences in metabolites levels between studied genotypes, but the meal-challenge-tests uncovered several postprandial alterations. We noted some differences in the postprandial phospholipid levels. Altered PCs and LPCs plasma profiles were associated with T2DM [24]. LPCs were reduced in subjects with diabetes [25] and with insulin resistance [26]. Our participants were free from T2DM and prediabetes states, and HR-genotype carriers did not differ in insulin sensitivity from the men carrying the LR-genotype. The changes in postprandial LPCs levels, typical for insulin resistance and T2DM, were induced mostly by the HC-meal consumption, but after the NC-meal intake, the HR-genotype carriers presented significantly higher AUCs of some postprandial LPCs levels. Yea K. et al. [27] showed that LPCs could stimulate glucose uptake via an insulin-independent mechanism. This is consistent with the results from our previous study, which showed that genotype CC carriers who presented lower AUC of postprandial LPCs after a HC-meal intake in this study also presented lower postprandial glucose utilization and higher blood glucose concentrations after the HC-meal intake in our previous experiment [11].

In HR-genotype men after the NC-meal intake, we also noticed higher AUCs of postprandial LA and lower AUCs of postprandial levels of long-chain fatty acids (LCFA) esters derived from arachidonic acid (AA), HETE, and from docosahexaenoic acid (DHA), the HDoHe, after both meal intakes. Some of the oxidized fatty acids had a biological activity and could signal through their own receptors to evoke a variety of physiological changes. It has been shown that reduced glucose-induced 20-HETE formations and release contribute to inefficient glucose-stimulated insulin secretion in islets isolated from T2DM humans and mice [28]. Moreover, after NC-meal intake, we noted the HR-genotype men had lower AUCs of postprandial levels of another hydroxy fatty acid—HODE. The HODEs are likely to be exogenous activators and natural ligands for the nuclear receptor peroxisome proliferator-activated receptors α (PPARα) [29] and PPARγ [30]. The PPARα is an important mediator of metabolic response to nutritional factors since it is involved in fasting and postprandial lipid metabolism regulation, as well as in the mechanisms associated with body energy production. However, it also modulates the transcription of genes involved in pathways of inflammatory responses [31]. PPARγ receptors play a key role in the insulin sensitization, adipocyte differentiation, and adipose tissue lipid metabolism dependent on nutritional state—the highest postprandial expression and activation leads to the upregulation of genes that mediate fatty acids trapping and uptake [32,33]. Adipose PPARγ protects nonadipose tissue against lipid overload [34], and the use of PPARγ agonists has been shown to cause a shift of fat distribution from visceral to subcutaneous adipose depots, which is associated with improvements in hepatic and peripheral tissue insulin sensitivity [35]. It has been found that the activation of PPARα and PPARγ attenuates total free fatty acid and triglyceride accumulation, which may reduce the risk of obesity, diabetes, and atherosclerosis [36]. Therefore, as was noted in our study, lower postprandial HODE levels (which are natural ligands for the PPARα and PPARγ receptors) in the HR-genotype men may have disadvantageous effects. Results from our larger cohort population have indicated that the PROX1 HR-genotype carriers present significantly higher visceral fat accumulation [11].

The HR-genotype men also presented higher AUCs of postprandial tetradecanedioic acid levels after the HC meal intake, which may suggest an altered peroxisomal beta-oxidation since the oxidation of tetradecanedioic acid has been found to be reduced by more than 75% in peroxisome deficient hepatocytes [37].

Our metabolomics analysis showed lower AUCs of postprandial leukotriene A4 (LTA4) plasma levels in the HR-genotype carriers after both meal intakes. The LTA4 could be further metabolized to form LTB4, which plays an important role in metabolic disruptions [38]. Therefore, as was noted in our study, lower LTA4 may be a beneficial symptom or may indicate the higher conversion into LTB4. It has been already shown that PROX1 is associated with defects affecting lymphatic vascular structure and function, which may lead to lymphedema and imbalanced eicosanoid metabolism [39,40].

After both meal intakes, the HR-risk genotype carriers presented higher AUCs of postprandial acylcarnitine levels. Increased plasma acylcarnitines levels have been reported in insulin-resistant and T2DM subjects as products of incomplete or inefficient β-oxidation, and tissue accumulation of acylcarnitine molecules may lead to activation of proinflammatory pathways, which are implicated in insulin resistance and T2DM development [41].

Furthermore, in the HR-genotype men, we also noticed lower AUCs of postprandial levels of two fatty acid amides (FAAs)—dodecanamide after both meals and linoleamide after the HC-meal intake. The FAAs may play roles as endogenous brain cannabinoid receptor ligands and may be involved in T2DM pathogenesis [42]. Moreover, linoleamide inhibits phospholipase A2 (PLA2) [43], the suppression of which protects against diet-induced obesity and diabetes, and PLA2-deficient mice presented increased postprandial hepatic fatty acid oxidation (FAO) [44].

We also observed lower AUCs of postprandial sphingosine levels after both meals in people in the HR-genotype group. Sphingosine is a breakdown product of ceramide degradation, and free sphingosine can be trapped for ceramide regeneration or for sphingosine-1-phosphate (S1P) formation, both of which have been associated with obesity, insulin resistance, and T2DM [45–47]. Lower plasma sphingosine levels observed in our study could have been a result of decreased release to the circulation (from ceramide degradation, etc.,) or increased rate of its intracellular acylation or phosphorylation, and both possibilities may have had a negative effect—the increase of cellular ceramide and S1P levels. Further studies are needed to elucidate the possible associations between the PROX1 HR-genotype and the sphingomyelin pathway.

The very interesting finding of our study is that the PROX1 gene may be involved in the postprandial bile acids signaling. After the HC-meal intake in the HR-genotype men, we noticed lower AUCs of postprandial taurocholic acid and higher AUCs of postprandial deoxycholic acid glycine conjugate levels after the NC-meal. It has been found that PROX1 suppress the transcription of the CYP7A1 gene, which codes the key enzyme of bile acid synthesis and may negatively modulate the bile acids synthesis [48]. Bile acids are metabolic regulating factors that act as signaling molecules through receptor-independent and receptor-dependent pathways, including nuclear farnesoid X receptor (FXR) and the membrane Takeda G protein-coupled receptor (TGR), which are implicated in the regulation of glucose, lipid, and energy metabolism. Dysregulation of these pathways may contribute to the metabolic disturbances and T2DM development [49–51]. The mechanisms by which bile acids are involved in glucose homeostasis regulation remain undefined. Many different subtypes of bile acids differ widely in their chemical composition as well as in their overall impact on health. Zaborska et al. [52] found that dietary supplementation of deoxycholic acid impairs whole body glucose regulation in mice by disrupting hepatic endoplasmic reticulum homeostasis, and in our experiment, the HR-genotype carriers presented higher AUCs of postprandial deoxycholic acid glycine conjugate levels after the NC-meal intake.

The carriers of the PROX1 HR-genotype also presented lower AUCs of postprandial ornithine levels after HC-meal intake. Increased ornithine levels as a product of arginine catabolism are associated with hyperglycemia and can be involved in the pathogenesis of T2DM [53,54], but lower ornithine levels may be an effect of an increased plasma arginase activity, which is increased in diabetic subjects and may be associated with vascular complications [54].

The PROX1 gene has been shown, thus far, to confer the susceptibility to T2DM mostly by its associations with fasting and glucose-stimulated insulin secretion [5] as well as fasting [9] and OGTT 2-h glucose levels [55]. Our study revealed other postprandial disruptions in the high-risk PROX1 genotype carriers, which may be a part of potential type 2 diabetes disease pathways. The summarizing of all metabolic alterations mentioned above is presented in Figure S2. Most of the alterations we found were observed after HC-meal intake, but the differences between studied genotypes in postprandial levels of molecules involved in pathways of inflammatory and oxidative stress responses were more pronounced after NC-meal intake. Oxidative stress impacts progressive disorders and is linked to metabolic disorders such as T2DM, since the activation of stress pathways plays a key role in the development of the insulin resistance and impaired insulin secretion [56]. We observed the differences between genotypes mostly by the NC-meal intake. This was perhaps due to the fact that the HC-meals induced a strong inflammatory response by themselves [57], and therefore the impact of the genetic risk could have been blurred—especially with a small sample size, which was a major limitation of our study. The main reasons for the small study sample were that a non-targeted LC-MS-based metabolomics approach could be performed in a limited set of samples, and, moreover, the presented study is a part of our larger project with very long and laborious protocol and procedures, which limited the number of volunteers participating.

5. Conclusions

In conclusion, our results showed an altered postprandial metabolite profile in the PROX1 HR-genotype carriers. Our observations indicate that one of the pathways involved in the T2DM development in subjects with the PROX1 CC genotype may be postprandial alterations, but further functional studies are required to extrapolate implications from our findings for the biochemical pathways associated with PROX1 SNPs and T2DM development. It may allow identifying the pathways and factors that interact with some dietary nutrients, leading to particular metabolic responses that are associated with the development of metabolic diseases.

Supplementary Materials: The following are available online at http://www.mdpi.com/2072-6643/11/4/882/s1, Metabolomics analysis- methods detailed description, Figure S1: The QC of performed analyses- PCA plots with marked QC samples, Figure S2: The summary of metabolic alterations observed after NC- and HC-meal intake, Table S1: Detailed information about compounds identification.

Author Contributions: Conceptualization and Methodology, E.A.-P., M.C., M.G., C.B., A.K.; Investigation and Formal Analysis, E.A.-P., J.G., P.S., M.C.; Writing—Original Draft Preparation, E.A.-P., J.G.; Statistical Analysis, J.G., P.S., M.C., W.B.; Supervision, M.G., K.S., C.B., A.K.; all authors approved the final version of the manuscript.

Funding: This research was funded by funds from the Medical University of Bialystok.

Acknowledgments: The authors would like to thank the Study Team of the Clinical Research Centre and Department of Endocrinology, Diabetology and Internal Medicine of Medical University of Bialystok for technical support.

Conflicts of Interest: The authors declare no conflict of interest.

References

1. International Diabetes Federation Diabetes Atlas, 7th ed. 2015. Available online: http://www.diabetesatlas.org/ (accessed on 1 December 2018).
2. Chamnan, P.; Simmons, R.K.; Forouhi, N.G.; Luben, R.N.; Khaw, K.T.; Wareham, N.J.; Griffin, S.J. Incidence of type 2 diabetes using proposed HbA1c diagnostic criteria in the european prospective investigation of cancer-norfolk cohort: Implications for preventive strategies. *Diabetes Care* **2011**, *34*, 950–956. [CrossRef] [PubMed]
3. Ferrannini, E.; Camastra, S. Relationship between impaired glucose tolerance, non-insulin-dependent diabetes mellitus and obesity. *Eur J. Clin. Investig.* **1998**, *28*, 3–6. [CrossRef]
4. Dupuis, J.; Langenberg, C.; Prokopenko, I.; Saxena, R.; Soranzo, N.; Jackson, A.U.; Wheeler, E.; Glazer, N.L.; Bouatia-Naji, N.; Gloyn, A.L.; et al. New genetic loci implicated in fasting glucose homeostasis and their impact on type 2 diabetes risk. *Nat. Genet.* **2010**, *42*, 105–116. [CrossRef] [PubMed]
5. Lecompte, S.; Pasquetti, G.; Hermant, X.; Grenier-Boley, B.; Gonzalez-Gross, M.; De Henauw, S.; Molnar, D.; Stehle, P.; Béghin, L.; Moreno, L.A.; et al. Genetic and molecular insights into the role of PROX1 in glucose metabolism. *Diabetes* **2013**, *62*, 1738–1745. [CrossRef]
6. Hamet, P.; Haloui, M.; Harvey, F.; Marois-Blanchet, F.C.; Sylvestre, M.P.; Tahir, M.R.; Simon, P.H.; Kanzki, B.S.; Raelson, J.; Long, C.; et al. PROX1 gene CC genotype as a major determinant of early onset of type 2 diabetes in slavic study participants from Action in Diabetes and Vascular Disease: Preterax and Diamicron MR Controlled Evaluation study. *J. Hypertens.* **2017**, *35*, S24–S32. [CrossRef] [PubMed]
7. Boesgaard, T.W.; Grarup, N.; Jørgensen, T.; Borch-Johnsen, K.; Hansen, T.; Pedersen, O.; Meta-Analysis of Glucose and Insulin-Related Trait Consortium (MAGIC). Variants at DGKB/TMEM195, ADRA2A, GLIS3 and C2CD4B loci are associated with reduced glucose-stimulated beta cell function in middle-aged Danish people. *Diabetologia* **2010**, *53*, 1647–1655. [CrossRef]
8. Wagner, R.; Dudziak, K.; Herzberg-Schäfer, S.A.; Machicao, F.; Stefan, N.; Staiger, H.; Häring, H.U.; Fritsche, A. Glucose-raising genetic variants in MADD and ADCY5 impair conversion of proinsulin to insulin. *PLoS ONE* **2011**, *6*, e23639. [CrossRef]
9. Barker, A.; Sharp, S.J.; Timpson, N.J.; Bouatia-Naji, N.; Warrington, N.M.; Kanoni, S.; Beilin, L.J.; Brage, S.; Deloukas, P.; Evans, D.M.; et al. Association of genetic Loci with glucose levels in childhood and adolescence: A meta-analysis of over 6000 children. *Diabetes* **2011**, *60*, 1805–1812. [CrossRef]
10. Wang, J.; Kilic, G.; Aydin, M.; Burke, Z.; Oliver, G.; Sosa-Pineda, B. Prox1 activity controls pancreas morphogenesis and participates in the production of "secondary transition" pancreatic endocrine cells. *Dev. Biol.* **2005**, *286*, 182–194. [CrossRef] [PubMed]

11. Kretowski, A.; Adamska, E.; Maliszewska, K.; Wawrusiewicz-Kurylonek, N.; Citko, A.; Goscik, J.; Bauer, W.; Wilk, J.; Golonko, A.; Waszczeniuk, M.; et al. The rs340874 PROX1 type 2 diabetes mellitus risk variant is associated with visceral fat accumulation and alterations in postprandial glucose and lipid metabolism. *Genes Nutr.* **2015**, *10*, 454. [CrossRef]
12. Bell, D.S.; O'Keefe, J.H.; Jellinger, P. Postprandial dysmetabolism: The missing link between diabetes and cardiovascular events? *Endocr. Pract.* **2008**, *14*, 112–124. [CrossRef]
13. Adamska-Patruno, E.; Ostrowska, L.; Goscik, J.; Fiedorczuk, J.; Moroz, M.; Kretowski, A.; Gorska, M. The Differences in Postprandial Serum Concentrations of Peptides That Regulate Satiety/Hunger and Metabolism after Various Meal Intake, in Men with Normal vs. Excessive BMI. *Nutrients* **2019**, *11*, 493. [CrossRef]
14. Adamska, E.; Ostrowska, L.; Gościk, J.; Waszczeniuk, M.; Krętowski, A.; Górska, M. Intake of Meals Containing High Levels of Carbohydrates or High Levels of Unsaturated Fatty Acids Induces Postprandial Dysmetabolism in Young Overweight/Obese Men. *Biomed. Res. Int.* **2015**, *2015*, 147196. [CrossRef]
15. Adamska-Patruno, E.; Ostrowska, L.; Goscik, J.; Pietraszewska, B.; Kretowski, A.; Gorska, M. The relationship between the leptin/ghrelin ratio and meals with various macronutrient contents in men with different nutritional status: A randomized crossover study. *Nutr. J.* **2018**, *17*, 118. [CrossRef]
16. Adamska, E.; Kretowski, A.; Goscik, J.; Citko, A.; Bauer, W.; Waszczeniuk, M.; Maliszewska, K.; Paczkowska-Abdulsalam, M.; Niemira, M.; Szczerbinski, L.; et al. The type 2 diabetes susceptibility TCF7L2 gene variants affect postprandial glucose and fat utilization in non-diabetic subjects. *Diabetes Metab.* **2018**, *44*, 379–382. [CrossRef]
17. Adamska-Patruno, E.; Goscik, J.; Czajkowski, P.; Maliszewska, K.; Ciborowski, M.; Golonko, A.; Wawrusiewicz-Kurylonek, N.; Citko, A.; Waszczeniuk, M.; Kretowski, A.; et al. The MC4R genetic variants are associated with lower visceral fat accumulation and higher postprandial relative increase in carbohydrate utilization in humans. *Eur. J. Nutr.* **2019**. [CrossRef]
18. Adamska, E.; Waszczeniuk, M.; Gościk, J.; Golonko, A.; Wilk, J.; Pliszka, J.; Maliszewska, K.; Lipińska, D.; Milewski, R.; Wasilewska, A.; et al. The usefulness of glycated hemoglobin A1c (HbA1c) for identifying dysglycemic states in individuals without previously diagnosed diabetes. *Adv. Med. Sci.* **2012**, *57*, 296–301. [CrossRef]
19. Ostrowska, L.; Witczak, K.; Adamska, E. Effect of nutrition and atherogenic index on the occurrence and intensity of insulin resistance. *Pol. Arch. Med. Wewn.* **2013**, *123*, 289–296. [CrossRef]
20. Lu, J.; Varghese, R.T.; Zhou, L.; Vella, A.; Jensen, M.D. Glucose tolerance and free fatty acid metabolism in adults with variations in TCF7L2 rs7903146. *Metabolism* **2017**, *68*, 55–63. [CrossRef]
21. Adamska-Patruno, E.; Ostrowska, L.; Golonko, A.; Pietraszewska, B.; Goscik, J.; Kretowski, A.; Gorska, M. Evaluation of Energy Expenditure and Oxidation of Energy Substrates in Adult Males after Intake of Meals with Varying Fat and Carbohydrate Content. *Nutrients* **2018**, *10*, 627. [CrossRef]
22. Samczuk, P.; Luba, M.; Godzien, J.; Mastrangelo, A.; Hady, H.R.; Dadan, J.; Barbas, C.; Gorska, M.; Kretowski, A.; Ciborowski, M. "Gear mechanism" of bariatric interventions revealed by untargeted metabolomics. *J. Pharm. Biomed. Anal.* **2018**, *151*, 219–226. [CrossRef]
23. Matthews, D.R.; Hosker, J.P.; Rudenski, A.S.; Naylor, B.A.; Treacher, D.F.; Turner, R.C. Homeostasis model assessment: Insulin resistance and beta-cell function from fasting plasma glucose and insulin concentrations in man. *Diabetologia* **1985**, *28*, 412–419. [CrossRef]
24. Floegel, A.; Stefan, N.; Yu, Z.; Mühlenbruch, K.; Drogan, D.; Joost, H.G.; Fritsche, A.; Häring, H.U.; Hrabě de Angelis, M.; Peters, A.; et al. Identification of serum metabolites associated with risk of type 2 diabetes using a targeted metabolomic approach. *Diabetes* **2013**, *62*, 639–648. [CrossRef]
25. Barber, M.N.; Risis, S.; Yang, C.; Meikle, P.J.; Staples, M.; Febbraio, M.A.; Bruce, C.R. Plasma lysophosphatidylcholine levels are reduced in obesity and type 2 diabetes. *PLoS ONE* **2012**, *7*, e41456. [CrossRef]
26. Tonks, K.T.; Coster, A.C.; Christopher, M.J.; Chaudhuri, R.; Xu, A.; Gagnon-Bartsch, J.; Chisholm, D.J.; James, D.E.; Meikle, P.J.; Greenfield, J.R.; et al. Skeletal muscle and plasma lipidomic signatures of insulin resistance and overweight/obesity in humans. *Obesity* **2016**, *24*, 908–916. [CrossRef]
27. Yea, K.; Kim, J.; Yoon, J.H.; Kwon, T.; Kim, J.H.; Lee, B.D.; Lee, H.J.; Lee, S.J.; Kim, J.I.; Lee, T.G.; et al. Lysophosphatidylcholine activates adipocyte glucose uptake and lowers blood glucose levels in murine models of diabetes. *J. Biol. Chem.* **2009**, *284*, 33833–33840. [CrossRef]

28. Tunaru, S.; Bonnavion, R.; Brandenburger, I.; Preussner, J.; Thomas, D.; Scholich, K.; Offermanns, S. 20-HETE promotes glucose-stimulated insulin secretion in an autocrine manner through FFAR1. *Nat. Commun.* **2018**, *9*, 177. [CrossRef]
29. Nagy, L.; Tontonoz, P.; Alvarez, J.G.; Chen, H.; Evans, R.M. Oxidized LDL regulates macrophage gene expression through ligand activation of PPARgamma. *Cell* **1998**, *93*, 229–240. [CrossRef]
30. Itoh, T.; Fairall, L.; Amin, K.; Inaba, Y.; Szanto, A.; Balint, B.L.; Nagy, L.; Yamamoto, K.; Schwabe, J.W. Structural basis for the activation of PPARgamma by oxidized fatty acids. *Nat. Struct. Mol. Biol.* **2008**, *15*, 924–931. [CrossRef]
31. Contreras, A.V.; Torres, N.; Tovar, A.R. PPAR-α as a key nutritional and environmental sensor for metabolic adaptation. *Adv. Nutr.* **2013**, *4*, 439–452. [CrossRef]
32. Semple, R.K.; Chatterjee, V.K.; O'Rahilly, S. PPAR gamma and human metabolic disease. *J. Clin. Investig.* **2006**, *116*, 581–589. [CrossRef]
33. Varga, T.; Czimmerer, Z.; Nagy, L. PPARs are a unique set of fatty acid regulated transcription factors controlling both lipid metabolism and inflammation. *Biochim. Biophys. Acta* **2011**, *1812*, 1007–1022. [CrossRef]
34. Sharma, A.M.; Staels, B. Review: Peroxisome proliferator-activated receptor gamma and adipose tissue-understanding obesity-related changes in regulation of lipid and glucose metabolism. *J. Clin. Endocrinol. Metab.* **2007**, *92*, 386–395. [CrossRef]
35. Miyazaki, Y.; Mahankali, A.; Matsuda, M.; Mahankali, S.; Hardies, J.; Cusi, K.; Mandarino, L.J.; DeFronzo, R.A. Effect of pioglitazone on abdominal fat distribution and insulin sensitivity in type 2 diabetic patients. *J. Clin. Endocrinol. Metab.* **2002**, *87*, 2784–2791. [CrossRef]
36. Ye, G.; Gao, H.; Wang, Z.; Lin, Y.; Liao, X.; Zhang, H.; Chi, Y.; Zhu, H.; Dong, S. PPARα and PPARγ activation attenuates total free fatty acid and triglyceride accumulation in macrophages via the inhibition of Fatp1 expression. *Cell Death Dis.* **2019**, *10*, 39. [CrossRef]
37. Dirkx, R.; Meyhi, E.; Asselberghs, S.; Reddy, J.; Baes, M.; Van Veldhoven, P.P. Beta-oxidation in hepatocyte cultures from mice with peroxisomal gene knockouts. *Biochem. Biophys. Res. Commun.* **2007**, *357*, 718–723. [CrossRef]
38. Filgueiras, L.R.; Serezani, C.H.; Jancar, S. Leukotriene B4 as a Potential Therapeutic Target for the Treatment of Metabolic Disorders. *Front. Immunol.* **2015**, *6*, 515. [CrossRef]
39. Escobedo, N.; Oliver, G. The Lymphatic Vasculature: Its Role in Adipose Metabolism and Obesity. *Cell Metab.* **2017**, *26*, 598–609. [CrossRef]
40. Tian, W.; Rockson, S.G.; Jiang, X.; Kim, J.; Begaye, A.; Shuffle, E.M.; Tu, A.B.; Cribb, M.; Nepiyushchikh, Z.; Feroze, A.H.; et al. Leukotriene B antagonism ameliorates experimental lymphedema. *Sci. Transl. Med.* **2017**, *9*. [CrossRef]
41. Adams, S.H.; Hoppel, C.L.; Lok, K.H.; Zhao, L.; Wong, S.W.; Minkler, P.E.; Hwang, D.H.; Newman, J.W.; Garvey, W.T. Plasma acylcarnitine profiles suggest incomplete long-chain fatty acid beta-oxidation and altered tricarboxylic acid cycle activity in type 2 diabetic African-American women. *J. Nutr.* **2009**, *139*, 1073–1081. [CrossRef]
42. Yamamoto, S.; Takehara, M.; Ushimaru, M. Inhibitory action of linoleamide and oleamide toward sarco/endoplasmic reticulum Ca^{2+}-ATPase. *Biochim. Biophys. Acta* **2017**, *1861*, 3399–3405. [CrossRef]
43. Jain, M.K.; Ghomashchi, F.; Yu, B.Z.; Bayburt, T.; Murphy, D.; Houck, D.; Brownell, J.; Reid, J.C.; Solowiej, J.E.; Wong, S.M. Fatty acid amides: Scooting mode-based discovery of tight-binding competitive inhibitors of secreted phospholipases A2. *J. Med. Chem.* **1992**, *35*, 3584–3586. [CrossRef]
44. Hollie, N.I.; Matlib, M.A.; Hui, D.Y. Direct inhibitory effects of phospholipase A2 enzymatic product lysophosphatidylcholine (LPC) on hepatic mitochondria. *Biochemistry* **2011**, *25*, 527. [CrossRef]
45. Kitatani, K.; Idkowiak-Baldys, J.; Hannun, Y.A. The sphingolipid salvage pathway in ceramide metabolism and signaling. *Cell Signal.* **2008**, *20*, 1010–1018. [CrossRef]
46. Kowalski, G.M.; Carey, A.L.; Selathurai, A.; Kingwell, B.A.; Bruce, C.R. Plasma sphingosine-1-phosphate is elevated in obesity. *PLoS ONE* **2013**, *8*, e72449. [CrossRef]
47. Haus, J.M.; Kashyap, S.R.; Kasumov, T.; Zhang, R.; Kelly, K.R.; Defronzo, R.A.; Kirwan, J.P. Plasma ceramides are elevated in obese subjects with type 2 diabetes and correlate with the severity of insulin resistance. *Diabetes* **2009**, *58*, 337–343. [CrossRef]

48. Qin, J.; Gao, D.M.; Jiang, Q.F.; Zhou, Q.; Kong, Y.Y.; Wang, Y.; Xie, Y.H. Prospero-related homeobox (Prox1) is a corepressor of human liver receptor homolog-1 and suppresses the transcription of the cholesterol 7-alpha-hydroxylase gene. *Mol. Endocrinol.* **2004**, *18*, 2424–2439. [CrossRef]
49. Prawitt, J.; Caron, S.; Staels, B. Bile acid metabolism and the pathogenesis of type 2 diabetes. *Curr. Diab. Rep.* **2011**, *11*, 160–166. [CrossRef]
50. Tomkin, G.H.; Owens, D. Obesity diabetes and the role of bile acids in metabolism. *J. Transl. Int. Med.* **2016**, *4*, 73–80. [CrossRef]
51. Kuipers, F.; Bloks, V.W.; Groen, A.K. Beyond intestinal soap–bile acids in metabolic control. *Nat. Rev. Endocrinol.* **2014**, *10*, 488–498. [CrossRef]
52. Zaborska, K.E.; Lee, S.A.; Garribay, D.; Cha, E.; Cummings, B.P. Deoxycholic acid supplementation impairs glucose homeostasis in mice. *PLoS ONE* **2018**, *13*, e0200908. [CrossRef] [PubMed]
53. Ramírez-Zamora, S.; Méndez-Rodríguez, M.L.; Olguín-Martínez, M.; Sánchez-Sevilla, L.; Quintana-Quintana, M.; García-García, N.; Hernández-Muñoz, R. Increased erythrocytes by-products of arginine catabolism are associated with hyperglycemia and could be involved in the pathogenesis of type 2 diabetes mellitus. *PLoS ONE* **2013**, *8*, e66823. [CrossRef] [PubMed]
54. Kashyap, S.R.; Lara, A.; Zhang, R.; Park, Y.M.; DeFronzo, R.A. Insulin reduces plasma arginase activity in type 2 diabetic patients. *Diabetes Care* **2008**, *31*, 134–139. [CrossRef] [PubMed]
55. Hu, C.; Zhang, R.; Wang, C.; Wang, J.; Ma, X.; Hou, X.; Lu, J.; Yu, W.; Jiang, F.; Bao, Y.; et al. Variants from GIPR, TCF7L2, DGKB, MADD, CRY2, GLIS3, PROX1, SLC30A8 and IGF1 are associated with glucose metabolism in the Chinese. *PLoS ONE* **2010**, *5*, e15542. [CrossRef] [PubMed]
56. Evans, J.L.; Goldfine, I.D.; Maddux, B.A.; Grodsky, G.M. Are oxidative stress-activated signaling pathways mediators of insulin resistance and beta-cell dysfunction? *Diabetes* **2003**, *52*, 1–8. [CrossRef] [PubMed]
57. Gregersen, S.; Samocha-Bonet, D.; Heilbronn, L.K.; Campbell, L.V. Inflammatory and oxidative stress responses to high-carbohydrate and high-fat meals in healthy humans. *J. Nutr. Metab.* **2012**, *2012*, 238056. [CrossRef] [PubMed]

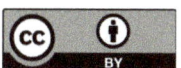

© 2019 by the authors. Licensee MDPI, Basel, Switzerland. This article is an open access article distributed under the terms and conditions of the Creative Commons Attribution (CC BY) license (http://creativecommons.org/licenses/by/4.0/).

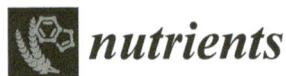

Review

Can Gut Microbiota Composition Predict Response to Dietary Treatments?

Jessica R Biesiekierski [1],*, Jonna Jalanka [2,3] and Heidi M Staudacher [4]

[1] Department of Dietetics, Nutrition & Sport, School of Allied Health Human Services & Sport, La Trobe University, 3086 Melbourne, Australia
[2] Human Microbiome Research Program, Faculty of Medicine, University of Helsinki, 00014 HY Helsinki, Finland; jonna.jalanka@helsinki.fi
[3] Nottingham Digestive Diseases Centre and NIHR Nottingham Biomedical Research Centre at Nottingham University Hospitals NHS Trust, the University of Nottingham, Nottingham NG7 2RD, UK
[4] Food and Mood Centre, IMPACT SRC, Deakin University, Geelong, VIC 3216, Australia; heidi.staudacher@deakin.edu.au
* Correspondence: j.biesiekierski@latrobe.edu.au; Tel.: +61-3-9479-5601

Received: 18 April 2019; Accepted: 20 May 2019; Published: 22 May 2019

Abstract: Dietary intervention is a challenge in clinical practice because of inter-individual variability in clinical response. Gut microbiota is mechanistically relevant for a number of disease states and consequently has been incorporated as a key variable in personalised nutrition models within the research context. This paper aims to review the evidence related to the predictive capacity of baseline microbiota for clinical response to dietary intervention in two specific health conditions, namely, obesity and irritable bowel syndrome (IBS). Clinical trials and larger predictive modelling studies were identified and critically evaluated. The findings reveal inconsistent evidence to support baseline microbiota as an accurate predictor of weight loss or glycaemic response in obesity, or as a predictor of symptom improvement in irritable bowel syndrome, in dietary intervention trials. Despite advancement in quantification methodologies, research in this area remains challenging and larger scale studies are needed until personalised nutrition is realistically achievable and can be translated to clinical practice.

Keywords: personalised nutrition; microbiota; dietary intervention; obesity; irritable bowel syndrome; gastrointestinal symptoms

1. Introduction

Diet is a modifiable risk factor for many non-communicable diseases and there is a high level of evidence supporting the efficacy of dietary interventions for both influencing disease risk and improving disease outcomes. For example, dietary intervention can reduce cardiovascular disease risk by 60% [1] and can successfully reduce gastrointestinal (GI) symptoms in at least 50% of patients with irritable bowel syndrome (IBS) [2]. However, individual variability in response to treatment is increasingly recognised, and this is reflected in the highly variable response rates in clinical trials of dietary interventions, particularly in obesity [3], cardiovascular disease [4] and IBS [2].

Personalised nutrition essentially enables the tailoring of dietary advice to the individual level through the incorporation of data related to specific biological pathways driving that individual's health or disease status, ultimately optimising the effectiveness of the advice. A comprehensive understanding of clinical conditions and underlying disease mechanisms is often required, including the genetic variants of the patient and the extent to which these variants interact with diet to affect disease risk and treatment in diverse populations.

Personalised nutrition models integrate a variety of host-specific variables including current diet, biological or phenotypical characteristics of the individual (age, stage of life, gender, body mass index (BMI), disease or health status) and genotypic characteristics. An understanding of epigenetics (regulation of gene expression) is also often included. Models will vary with the clinical condition and its underlying mechanisms, and with the research hypothesis, where different combinations of characteristics are possible. Most evidence supporting personalised nutrition has come from observational studies with disease risk factors as outcomes (e.g., postprandial glucose response). However, there are some trials using clinical endpoints that have incorporated participant information to test prediction of responses [5] and large-scale studies collecting multi-dimensional data to predict response to acute diet challenges [6].

Gut microbiota is one variable shown to be mechanistically relevant for a number of disease states and therefore has a potential role in the development of personalised dietary advice. Microbiota has a profound impact on our health, and alterations to its composition and its dysfunction have been associated with several chronic diseases [7]. Despite the lack of a clear definition of a "healthy microbiota", its general hallmarks include its resistance to compositional change and its responsiveness to environmental challenges [8]. This allows continuous operation of essential metabolic and immune functions including host nutrient metabolism, maintenance of structural integrity of the gut mucosal barrier, immunomodulation and protection against pathogens.

Diet is well known as one of the major drivers of microbiota composition [9] and conversely, the microbiota response to dietary intervention varies between individuals [10]. In the last decade, efforts have been directed to beginning to understand how biological response may be influenced by the baseline microbiota [11]. Much of the research investigating the predictive capacity of baseline microbiota for clinical response to dietary intervention has been reported in two specific health conditions, namely, obesity and IBS.

1.1. Clinical Condition 1: Obesity

Overweight and obesity rates continue to rise worldwide. In 2013, among adults (age ≥20 years), 37% of men and 30% of women were considered overweight (BMI 25–29.9) or obese (BMI ≥30) [12]. Obesity is associated with numerous chronic diseases and increases the risk for type 2 diabetes, metabolic disorder and cancer [13,14]. The pathogenesis of obesity is complex, with environmental, sociocultural, behavioural, physiological, genetic and epigenetic factors known to be contributors. Treatment often requires significant behaviour modification including dietary change and physical activity. Common dietary approaches include a low-fat diet, a high-protein diet or the DASH (Dietary Approaches to Stop Hypertension) diet [15,16]. Pharmacotherapy, medical devices and bariatric surgery are other treatment options for patients requiring additional intervention. Given the multifaceted nature of obesity, there is no single nor simple treatment solution, and therefore novel, and most likely personalised, interventions may be necessary for effective treatment.

1.2. Clinical Condition 2: Irritable Bowel Syndrome

Irritable bowel syndrome (IBS), a chronic functional bowel disorder characterised by abdominal pain and altered bowel habit [17], affects 11% of individuals globally [18]. Positive diagnosis is based on the symptom profile meeting Rome IV criteria, and patients are classified into one of four IBS subtypes (diarrhoea-predominant, constipation-predominant, mixed and unsubtyped) [17]. The pathophysiology of IBS is not completely elucidated. Most factors proposed are embodied with the concept of a disturbed bidirectional brain–gut axis, including alterations in the central nervous system (e.g., high prevalence of anxiety and depression), visceral hypersensitivity, increased gut epithelial permeability, low grade inflammation and an altered microbiome.

Lifestyle advice, including healthy diet and exercise, is usually considered as first line therapy, followed by symptom-directed pharmacotherapies (anti-spasmodics, laxatives, pro-secretory agents) which have varying efficacy and safety profile [19]. The low FODMAP diet, an approach restricting the intake of specific fermentable carbohydrates (i.e., oligo-, di-, mono-saccharides and polyols) is a second-line dietary intervention [20] and, although successful in inducing global symptom response in many, is often not effective for up to 50% of patients [2].

1.3. Purpose of Review

Recent research suggests that dietary advice could be revolutionised towards a more personalised approach for a spectrum of disease states. Accurate prediction of clinical response, such as weight loss in obesity or symptom improvement in IBS, may not only improve short-term clinical response but also long-term treatment efficacy and overall health outcomes in response to dietary intervention. This paper aims to review the current state of evidence related to how knowledge of gut microbiota may facilitate personalised dietary treatments in obesity and in IBS, with a focus on human dietary intervention trials. In addition, the article aims to identify the knowledge gaps and address the implications of research to date. Studies were selected for inclusion if they assessed baseline microbiota composition as a prediction tool for the clinical response after dietary intervention in human cohorts with IBS and obesity. Can gut microbiota composition predict response to dietary treatments?

1.4. Role of Intestinal Microbiota in Obesity

Several lines of evidence support a role for microbiota in the pathophysiology of obesity. The obese mouse model is characterised by a 50% decrease in *Bacteroidetes* abundance, an increase in *Firmicutes* [21] and a lower abundance of *Akkermansia muciniphila* [22] compared with lean mice. Clinical research in humans supports this, with evidence of fewer *Bacteroides* and more *Firmicutes* [21], as well as a lower abundance of *Bifidobacteria* [23] compared with lean controls. Obesity is also associated with a lower bacterial richness (where richness is defined as the number of different species in an ecosystem) and those with a lower bacterial richness gain more weight over time [24]. Efficacy of probiotics [25] and faecal microbiota transplantation (FMT) [26] (via colonisation with "lean microbiota") to induce weight loss in obese individuals implies that attempts at "correcting" the microbial equilibrium can influence body weight and adiposity in obesity.

Although the underlying mechanisms by which gut microbiota contributes to obesity are not fully understood, evidence suggests contributing pathways include activity of the fermentation by-product short-chain fatty acids (SCFAs) in regulating gut hormones and influencing energy harvest [27]. Gut microbiota may also suppress the production of fasting-induced adipose factors [28] and be linked to inflammatory responses [29], regulation of lipogenesis pathways of triglyceride synthesis [30] and impaired innate immune interactions [31].

1.5. Impact of Dietary Treatment on the Microbiome in Obesity

Energy restriction is the staple dietary intervention in obesity. When obese humans are assigned to either a fat-restricted or carbohydrate-restricted diet, the resulting increase in abundance of *Bacteroidetes* correlates with percentage loss of body weight [21]. Others demonstrate that three months of a formula-based very low-calorie diet (800 kcal/day) in 18 obese adults led to 21 kg average weight loss with concomitant changes in microbiota and bacterial metabolism [32]. The indicative taxa for the microbial diversity change involved the increase in *Acinetobacter*. Furthermore, a six-week energy-restricted high-protein diet in 38 obese adults improved low gene richness (i.e., number of detected bacterial genes) and increased the abundance of most gene clusters [33]. Another study assessed the impact of a Mediterranean diet compared with a low-fat diet in 20 obese men. There were no significant differences in the metabolic variables measured (weight change was not reported) between the diets after one year of dietary intervention. However, the low-fat diet group demonstrated an increased relative abundance of *Prevotella* and decreased *Roseburia* genera from baseline, whereas the Mediterranean diet led to the reverse, a decreased abundance of *Prevotella* and increased abundances of the *Roseburia* and *Oscillospira* genera from baseline [34]. These diets led to differential alterations in gut microbiota due to changes in food groups.

In addition to energy restriction, dietary interventions designed to target gut microbiota have used a range of potential modulators and have assessed various obesity risk factors. For example, one prebiotic supplementation study showed that a 16-week intervention of oligofructose-enriched inulin in overweight or obese children (7–12 years) led to a greater abundance of *Bifidobacteria* compared with controls who received maltodextrin [35]. Many other within-group changes were observed for microbiota, but importantly, changes in gut microbial abundance coincided with beneficial changes in body composition and biological parameters of interleukin-6 and serum triglycerides compared with controls. Others have studied the effect of prebiotics through food or whole diet interventions. One uncontrolled trial delivered a diet rich in non-digestible carbohydrates (based on whole grains, traditional Chinese medicinal foods and prebiotics) via hospitalised intervention in 21 morbidly obese children (3–16 years) for 30 days [36]. Microbiota composition, which had been enriched with potentially pathogenic bacteria at baseline, was much higher post-intervention in beneficial groups of bacteria, such as *Bifidobacterium* spp. Structural changes at the individual bacterial genome level were also significantly associated with improvements in host metabolic health (e.g., serum antigen load, alleviation of inflammation) alongside the 9.5% loss of initial bodyweight [36].

1.6. Microbiome as a Predictor for Dietary Treatment Response in Obesity

In the last five years, there have been four relatively small dietary trials that assessed the association of baseline microbiota with either weight response in obese cohorts or the response of postprandial hyperglycaemia in healthy individuals, an independent risk factor for obesity. Furthermore, there have been two studies that used microbiota as a prediction tool to model weight response in obesity cohorts and two to predict glycaemic response in healthy individuals (Table 1).

First, a summary of the studies assessing weight response in obesity is presented. Two unrandomised trials have demonstrated the utility of baseline microbiota in predicting bodyweight response to dietary intervention. One showed that a higher gene richness at baseline was associated with a greater reduction in adipose tissue and systemic inflammation after a six-week energy-restricted high-protein diet ($n = 38$) [33]. The other reported that higher baseline abundance of *Akkermansia muciniphila* was associated with greater improvement in insulin sensitivity and body fat distribution after a six-week energy-restricted diet ($n = 49$) [37]. The first of two modelling studies implemented a six-week energy-restricted, high-protein diet followed by a six-week period of weight maintenance in obese or overweight individuals ($n = 50$) [38]. A combination of biological, gut microbiota and environmental factors were used to predict individual weight loss trajectory using a graphical Bayesian network framework. Those who lost the least weight and regained the most were characterised by higher abundances of *Lactobacillus, Leuconostoc and Pediococcus* genera. The overall microbiota composition at baseline was not identified by the framework as a predictor for weight loss. In another modelling study, the likelihood of weight loss in 78 obese adults undertaking high-fibre dietary interventions was related to the abundance of *Firmicutes* at baseline [39].

Key studies in the personalised nutrition field have investigated postprandial glycaemic responses (PPGR) to dietary intervention. One crossover randomised clinical trial (RCT) randomised 39 healthy participants to a three-day intervention of barley kernel-based bread or white wheat flour bread (100 g starch/day). The 10 participants demonstrating the most pronounced improvement in glucose and insulin response after a standardised breakfast following the barley kernel-based bread intervention were classified as responders. Responders were characterised by a higher *Prevotella/Bacteroides* ratio, higher relative abundance of *Dorea* and greater microbial potential to ferment complex oligosaccharides at baseline compared with non-responders [40]. Also implementing a bread intervention, a second RCT provided 20 healthy participants with three portions of 145 g sourdough-leavened whole-grain bread or 110 g white bread per day for one week. The interpersonal variability in glycaemic response to the different bread types could be reliably predicted with baseline microbiome data (accuracy ROC curve of 0.83) [41].

Table 1. Summary of recent trials reporting on the association between baseline gut microbiota composition and association with clinical response in obesity.

Study	Study Design	No. of Subjects	Clinical Condition	Dietary Intervention	Control	Key Findings	Ref.
Controlled trials – weight response							
Cotillard et al., 2013	Non-randomised clinical trial	49 (f = 41, m = 8)	Obesity (n = 38, and n = 11 overweight)	6-week energy-restricted high-protein diet followed by a 6-week weight-maintenance diet	-	Responders: Higher gene richness (where responders were those with marked improvement of adipose tissue and systemic inflammation).	[33]
Dao et al., 2016	Non-randomised clinical trial	49 (f = 41, m = 8)	Obesity and overweight	3-week calorie restriction	-	Responders: Higher gene richness and *Akkermansia muciniphila* abundance was associated with most improved body fat distribution, fasting plasma glucose, plasma triglycerides, improvement in insulin sensitivity.	[37]
Modelling studies – weight response							
Kong et al., 2013	Network modelling	50 (f = 42, m = 8)	Obesity and overweight	6-week energy-restricted, high-protein diet followed by maintenance phase	-	Responders: Baseline microbiota not identified as a predictor. Non-responders: High *Lactobacillus*/*Leuconostoc*/*Pediococcus*.	[38]
Korpela et al., 2014	Predictive modelling	78 (f = 40, m = 38)	3 cohorts with obesity	3 different types of dietary interventions varying in carbohydrate quality and quantity	-	Responders: High abundance of *Firmicutes*, where the microbiota composition was associated with change in serum cholesterol levels.	[39]
Controlled trials – glycaemic response							
Kovatcheva-Datchary et al., 2015	RCT, crossover	39 (f = 33, m = 6)	Healthy	3-day barley kernel-based bread	3-day white wheat flour bread	Responders: Higher *Prevotella*/*Bacteroides* ratio and increased *Dorea* that could predict PPGR to barley kernel-based bread.	[40]
Korem et al., 2017	RCT, crossover	20 (f = 11, m = 9)	Healthy	1 week of 3× 145 g whole-grain sourdough/day	1 week of 3× 110 g refined white bread/day	Responders: Specific microbial signature (especially abundances of *Coprobacter fastidiosus* and *Lachnospiraceae bacterium*) could predict PPGR to either bread.	[41]
Modelling studies – glycaemic response							
Zeevi et al., 2015	Machine learning algorithm	800 (f = 480, m = 320)	Healthy (assessing glycaemic response)	1-week usual diet with one standardised meal with 50 g available carbohydrate/day	-	Responders: Proteobacteria, Enterobacteriaceae and Actinobacteria were associated with elevated PPGRs. Non-responders: Clostridia and Prevotellaceae associated with lower PPGRs.	[6]
Mendes-Soares et al., 2019	Same modelling framework as Zeevi et al., 2015 [6]	327 (f = 255, m = 72)	Healthy (assessing glycaemic response)	6-day usual diet including four standardised meals with 50 g available carbohydrate	-	Baseline microbiota combined with other physiological characteristics was more predictive of PPGR than using only calorie or carbohydrate content of foods.	[42]

PPGR, postprandial glycaemic response; RCT, randomised clinical trial.

The most impressive study that has investigated predictors of biological responses to diet to date is a large predictive modelling study. Participants' (n = 800) blood glucose was continuously monitored for one week whilst they recorded daily activities and dietary intake [6]. The PPGR to the first meal of every day, which was one of four different standardised meals (equivalent to 50 g carbohydrate), was a key component of a large dataset of clinical, anthropometric, dietary and biological information. PPGR variability was associated with a variety of clinical factors (HbA1c%, BMI, systolic blood pressure and alanine aminotransferase (ALT) activity). However, intriguingly, Proteobacteria and Enterobacteriaceae were positively associated with some of the PPGR to the standardised meal; associations with glycaemic response were also evident for certain microbial pathways at the functional level. From these data, a prediction model using thousands of decision trees based on 137 features representing meal content, daily activity, blood parameters and microbiome features was then validated in a separate 100-person cohort [6]. Similarly, others have used six-day PPGR data in 327 healthy participants to demonstrate that baseline microbiome combined with other physiological characteristics is highly predictive of postprandial responses. This was more predictive than standard clinical approaches that incorporate calorie or carbohydrate content alone [42].

Together, the findings from the obesity cohorts and glycaemic response studies highlight that microbiota composition and abundance of specific taxa present an exciting opportunity to enable predicting responsiveness to diet. However, challenges in interpreting the evidence exist, including the heterogeneity of studies, such as the length of dietary challenge (three to six weeks in obesity, three days to one week in PPGR), the type and intensity of intervention (level of caloric restriction, types of carbohydrate) and the number of taxa analysed. Most studies defined their subject cohort, including presence of comorbidity and medication use; however, many did not report on other external factors that could influence microbiota composition (e.g., probiotics), which may have contributed to the heterogeneity of findings.

1.7. Role of Intestinal Microbiota in IBS

Evidence for microbiota in the development and/or as a driving force of symptom severity in IBS has been accumulating for some 35 years. The line of evidence that is most well supported in the literature is the observation that the faecal microbiota composition of patients differs from that of healthy controls, although there is little consistency in findings across studies [43,44]. Reported differences include a higher *Firmicutes/Bacteroidetes* ratio [45–49], a lower *Bifidobacteria* abundance [48,50–55] and instability in response to dietary change [56] in IBS compared with healthy controls. Differences have not been limited to the luminal compartment; colonic mucosal microbial composition also deviates from healthy controls [46,51,57]. Distinct microbial profiles associated with severity of gut symptoms [47–49,57,58] or presence of psychological morbidity [47,57–59] support a potential role for microbiota in perpetuating symptoms. Although one of the most recent investigations of microbiota in IBS identified a distinct faecal and mucosal signature associated with categories of symptom severity in IBS [49], a unique and consistent microbial signature differentiating IBS from non-IBS has not been identified.

A number of other lines of evidence supporting the important role of microbiota in the pathophysiology of IBS come from animal models. The presence of transplanted microbiota from individuals with IBS in germ-free mice leads to the transfer of the disease state, including altered microbiota composition, visceral hypersensitivity, altered transit, immune activation and behavioural manifestations of the condition [60,61]. Other animal data suggest microbial metabolites, such as SCFAs, induce visceral hypersensitivity, a key feature of IBS [62]. In humans, additional support for the involvement of microbiota in IBS aetiology is the presence of systemic and mucosal immune activation, with the altered gut microbiota a potential key driver of this dysregulation [63]. Finally, although it is still unclear whether a divergent microbiota is a primary phenomenon, the efficacy of therapies such as probiotics and FMT implies that attempts at "correcting" the abnormality lead to at least partial restoration of microbial and GI equilibrium [64,65].

1.8. Impact of Dietary Treatment on the Microbiome in IBS

Over the past 10 years, clinical trials of the low FODMAP diet have vastly outnumbered studies of other "whole diet" interventions in IBS. Response rates of 50–80% are reported in RCTs in which the advice is dietitian-led [2]. The impact of short-term FODMAP restriction on the faecal microbiota has been reported in a number of trials of dietary advice in free-living individuals with IBS [65–69] and in a highly controlled feeding trial [70]. A variety of taxonomic changes have been reported, of which the most consistent finding is a lower relative or absolute abundance of *Bifidobacteria* compared with controls and/or pre-intervention [65–67,69–71]. Interestingly, those individuals with greater *Bifidobacteria* abundance at baseline exhibit the greatest depletion in response to FODMAP restriction [65]. Altered metabolomic profile in response to FODMAP restriction has also been reported in IBS, suggesting there is a change in metabolic activity of microbes in response to reduced availability of fermentable carbohydrates or increased availability of alternative dietary substrates [67,71]. Whether these microbial changes are key to inducing symptomatic response to a low FODMAP diet is not known from the current evidence. The anti-bifidogenic effect of the low FODMAP diet is inconsistent with a "more is better" hypothesis that could be postulated from the inverse correlation between *Bifidobacteria* and symptom severity [48,57] and the trend toward efficacy of *Bifidobacteria*-containing probiotic supplements in IBS [72].

1.9. Microbiome as a Predictor for Dietary Treatment Response in IBS

The ability to predict symptomatic response to the low FODMAP diet has been of recent interest, particularly considering the diet is intensive to implement and requires dietetic supervision [73], and that up to half of individuals may not benefit. There is limited but consistent evidence that baseline demographic or clinical characteristics do not differentiate responders from non-responders to the low FODMAP diet [68,74–76].

Five studies have investigated whether baseline microbiota could predict symptomatic response to the low FODMAP diet (Table 2). One four-week RCT (19/33 responders, 61%) [5] and a four-week uncontrolled trial (32/61 responders, 52%) [77] of low FODMAP dietary advice propose baseline microbial profile to be predictive of response, using a microbial mapping technique based on selected DNA probes [78]. Of the 45 bacterial markers at baseline in the latter trial, 10 differentiated responders from non-responders with a positive predictive value of 76.0 (95% CI 61–87) using scores based on an arbitrary microbial "response index". A third study, a small uncontrolled one-week trial in children (4/8 responders, 50%), reported that a lower abundance of saccharolytic *Bacteroides* and Bacteroidales was predictive of dietary response [68]. This was followed by a crossover RCT (8/33 responders, 24%) that reported baseline enrichment of a range of saccharolytic taxa including *Bacteroides* and *Faecalibacterium prausnitzii* in responders compared with non-responders [79]. However, not all studies report positive findings; one trial found no predictive value of baseline microbiota in determining clinical response to a low FODMAP diet, although the highly controlled four-week feeding RCT in adults (11/27 responders, 41%) based findings on abundances of a select few taxa using qPCR analysis. It must also be noted that both trials of crossover design may have influenced microbial composition of those receiving low FODMAP diet as the second intervention [68,70].

Table 2. Summary of recent trials reporting on the association between baseline gut microbiota composition and association with clinical response in IBS.

Study	Study Design	No. of Subjects	IBS Sub-Type	Dietary Intervention	Control	Key Findings	Ref.
Chumpitazi et al., 2014	Dietary advice uncontrolled trial	8 children (f = 4, m = 4)	Paediatric Rome III; all IBS subtypes included	Low FODMAP	-	Responders: Greater richness and diversity compared at baseline compared with non-responders. Greater abundance of *Bacteroides*, unclassified Ruminococcaceae and *Faecalibacterium prausnitzii* at baseline compared with non-responders.	[68]
Halmos et al., 2015	Crossover feeding RCT	27 (f = 21, m = 6)	Rome III, all IBS subtypes included	Low FODMAP	Typical Australian diet	No baseline microbiota differences identified between responders and non-responders.	[70]
Chumpitazi et al., 2015	Crossover feeding RCT	33 children (f = 22, m = 11)	Paediatric Rome III; all IBS subtypes included	Low FODMAP	American childhood diet	Responders: Greater abundances for a range of saccharolytic taxa including within the family Bacteroidoidaceae and order Clostridiales (e.g., *F. Prausnitzii*) compared with non-responders.	[79]
Bennet et al., 2018	Dietary advice RCT	61 (f = 51, m = 10), 33 low FODMAP	Rome III; all IBS subtypes included	Low FODMAP	Traditional IBS diet	Responders: Increased abundance of *Streptococcus*, *Dorea* and *Ruminococcus gnavus* at baseline compared with non-responders. Lower dysbiosis index at baseline compared with non-responders.	[5]
Valeur et al., 2018	Dietary advice uncontrolled trial	61 (f = 54, m = 7)	Rome III, all IBS subtypes included	Low FODMAP	-	Responders: Greater abundance of *Bacteroides fragilis*, *Acinetobacter*, *Ruminiclostridium*, *Streptococcus* and *Eubacterium* at baseline compared with non-responders. Lower abundance of *Clostridia*, *Actinomycetales*, *Anaerotruncus* and *Escherichia* at baseline compared with non-responders.	[77]

IBS, irritable bowel syndrome; RCT, randomised clinical trial.

There are obvious challenges in interpreting the evidence from these trials. Pre-intervention environmental factors (e.g., medication, probiotic intake) that could impact on baseline microbiota composition are not always reported or controlled. Heterogeneity in baseline stool consistency and psychological comorbidity, both associated with altered microbiota composition [47,80,81], also complicate the identification of a distinct "responder" microbiota. Second, the stringency of low FODMAP dietary advice varies between studies. Insufficient FODMAP restriction could lead to an underestimation of true responders. Furthermore, clinical response criteria vary across studies, ranging from validated criteria [5,77] through to arbitrary cut-offs [70], leading to a sizable range of symptom severities in "responders" after low FODMAP treatment. Finally, no two studies so far have utilised the same statistical modelling techniques to explore the potential of microbiota as a predictor; ideally, the choice of statistical approach should be made by an independent blinded researcher to enable objective and statistically rigorous findings.

Based on the literature thus far, there is inconsistent evidence to support the use of one baseline microbiota signature to accurately predict response to a low FODMAP diet. Evidence that a baseline bacterial volatile organic compound profile may very accurately select responders [82] suggests the possibility that the metabolic function of bacteria may be important in determining response. Validation studies in well-controlled studies of specific IBS subtypes are warranted.

2. General Discussion and Limitations

Few human studies (summarised in Tables 1 and 2) have been conducted investigating whether specific microbial signatures predict response to dietary interventions. The conditions of obesity and IBS represent the best examples of preliminary work conducted in this area. Based on this review, there is inconsistent evidence to support the existence of specific microbiota signatures to accurately predict clinical response to dietary intervention in obesity and IBS. A number of limitations still impede progress in this sphere of research.

First, microbial sampling (i.e., faecal or biopsy) and quantification methodologies applied across studies thus far have been inconsistent. The increasing power and sensitivity of modern sequencing techniques has led to the rapid development of high-throughput methods for assessing genome-wide genetic variations. However, the approaches used to characterise the human microbiota still vary widely. Furthermore, technical accuracy is crucial throughout processing and analysis. For example, the suboptimal mechanical lysis during extraction of the microbiota DNA from faecal or biopsy samples, a key step in the analysis pipeline [83], will distort the downstream analysis more than any other analysis step.

Second, there are several shortcomings in the predictive modelling analysis methods utilised. Therefore, it is important that consistent analysis pipelines be adopted worldwide enabling comparison of data between studies. Studies may be limited to exploratory statistical analysis until clinical studies can be adequately designed and powered for primary analysis.

Third, there are many problematic confounding factors that can impact on baseline microbiota composition. These factors include, but are not limited to, the host genetic makeup, long-term dietary habits, ethnicity, sanitation, geographical location, exercise and lifestyle habits, and antibiotic use. This further highlights the conclusion that any personalised predictive model incorporating gut microbial composition must consider multiple additional relevant individual datapoints, which may vary with disease state. It is also acknowledged that some chronic diseases, although benefiting from dietary intervention, may never be amenable to a microbiota-based personalised nutrition approach due to inherent heterogeneity in microbiota composition across individuals.

Finally, for ultimate translation into clinical practice, there is a need to understand if the results gained from short-term studies predicting host response can be translated into durable responses over time, leading to long-term positive health outcomes. Longer duration of studies and intervention periods are also needed.

3. Conclusions

Diet is one of the most important determinants of the gut microbiota composition. However, the relationship between diet and microbiota is complex and not completely understood. Consequently, personalised nutrition models that predict clinical response to dietary treatment based on the microbial composition are still extremely challenging to test in the research context. Some evidence of associations between gut microbiota and response to dietary treatments for both obesity and IBS suggests that links exist between microbiota composition and inter-individuality in host response to diet. However, personalised nutrition research is in its infancy and specific microbiota signatures that predict individualised responses to dietary treatment are still elusive; advancements in analysis technologies and consistent bioinformatic approaches will be important for progress.

Author Contributions: Conceptualisation, writing, draft preparation, review and editing: J.R.B., J.J. and H.M.S.

Funding: Jonna Jalanka was supported by a Fellowship from the Finnish Academy (Grant No. 0313471-7). Heidi Staudacher was supported by an Alfred Deakin Postdoctoral Fellowship.

Conflicts of Interest: The authors declare no conflict of interest.

Abbreviations

ALT	Alanine aminotransferase
FMT	Faecal microbiota transplant
FODMAP	Fermentable oligo-, di-, monosaccharides and polyols
IBS	Irritable bowel syndrome
PPGR	Postprandial glycaemic response
RCT	Randomised clinical trial
RNA	Ribonucleic acid
SCFA	Short-chain fatty acid

References

1. Kris-Etherton, P.M.; Etherton, T.D.; Carlson, J.; Gardner, C. Recent discoveries in inclusive food-based approaches and dietary patterns for reduction in risk for cardiovascular disease. *Curr. Opin. Lipidol.* **2002**, *13*, 397–407. [CrossRef]
2. Staudacher, H.M.; Whelan, K. The low FODMAP diet: Recent advances in understanding its mechanisms and efficacy in IBS. *Gut* **2017**, *66*, 1517–1527. [CrossRef]
3. Seganfredo, F.B.; Blume, C.A.; Moehlecke, M.; Giongo, A.; Casagrande, D.S.; Spolidoro, J.V.N.; Padoin, A.V.; Schaan, B.D.; Mottin, C.C. Weight-loss interventions and gut microbiota changes in overweight and obese patients: A systematic review. *Obes. Rev.* **2017**, *18*, 832–851. [CrossRef]
4. McMillan-Price, J.; Petocz, P.; Atkinson, F.; O'Neill, K.; Samman, S.; Steinbeck, K.; Caterson, I.; Brand-Miller, J.J. Comparison of 4 diets of varying glycemic load on weight loss and cardiovascular risk reduction in overweight and obese young adults: A randomized controlled trial. *Arch. Intern. Med.* **2006**, *166*, 1466–1475. [CrossRef]
5. Bennet, S.M.P.; Bohn, L.; Storsrud, S.; Liljebo, T.; Collin, L.; Lindfors, P.; Tornblom, H.; Ohman, L.; Simren, M. Multivariate modelling of faecal bacterial profiles of patients with IBS predicts responsiveness to a diet low in FODMAPs. *Gut* **2018**, *67*, 872–881. [CrossRef]
6. Zeevi, D.; Korem, T.; Zmora, N.; Israeli, D.; Rothschild, D.; Weinberger, A.; Ben-Yacov, O.; Lador, D.; Avnit-Sagi, T.; Lotan-Pompan, M.; et al. Personalized Nutrition by Prediction of Glycemic Responses. *Cell* **2015**, *163*, 1079–1094. [CrossRef]
7. de Vos, W.M.; de Vos, E.A. Role of the intestinal microbiome in health and disease: From correlation to causation. *Nutr. Rev.* **2012**, *70*, S45–S56. [CrossRef]
8. Gonze, D.; Coyte, K.Z.; Lahti, L.; Faust, K. Microbial communities as dynamical systems. *Curr. Opin. Microbiol.* **2018**, *44*, 41–49. [CrossRef]
9. Faith, J.J.; McNulty, N.P.; Rey, F.E.; Gordon, J.I. Predicting a human gut microbiota's response to diet in gnotobiotic mice. *Science* **2011**, *333*, 101–104. [CrossRef]

10. Salonen, A.; Lahti, L.; Salojärvi, J.; Holtrop, G.; Korpela, K.; Duncan, S.H.; Date, P.; Farquharson, F.; Johnstone, A.M.; E Lobley, G.; et al. Impact of diet and individual variation on intestinal microbiota composition and fermentation products in obese men. *ISME J.* **2014**, *8*, 2218–2230. [CrossRef]
11. Tuohy, K.M.; Kolida, S.; Lustenberger, A.M.; Gibson, G.R.; Tuohy, K. The prebiotic effects of biscuits containing partially hydrolysed guar gum and fructo-oligosaccharides- a human volunteer study. *Br. J. Nutr.* **2001**, *86*, 341–348. [CrossRef]
12. Ng, M.; Fleming, T.; Robinson, M.; Thomson, B.; Graetz, N.; Margono, C.; Mullany, E.C.; Biryukov, S.; Abbafati, C.; Abera, S.F.; et al. Global, regional, and national prevalence of overweight and obesity in children and adults during 1980-2013: A systematic analysis for the Global Burden of Disease Study 2013. *Lancet* **2014**, *384*, 766–781. [CrossRef]
13. Meigs, J.B.; Wilson, P.W.F.; Fox, C.S.; Vasan, R.S.; Nathan, D.M.; Sullivan, L.M.; D'Agostino, R.B. Body mass index, metabolic syndrome, and risk of type 2 diabetes or cardiovascular disease. *J. Clin. Endocrinol. Metab.* **2006**, *91*, 2906–2912. [CrossRef]
14. Lauby-Secretan, B.; Grosse, Y.; Bianchini, F.; Loomis, D.; Straif, K.; Scoccianti, C. Body Fatness and Cancer–Viewpoint of the IARC Working Group. *N. Engl. J. Med.* **2016**, *375*, 794–798. [CrossRef]
15. Sackner-Bernstein, J.; Kanter, D.; Kaul, S. Dietary Intervention for Overweight and Obese Adults: Comparison of Low-Carbohydrate and Low-Fat Diets. A Meta-Analysis. *PLoS ONE* **2015**, *10*, e0139817. [CrossRef]
16. Soltani, S.; Shirani, F.; Chitsazi, M.J.; Salehi-Abargouei, A. The effect of dietary approaches to stop hypertension (DASH) diet on weight and body composition in adults: A systematic review and meta-analysis of randomized controlled clinical trials. *Obes. Rev.* **2016**, *17*, 442–454. [CrossRef]
17. Lacy, B.E.; Mearin, F.; Chang, L.; Chey, W.D.; Lembo, A.J.; Simrén, M.; Spiller, R. Bowel Disorders. *Gastroenterology* **2016**, *150*, 1393–1407. [CrossRef]
18. Lovell, R.M.; Ford, A.C. Global prevalence of and risk factors for irritable bowel syndrome: A meta-analysis. *Clin. Gastroenterol. Hepatol.* **2012**, *10*, 712–721. [CrossRef]
19. Ford, A.C.; Moayyedi, P.; Chey, W.D.; Harris, L.A.; Lacy, B.E.; Saito, Y.A.; Quigley, E.M.M. American College of Gastroenterology Monograph on Management of Irritable Bowel Syndrome. *Am. J. Gastroenterol.* **2018**, *113* (Suppl. S2), 1–18. [CrossRef]
20. McKenzie, Y.A.; Bowyer, R.K.; Leach, H.; Gulia, P.; Horobin, J.; O'Sullivan, N.A.; Pettitt, C.; Reeves, L.B.; Seamark, L.; Williams, M.; et al. British Dietetic Association systematic review and evidence-based practice guidelines for the dietary management of irritable bowel syndrome in adults. *J. Hum. Nutr. Diet.* **2016**, *29*, 549–575. [CrossRef]
21. Ley, R.E.; Turnbaugh, P.J.; Klein, S.; Gordon, J.I. Microbial ecology: Human gut microbes associated with obesity. *Nature* **2006**, *444*, 1022–1023. [CrossRef]
22. Plovier, H.; Everard, A.; Druart, C.; Depommier, C.; Van Hul, M.; Geurts, L.; Chilloux, J.; Ottman, N.; Duparc, T.; Lichtenstein, L.; et al. A purified membrane protein from Akkermansia muciniphila or the pasteurized bacterium improves metabolism in obese and diabetic mice. *Nat. Med.* **2017**, *23*, 107–113. [CrossRef]
23. Singh, R.K.; Chang, H.-W.; Yan, D.; Lee, K.M.; Ucmak, D.; Wong, K.; Abrouk, M.; Farahnik, B.; Nakamura, M.; Zhu, T.H.; et al. Influence of diet on the gut microbiome and implications for human health. *J. Transl. Med.* **2017**, *15*, 73. [CrossRef]
24. Le Chatelier, E.; MetaHIT Consortium; Nielsen, T.; Qin, J.; Prifti, E.; Hildebrand, F.; Falony, G.; Almeida, M.; Arumugam, M.; Batto, J.-M.; et al. Richness of human gut microbiome correlates with metabolic markers. *Nature* **2013**, *500*, 541–546.
25. Borgeraas, H.; Johnson, L.K.; Skattebu, J.; Hertel, J.K.; Hjelmesaeth, J. Effects of probiotics on body weight, body mass index, fat mass and fat percentage in subjects with overweight or obesity: A systematic review and meta-analysis of randomized controlled trials. *Obes. Rev.* **2018**, *19*, 219–232. [CrossRef]
26. Vrieze, A.; Van Nood, E.; Holleman, F.; Salojärvi, J.; Kootte, R.S.; Bartelsman, J.F.; Dallinga–Thie, G.M.; Ackermans, M.T.; Serlie, M.J.; Oozeer, R.; et al. Transfer of Intestinal Microbiota from Lean Donors Increases Insulin Sensitivity in Individuals with Metabolic Syndrome. *Gastroenterology* **2012**, *143*, 913–916. [CrossRef]
27. Lin, H.V.; Frassetto, A.; Kowalik, E.J., Jr.; Nawrocki, A.R.; Lu, M.M.; Kosinski, J.R.; Hubert, J.A.; Szeto, D.; Yao, X.; Forrest, G.; et al. Butyrate and propionate protect against diet-induced obesity and regulate gut hormones via free fatty acid receptor 3-independent mechanisms. *PLoS ONE* **2012**, *7*, e35240. [CrossRef]

28. Bäckhed, F.; Manchester, J.K.; Semenkovich, C.F.; Gordon, J.I. Mechanisms underlying the resistance to diet-induced obesity in germ-free mice. *Proc. Natl. Acad. Sci. USA* **2007**, *104*, 979–984. [CrossRef]
29. Wellen, K.E.; Hotamisligil, G.S. Inflammation, stress, and diabetes. *J. Clin. Investig.* **2005**, *115*, 1111–1119. [CrossRef]
30. Go, G.W.; Oh, S.; Park, M.; Gang, G.; McLean, D.; Yang, H.S.; Song, M.H.; Kim, Y. t10,c12 conjugated linoleic acid upregulates hepatic de novo lipogenesis and triglyceride synthesis via mTOR pathway activation. *J. Microbiol. Biotechnol.* **2013**, *23*, 1569–1576. [CrossRef]
31. Vijay-Kumar, M.; Aitken, J.D.; Carvalho, F.A.; Cullender, T.C.; Mwangi, S.; Srinivasan, S.; Sitaraman, S.V.; Knight, R.; Ley, R.E.; Gewirtz, A.T. Metabolic syndrome and altered gut microbiota in mice lacking Toll-like receptor 5. *Science* **2010**, *328*, 228–231. [CrossRef]
32. Heinsen, F.-A.; Fangmann, D.; Müller, N.; Schulte, D.M.; Rühlemann, M.C.; Türk, K.; Settgast, U.; Lieb, W.; Baines, J.F.; Schreiber, S.; et al. Beneficial Effects of a Dietary Weight Loss Intervention on Human Gut Microbiome Diversity and Metabolism Are Not Sustained during Weight Maintenance. *Obes. Facts* **2016**, *9*, 379–391. [CrossRef]
33. Cotillard, A.; ANR MicroObes Consortium; Kennedy, S.P.; Kong, L.C.; Prifti, E.; Pons, N.; Le Chatelier, E.; Almeida, M.; Quinquis, B.; Levenez, F.; et al. Dietary intervention impact on gut microbial gene richness. *Nature* **2013**, *500*, 585–588.
34. Haro, C.; Montes-Borrego, M.; Rangel-Zúñiga, O.A.; Alcala-Diaz, J.F.; Gomez-Delgado, F.; Perez-Martinez, P.; Delgado-Lista, J.; Quintana-Navarro, G.M.; Tinahones, F.J.; Landa, B.B.; et al. Two Healthy Diets Modulate Gut Microbial Community Improving Insulin Sensitivity in a Human Obese Population. *J. Clin. Endocrinol. Metab.* **2016**, *101*, 233–242. [CrossRef]
35. Nicolucci, A.C.; Hume, M.P.; Martínez, I.; Mayengbam, S.; Walter, J.; Reimer, R.A. Prebiotics Reduce Body Fat and Alter Intestinal Microbiota in Children Who Are Overweight or with Obesity. *Gastroenterology* **2017**, *153*, 711–722. [CrossRef]
36. Zhang, C.; Yin, A.; Li, H.; Wang, R.; Wu, G.; Shen, J.; Zhang, M.; Wang, L.; Hou, Y.; Ouyang, H.; et al. Dietary Modulation of Gut Microbiota Contributes to Alleviation of Both Genetic and Simple Obesity in Children. *EBioMedicine* **2015**, *2*, 968–984. [CrossRef]
37. Dao, M.C.; Everard, A.; Aron-Wisnewsky, J.; Sokolovska, N.; Prifti, E.; Verger, E.O.; Kayser, B.D.; Levenez, F.; Chilloux, J.; Hoyles, L.; et al. Akkermansia muciniphila and improved metabolic health during a dietary intervention in obesity: Relationship with gut microbiome richness and ecology. *Gut* **2016**, *65*, 426–436. [CrossRef]
38. Kong, L.C.; Wuillemin, P.-H.; Bastard, J.-P.; Sokolovska, N.; Gougis, S.; Fellahi, S.; Darakhshan, F.; Bonnefont-Rousselot, D.; Bittar, R.; Doré, J.; et al. Insulin resistance and inflammation predict kinetic body weight changes in response to dietary weight loss and maintenance in overweight and obese subjects by using a Bayesian network approach. *Am. J. Clin. Nutr.* **2013**, *98*, 1385–1394. [CrossRef]
39. Korpela, K.; Flint, H.J.; Johnstone, A.M.; Lappi, J.; Poutanen, K.; Dewulf, E.; Delzenne, N.; De Vos, W.M.; Salonen, A. Gut Microbiota Signatures Predict Host and Microbiota Responses to Dietary Interventions in Obese Individuals. *PLoS ONE* **2014**, *9*, e90702. [CrossRef]
40. Kovatcheva-Datchary, P.; Nilsson, A.; Akrami, R.; Lee, Y.S.; De Vadder, F.; Arora, T.; Hallén, A.; Martens, E.; Björck, I.; Bäckhed, F. Dietary Fiber-Induced Improvement in Glucose Metabolism Is Associated with Increased Abundance of Prevotella. *Cell Metab.* **2015**, *22*, 971–982. [CrossRef]
41. Korem, T.; Zeevi, D.; Zmora, N.; Weissbrod, O.; Bar, N.; Lotan-Pompan, M.; Avnit-Sagi, T.; Kosower, N.; Malka, G.; Rein, M.; et al. Bread Affects Clinical Parameters and Induces Gut Microbiome-Associated Personal Glycemic Responses. *Cell Metab.* **2017**, *25*, 1243–1253. [CrossRef]
42. Mendes-Soares, H.; Raveh-Sadka, T.; Azulay, S.; Edens, K.; Ben-Shlomo, Y.; Cohen, Y.; Ofek, T.; Bachrach, D.; Stevens, J.; Colibaseanu, D.; et al. Assessment of a Personalized Approach to Predicting Postprandial Glycemic Responses to Food Among Individuals Without Diabetes. *JAMA Netw. Open* **2019**, *2*, e188102. [CrossRef]
43. Rajilić-Stojanović, M.; Jonkers, D.M.; Salonen, A.; Hanevik, K.; Raes, J.; Jalanka, J.; De Vos, W.M.; Manichanh, C.; Golic, N.; Enck, P.; et al. Intestinal microbiota and diet in IBS: Causes, consequences, or epiphenomena? *Am. J. Gastroenterol.* **2015**, *110*, 278–287. [CrossRef]
44. Pittayanon, R.; Lau, J.T.; Yuan, Y.; Leontiadis, G.I.; Tse, F.; Surette, M.; Moayyedi, P. Gut Microbiota in Patients with Irritable Bowel Syndrome-a Systematic Review. *Gastroenterology* **2019**. [CrossRef]

45. Sundin, J.; Rangel, I.; Fuentes, S.; Heikamp-de Jong, I.; Hultgren-Hornquist, E.; de Vos, W.M.; Brummer, R.J. Altered faecal and mucosal microbial composition in post-infectious irritable bowel syndrome patients correlates with mucosal lymphocyte phenotypes and psychological distress. *Aliment. Pharmacol. Ther.* **2015**, *41*, 342–351. [CrossRef]
46. Rangel, I.; Sundin, J.; Fuentes, S.; Repsilber, D.; De Vos, W.M.; Brummer, R.J. The relationship between faecal-associated and mucosal-associated microbiota in irritable bowel syndrome patients and healthy subjects. *Aliment. Pharmacol. Ther.* **2015**, *42*, 1211–1221. [CrossRef]
47. Jeffery, I.B.; O'Toole, P.W.; Ohman, L.; Claesson, M.J.; Deane, J.; Quigley, E.M.; Simren, M. An irritable bowel syndrome subtype defined by species-specific alterations in faecal microbiota. *Gut* **2012**, *61*, 997–1006. [CrossRef]
48. Rajilić–Stojanović, M.; Biagi, E.; Heilig, H.G.; Kajander, K.; Kekkonen, R.A.; Tims, S.; De Vos, W.M. Global and deep molecular analysis of microbiota signatures in fecal samples from patients with irritable bowel syndrome. *Gastroenterology* **2011**, *141*, 1792–1801. [CrossRef]
49. Tap, J.; Derrien, M.; Törnblom, H.; Brazeilles, R.; Cools-Portier, S.; Doré, J.; Störsrud, S.; Le Nevé, B.; Öhman, L.; Simrén, M. Identification of an Intestinal Microbiota Signature Associated with Severity of Irritable Bowel Syndrome. *Gastroenterology* **2017**, *152*, 111–123. [CrossRef]
50. Si, J.-M.; Yu, Y.-C.; Fan, Y.-J.; Chen, S.-J. Intestinal microecology and quality of life in irritable bowel syndrome patients. *World J. Gastroenterol.* **2004**, *10*, 1802–1805. [CrossRef]
51. Kerckhoffs, A.P.; Samsom, M.; Van Der Rest, M.E.; De Vogel, J.; Knol, J.; Ben-Amor, K.; Akkermans, L.M. Lower Bifidobacteria counts in both duodenal mucosa-associated and fecal microbiota in irritable bowel syndrome patients. *World J. Gastroenterol.* **2009**, *15*, 2887–2892.
52. Balsari, A.; Ceccarelli, A.; Dubini, F.; Fesce, E.; Poli, G. The fecal microbial population in the irritable bowel syndrome. *Microbiologica* **1982**, *5*, 185–194.
53. Malinen, E.; Rinttilä, T.; Kajander, K.; Mättö, J.; Kassinen, A.; Krogius, L.; Saarela, M.; Korpela, R.; Palva, A. Analysis of the fecal microbiota of irritable bowel syndrome patients and healthy controls with real-time PCR. *Am. J. Gastroenterol.* **2005**, *100*, 373–382. [CrossRef]
54. Malinen, E.; Krogius-Kurikka, L.; Lyra, A.; Nikkilä, J.; Jääskeläinen, A.; Rinttilä, T.; Vilpponen-Salmela, T.; Von Wright, A.J.; Palva, A. Association of symptoms with gastrointestinal microbiota in irritable bowel syndrome. *World J. Gastroenterol.* **2010**, *16*, 4532–4540. [CrossRef]
55. Matto, J.; Maunuksela, L.; Kajander, K.; Palva, A.; Korpela, R.; Kassinen, A.; Saarela, M.; Mättö, J. Composition and temporal stability of gastrointestinal microbiota in irritable bowel syndrome- a longitudinal study in IBS and control subjects. *FEMS Immunol. Med. Microbiol.* **2005**, *43*, 213–222. [CrossRef]
56. Manichanh, C.; Eck, A.; Varela, E.; Roca, J.; Clemente, J.C.; Gonzalez, A.; Knights, D.; Knight, R.; Estrella, S.; Hernandez, C.; et al. Anal gas evacuation and colonic microbiota in patients with flatulence: Effect of diet. *Gut* **2014**, *63*, 401–408. [CrossRef] [PubMed]
57. Parkes, G.C.; Rayment, N.B.; Hudspith, B.N.; Petrovska, L.; Lomer, M.C.; Brostoff, J.; Whelan, K.; Sanderson, J.D. Distinct microbial populations exist in the mucosa-associated microbiota of sub-groups of irritable bowel syndrome. *Neurogastroenterol. Motil.* **2012**, *24*, 31–39. [CrossRef]
58. Jalanka-Tuovinen, J.; Salojarvi, J.; Salonen, A.; Immonen, O.; Garsed, K.; Kelly, F.M.; Zaitoun, A.; Palva, A.; Spiller, R.C.; de Vos, W.M. Faecal microbiota composition and host-microbe cross-talk following gastroenteritis and in postinfectious irritable bowel syndrome. *Gut* **2014**, *63*, 1737–1745. [CrossRef]
59. Peter, J.; Fournier, C.; Durdevic, M.; Knoblich, L.; Keip, B.; Dejaco, C.; Trauner, M.; Moser, G. A Microbial Signature of Psychological Distress in Irritable Bowel Syndrome. *Psychosom. Med.* **2018**, *80*, 698–709. [CrossRef]
60. De Palma, G.; Lynch, M.D.J.; Lu, J.; Dang, V.T.; Deng, Y.; Jury, J.; Umeh, G.; Miranda, P.M.; Pastor, M.P.; Sidani, S.; et al. Transplantation of fecal microbiota from patients with irritable bowel syndrome alters gut function and behavior in recipient mice. *Sci. Transl. Med.* **2017**, *9*, eaaf6397. [CrossRef] [PubMed]
61. Crouzet, L.; Gaultier, E.; Del'Homme, C.; Cartier, C.; Delmas, E.; Dapoigny, M.; Fioramonti, J.; Bernalier-Donadille, A. The hypersensitivity to colonic distension of IBS patients can be transferred to rats through their fecal microbiota. *Neurogastroenterol. Motil.* **2013**, *25*, e272–e282. [CrossRef]
62. Bourdu, S.; Dapoigny, M.; Chapuy, E.; Artigue, F.; Vasson, M.-P.; Déchelotte, P.; Bommelaer, G.; Eschalier, A.; Ardid, D. Rectal instillation of butyrate provides a novel clinically relevant model of noninflammatory colonic hypersensitivity in rats. *Gastroenterology* **2005**, *128*, 1996–2008. [CrossRef]

63. Ohman, L.; Tornblom, H.; Simren, M. Crosstalk at the mucosal border: Importance of the gut microenvironment in IBS. *Nat. Rev. Gastroenterol. Hepatol.* **2015**, *12*, 36–49. [CrossRef]
64. Johnsen, P.H.; Hilpüsch, F.; Cavanagh, J.P.; Leikanger, I.S.; Kolstad, C.; Valle, P.C.; Goll, R. Faecal microbiota transplantation versus placebo for moderate-to-severe irritable bowel syndrome: A double-blind, randomised, placebo-controlled, parallel-group, single-centre trial. *Lancet Gastroenterol. Hepatol.* **2018**, *3*, 17–24. [CrossRef]
65. Staudacher, H.M.; Lomer, M.C.E.; Anderson, J.L.; Barrett, J.S.; Muir, J.G.; Irving, P.M.; Whelan, K. Fermentable carbohydrate restriction reduces luminal bifidobacteria and gastrointestinal symptoms in patients with irritable bowel syndrome. *J. Nutr.* **2012**, *142*, 1510–1518. [CrossRef]
66. Staudacher, H.M.; Lomer, M.C.; Farquharson, F.M.; Louis, P.; Fava, F.; Franciosi, E.; Scholz, M.; Tuohy, K.M.; Lindsay, J.O.; Irving, P.M.; et al. A Diet Low in FODMAPs Reduces Symptoms in Patients with Irritable Bowel Syndrome and A Probiotic Restores Bifidobacterium Species: A Randomized Controlled Trial. *Gastroenterology* **2017**, *153*, 936–947. [CrossRef]
67. McIntosh, K.; Reed, D.E.; Schneider, T.; Dang, F.; Keshteli, A.H.; De Palma, G.; Madsen, K.; Bercik, P.; Vanner, S. FODMAPs alter symptoms and the metabolome of patients with IBS: A randomised controlled trial. *Gut* **2017**, *66*, 1241–1251. [CrossRef]
68. Chumpitazi, B.P.; Hollister, E.B.; Oezguen, N.; Tsai, C.M.; McMeans, A.R.; A Luna, R.; Savidge, T.C.; Versalovic, J.; Shulman, R.J. Gut microbiota influences low fermentable substrate diet efficacy in children with irritable bowel syndrome. *Gut Microbes* **2014**, *5*, 165–175. [CrossRef]
69. Huaman, J.-W.; Mego, M.; Manichanh, C.; Cañellas, N.; Cañueto, D.; Segurola, H.; Jansana, M.; Malagelada, C.; Accarino, A.; Vulevic, J.; et al. Effects of Prebiotics vs a Diet Low in FODMAPs in Patients with Functional Gut Disorders. *Gastroenterology* **2018**, *155*, 1004–1007. [CrossRef]
70. Halmos, E.P.; Christophersen, C.T.; Bird, A.R.; Shepherd, S.J.; Gibson, P.R.; Muir, J.G. Diets that differ in their FODMAP content alter the colonic luminal microenvironment. *Gut* **2015**, *64*, 93–100. [CrossRef]
71. Sloan, T.J.; Jalanka, J.; Major, G.A.D.; Krishnasamy, S.; Pritchard, S.; Abdelrazig, S.; Korpela, K.; Singh, G.; Mulvenna, C.; Hoad, C.L.; et al. A low FODMAP diet is associated with changes in the microbiota and reduction in breath hydrogen but not colonic volume in healthy subjects. *PLoS ONE* **2018**, *13*, e0201410. [CrossRef]
72. Ford, A.C.; Harris, L.A.; Lacy, B.E.; Quigley, E.M.M.; Moayyedi, P. Systematic review with meta-analysis: The efficacy of prebiotics, probiotics, synbiotics and antibiotics in irritable bowel syndrome. *Aliment. Pharmacol. Ther.* **2018**, *48*, 1044–1060. [CrossRef]
73. O'Keeffe, M.; Lomer, M.C. Who should deliver the low FODMAP diet and what educational methods are optimal: A review. *J. Gastroenterol. Hepatol.* **2017**, *32*, 23–26. [CrossRef]
74. Eswaran, S.L.; Chey, W.D.; Han-Markey, T.; Ball, S.; Jackson, K. A Randomized Controlled Trial Comparing the Low FODMAP Diet vs. Modified NICE Guidelines in US Adults with IBS-D. *Am. J. Gastroenterol.* **2016**, *111*, 1824–1832.
75. Wilder-Smith, C.H.; Materna, A.; Wermelinger, C.; Schuler, J. Fructose and lactose intolerance and malabsorption testing: The relationship with symptoms in functional gastrointestinal disorders. *Aliment. Pharmacol. Ther.* **2013**, *37*, 1074–1083. [CrossRef]
76. Böhn, L.; Störsrud, S.; Liljebo, T.; Collin, L.; Lindfors, P.; Törnblom, H.; Simrén, M. Diet low in FODMAPs Reduces Symptoms of Irritable Bowel Syndrome as Well as Traditional Dietary Advice: A Randomized Controlled Trial. *Gastroenterology* **2015**, *149*, 1399–1407. [CrossRef]
77. Valeur, J.; Småstuen, M.C.; Knudsen, T.; Lied, G.A.; Røseth, A.G. Exploring Gut Microbiota Composition as an Indicator of Clinical Response to Dietary FODMAP Restriction in Patients with Irritable Bowel Syndrome. *Dig. Dis. Sci.* **2018**, *63*, 429–436. [CrossRef]
78. Casén, C.; Vebø, H.C.; Sekelja, M.; Hegge, F.T.; Karlsson, M.K.; Ciemniejewska, E.; Dzankovic, S.; Frøyland, C.; Nestestog, R.; Engstrand, L.; et al. Deviations in human gut microbiota: A novel diagnostic test for determining dysbiosis in patients with IBS or IBD. *Aliment. Pharmacol. Ther.* **2015**, *42*, 71–83. [CrossRef]
79. Chumpitazi, B.P.; Cope, J.L.; Hollister, E.B.; Tsai, C.M.; McMeans, A.R.; Luna, R.A.; Versalovic, J.; Shulman, R.J. Randomised clinical trial: Gut microbiome biomarkers are associated with clinical response to a low FODMAP diet in children with the irritable bowel syndrome. *Aliment. Pharmacol. Ther.* **2015**, *42*, 418–427. [CrossRef]
80. Liu, Y.; Zhang, L.; Wang, X.; Jiang, R.; Xia, Z.; Xu, Z.; Nie, Y.; Lv, X.; Wu, X.; Zhu, H.; et al. Similar Fecal Microbiota Signatures in Patients with Diarrhea-Predominant Irritable Bowel Syndrome and Patients with Depression. *Clin. Gastroenterol. Hepatol.* **2016**, *14*, 1602–1611. [CrossRef]

81. Vandeputte, D.; Falony, G.; Vieira-Silva, S.; Tito, R.Y.; Joossens, M.; Raes, J. Stool Stool consistency is strongly associated with gut microbiota richness and composition, enterotypes and bacterial growth rates. *Gut* **2016**, *65*, 57–62. [CrossRef]
82. Rossi, M.; Aggio, R.; Staudacher, H.M.; Lomer, M.C.; Lindsay, J.O.; Irving, P.; Probert, C.; Whelan, K. Volatile Organic Compounds in Feces Associate with Response to Dietary Intervention in Patients with Irritable Bowel Syndrome. *Clin. Gastroenterol. Hepatol.* **2017**, *16*, 385–391. [CrossRef]
83. Costea, P.I.; Zeller, G.; Sunagawa, S.; Pelletier, E.; Alberti, A.; Levenez, F.; Tramontano, M.; Driessen, M.; Hercog, R.; Jung, F.-E.; et al. Towards standards for human fecal sample processing in metagenomic studies. *Nat. Biotechnol.* **2017**, *35*, 1069–1076. [CrossRef]

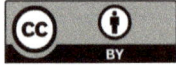
© 2019 by the authors. Licensee MDPI, Basel, Switzerland. This article is an open access article distributed under the terms and conditions of the Creative Commons Attribution (CC BY) license (http://creativecommons.org/licenses/by/4.0/).

MDPI
St. Alban-Anlage 66
4052 Basel
Switzerland
Tel. +41 61 683 77 34
Fax +41 61 302 89 18
www.mdpi.com

Nutrients Editorial Office
E-mail: nutrients@mdpi.com
www.mdpi.com/journal/nutrients

www.ingramcontent.com/pod-product-compliance
Lightning Source LLC
LaVergne TN
LVHW071955080526
838202LV00064B/6751